DEEP VEIN THROMBOSIS

Edited by **Gregory Cheng**

Deep Vein Thrombosis
Edited by Gregory Cheng

Published by InTech
Janeza Trdine 9, 51000 Rijeka, Croatia

Publishing Process Manager Masa Vidovic

Technical Editor Teodora Smiljanic

Cover Designer InTech Design Team

Additional hard copies can be obtained from orders@intechopen.com

Deep Vein Thrombosis, Edited by Gregory Cheng
p. cm.
978-953-51-0225-0

For EU product safety concerns:
IN TECH d.o.o., Prolaz Marije Krucifikse Kozulić 3, 51000 Rijeka, Croatia,
info@intechopen.com or visit our website at intechopen.com.

Meet the editor

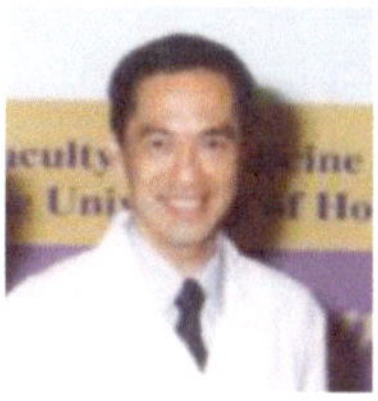

Gregory Cheng, MD, PhD is the deputy director of the Dr. Stanley Ho Medical Development Foundation, Macau. He is the former head of division of Hematology at the Chinese University of Hong Kong. He earned his medical degree and PhD degree from the University of Toronto in 1978 and 1989 respectively. His clinical practice and research focus on immune thrombocytopenia, deep vein thrombosis, transfusion medicine and hematologic malignancies, such as acute and chronic leukemia, myelodysplastic syndromes, myeloproliferative disorders, lymphomas, and myeloma. His research has resulted in publications in peer-reviewed journals such as the New England Journal of Medicine, Lancet, JAMA, Blood, and BMJ.

Contents

Preface XI

Chapter 1 **Risk Factors of Deep Vein Thrombosis 1**
Mustafa Sirlak, Mustafa Bahadir Inan, Demir Cetintas and Evren Ozcinar

Chapter 2 **Venous Stasis and Deep Vein Thrombosis Prevention in Laparoscopic Surgery 31**
Mindaugas Kiudelis, Dalia Adukauskienė and Rolandas Gerbutavičius

Chapter 3 **Vena Cava Malformations as an Emerging Etiologic Factor for Deep Vein Thrombosis in Young Patients 43**
Massimiliano Bianchi, Lorenzo Faggioni, Virna Zampa, Gina D'Errico, Paolo Marraccini and Carlo Bartolozzi

Chapter 4 **Endovascular Therapies in Acute DVT 59**
Jeff Tam and Jim Koukounaras

Chapter 5 **Radiological Imaging and Intervention in Venous Thrombosis 79**
Andrew Christie, Giles Roditi, Ananthakrishnan Ganapathy and Chris Cadman

Chapter 6 **Emerging Issues in Deep Vein Thrombosis; (DVT) in Liver Disease and in Developing Countries 99**
Farjah H. AlGahtani and Abdel Galil Abdel Gader

Chapter 7 **Venous Thromboembolism Prophylaxis in Cancer Patients 111**
Hikmat Abdel-Razeq

Chapter 8 **Deep Vein Thrombosis of the Arms 129**
Peter Marschang

Chapter 9 **The Post Thrombotic Syndrome 143**
Paolo Prandoni and Susan R Kahn

Chapter 10 **Venous Thromboembolism in Orthopaedic Surgery 159**
Justin R. Knight and Michael H. Huo

Chapter 11 **Deep Venous Thrombosis After Radical Pelvic Surgery 173**
Bedeir Ali-El-Dein

Preface

Venous thromboembolism (VTE) is a common disease with an incidence of over 1 in 1000 in Western countries. It is associated with significant morbidities and costs. Post-thrombotic syndrome may develop in one third of patients with deep vein thrombosis (DVT) with considerable socio-economic consequences. DVT is usually seen in patients with underlying risk factors and patients undergoing major pelvic and orthopaedic surgeries. Numerous guidelines suggest use of DVT thromboprophylaxis in these patients, but despite encouraging results of thromboprophylaxis, many studies showed low compliance rates with such guidelines. Also in regions with low DVT prevalence, the benefit of pharmacological prophylaxis is not clear. Patients undergoing laporoscopic operations are also at risks of VTE because of increased venous stasis caused by abdominal insufflation and prolonged reverse Trendelenburg position. Most DVT occur in the lower limbs, but DVT the arms may account for 5% of VTE cases. Cancer and its treatment are recognized risk factors for VTE and extended prophylaxis in ambulatory cancer patients may be required. Recent radiological advances have facilitated the diagnosis and management of DVT and have also identified vena cava malformations as a new etiologic factor in young DVT patients. Endovascular therapy is a potential treatment option in acute DVT. Chronic liver disease is recently recognised as a hypercoagulable state. All this issues will be addressed by various experts in this book.

Dr. Gregory Cheng
Department of Medicine and Therapeutics,
The Chinese University of Hong Kong, Shatin,
Hong Kong

1

Risk Factors of Deep Vein Thrombosis

Mustafa Sirlak, Mustafa Bahadir Inan,
Demir Cetintas and Evren Ozcinar
*Ankara University School of Medicine, Department of Cardiovascular Surgery,
Ankara,
Turkey*

1. Introduction

Deep vein thrombosis is a clinical challenge for doctors of all disciplines. It can complicate the course of a disease but might also be encountered in the absence of precipitating disorders. Thrombosis can take place in any section of the venous system, but arises most frequently in the deep veins of the leg. Long-term morbidity due to post-thrombotic syndrome is common and can be substantial. The major concern, however, is embolisation of the thrombus to the lung, which can be fatal. Deep vein thrombosis is highly prevalent and poses a burden on health economy. The disorder and its sequelae are also among the best examples of preventable diseases. Relevant data for the frequency of deep vein thrombosis derive from large community-based studies because they mainly reflect symptomatic rather than asymptomatic disease. In a systematic review, the incidence of first deep vein thrombosis in the general population was 0·5 per 1000 person-years.[1] The disorder is rare in children younger than 15 years,[2,3] but its frequency increases with age, with incidence per 1000 person-years of 1·8 at age 65–69 years and 3·1 at age 85–89 years.[4] Two-thirds of first-time episodes of deep vein thrombosis are caused by risk factors, including surgery, cancer, immobilisation, or admission for other reasons.[5,6] Risk for first deep vein thrombosis seems to be slightly higher in men than in women.[6,9] In a population-based cohort study, the age-adjusted incidence of first venous thromboembolism was 1·3 per 1000 person-years in men and 1·1 per 1000 person-years in women.[2] It is noteworthy that the risk for recurrence of this disorder is higher in men than in women.[6,10]

Conditions associated with increased risk for deep vein thrombosis
Advancing age
Obesity
Previous venous thromboembolism
Surgery
Trauma
Active cancer
Acute medical illnesses – eg, acute myocardial infarction, heart failure, respiratory failure, infection
Inflammatory bowel disease

Antiphospholiped syndrome
Dyslipoproteinaemia
Nephrotic syndrome
Paroxysmal nocturnal haemoglobinuria
Myeloproliferative diseases
Behçet's syndrome
Varicose veins
Superficial vein thrombosis
Congenital venous malformation
Long-distance travel
Prolonged bed rest
İmmobilisation
Limb paresis
Chronic care facility stay
Pregnancy/Puerperium
Oral contraceptives
Hormone replacement theraphy
Heparin-induced thrombocitopenia
Other drugs Chemotheraphy Tamoxifen Thalidomide Antipsychotics
Central Venous catheter
Vena cava filter
İntravenous drug abuse

Rudolph Virchow is recognized as the first person to link the development of VTE to the presence of at least 1 of 3 conditions: venous stasis, vascular injury, and/or hypercoagulability. 11 Each of these factors can alter the delicate hemostatic balance toward hypercoagulability and development of thrombosis. Several aspects of surgery can be linked to Virchow's triad. Coleridge-Smith et al12 reported in 1990 that venous stasis occurs during general surgery, with veins dilating 22% to 28% in patients undergoing general anesthesia and surgery and up to 57% in those who also received an infusion of 1 L of saline during surgery. The investigators suggested that it is this intraoperative venous distension that underlies the risk for DVT in patients undergoing surgery. They suggested that the venous distension is the result of loss of muscle tone that is caused by the muscle relaxants used during surgery. Muscle paralysis resulting from regional anesthesia also can lead to venous dilatation. These effects can be modified to some extent by the use of graduated compression stockings during surgery.13 In a study of 40 patients undergoing surgery of the abdomen or neck, the median vein diameter in the extremity studied was 2.6 mm at the beginning of surgery in both the control and intervention groups (control group, n = 20; median vein diameter, 2.6 mm; interquartile range [IQR], 2.1–3.3 mm; stocking group, n =20; median vein diameter, 2.6 mm; IQR, 2.1–3.7 mm). This decreased to a median vein diameter of 1.6 mm (IQR, 1.3–2.8 mm) after application of a stocking, whereas vein diameter increased from 2.6 to 2.9 mm (IQR, 2.3– 4.0 mm) in the control group.13 Comerota et al14 found that in patients undergoing total hip replacement surgery, handling of soft tissue (muscle) during surgery leads to venodilation, whereas bone manipulation leads to venoconstriction. The venous dilatation that occurs during surgery causes cracks in the endothelium, which provides a nidus for thrombosis as the blood coagulation system is activated. The researchers also showed that pharmacologic control of venodilation during surgery reduced postoperative DVT.14 Microscopic vessel wall damage, 15 such as that demonstrated in patients undergoing hip and knee replacement surgeries, also contributes to the development of VTE. 16,17 Tissue factor released from the blood vessel wall after injury drives thrombus formation,18 which may help explain the increased risk of VTE in patients undergoing surgery. The third factor in Virchow's triad, hypercoagulability, is linked to a number of factors, including certain genetic traits. Deficiencies of antithrombin, protein C, or protein S, or mutations of factor V Leiden or factor II (prothrombin) G20210A genes lead to hypercoagulable states.11 Although these genetic factors account for only a small percentage of the total cases of VTE, more than half of all patients with juvenile or idiopathic VTE have been identified with an inherited thrombophilic condition.11. Given that VTE is the leading preventable cause of in-hospital deaths,19 every patient should be screened before other lesser screens are performed (bedsores, risk of falls, nutritional evaluation, and so forth). Stated another way— every patient deserves a proper history and physical to uncover any possible factors that might increase their risk of a VTE.

	Deep vein thrombosis		**Pulmonary embolism**	
	Calf	Proximal	Clinical	Fatal
Low risk (minor surgery in patients < 40 years with no additional risk factors)	2%	0-4%	0-2%	<0,01%
Moderate risk (minor surgery and additional risk factor	10-20%	2-4%	1-2%	0,1-0,4%
High risk (surgery in patients > 60 years or age 40-60 years with additional risk factors (previous venous thromboembolism, cancer, thrombophilia)	20-40%	4-8%	2-4%	0,4-1,0%
Highest risk (surgery in patients with multiple risk factors [age > 40 years, cancer, previous venous thromboembolism]: hip or knee arthroplasty, hip fracture surgery; major trauma - spinal cord surgery)	40-80%	10-20%	4-10%	0,2-5%
Modified from reference 16 with permission of the American College of Chest Physicians.				

Table 1. Risk of venous thromboembolism in surgical patients without prophylaxis

In 1992, the Thromboembolic Risk Factors (THRIFT) Consensus Group identified acquired risk factors for VTE.20 Sixteen years later, the most recent update of the American College of Chest Physicians (ACCP) guidelines for VTE prophylaxis reveals essentially the same risk factors for VTE as those identified by THRIFT, with the addition of a few new ones, including acute medical illness, and the removal of smoking as a separate risk factor (Table

1). 19 The incidence of VTE increases dramatically in tandem with the number of risk factors identified in patients.11,21 Most hospitalized patients have at least one risk factor for VTE, and the most recent ACCP review of VTE estimated that approximately 40% have 3 or more risk factors.19 These include fracture (hip or leg), hip or knee replacement, major general surgery, major trauma, and spinal cord injury,11 as well as a history of VTE,11 thrombophilia, 11 inflammatory bowel disease,22 postoperative infection, 19 and cancer.23 Bed rest for more than 72 hours,11,24 use of hormones,11 and impaired mobility11 are additional risk factors. Many of these factors are not simple binary (ie, yes/no) risks. For example, age is a significant risk factor, with the risk approximately doubling with each decade beyond age 40.11,25 It is not sufficient to use a single age cut-off level to define high or low risk.11 Similarly, the incidence of VTE increases with length of surgery.26,27 In addition, Sugerman et al28 found higher rates of VTE in obese patients (mean body mass index, 61) who also had venous stasis syndrome; a simple cut-off level based on a definition of obesity would not capture this increased risk. In fact, Anderson and Spencer11 suggest that the association of risk of VTE and weight alone is a weak one. As noted earlier, hospitalized patients usually have at least 1 risk factor for VTE, and more than a third of hospitalized patients have 3 risk factors or more.19 Risk factor weighting can be used to calculate the risk for an individual patient, and the results may be used to determine several aspects of prophylaxis, such as the length of prophylaxis (including out-of-hospital prophylaxis), selection of prophylactic agent, timing of first dose, and the need for combined use of physical and pharmacologic methods.

Risk assessment typically has taken 1 of 2 approaches, group risk assessment or individual risk assessment. The group risk assessment approach assigns patients to one of a few broad risk categories, whereas individual risk assessment seeks to define risk more accurately by using individualized risk scores.19 The system recommended by the 2001 ACCP guidelines used a group risk assessment in which the type of surgery ("major" vs "minor"), age bracket, and presence of additional risk factors were used to assign patients to 1 of 4 risk groups29; however, this was based on older studies, arbitrary age cut-off levels, and inexact definitions.[19] The ACCP has refined this recommendation with a newer one in which patients are assigned 1 of 3 VTE risk levels based on type of surgery, patient mobility, overall risk of bleeding, and moderate/high risk of VTE based on the presence of additional risk factors 19 As the investigators note, this group risk assessment approach ignores the substantial variability in patient-specific risk factors, but it does take into account what they view as the principal risk factor (surgery vs acute medical illness). This approach is most appropriate for patients who fit the criteria of the randomized clinical trials that were used to develop the model; the investigators include a disclaimer for patient groups that have not been included in clinical trials or for types of patients who have not been tested.19 However, the group risk assessment approach recommended by the ACCP may not be appropriate for all individual patients.30 Out-of-hospital prophylaxis is not addressed except for a few very high risk groups (major cancer surgery, total joint replacement).19 It may be more appropriate to use the individual risk assessment approach to identify and evaluate all possible risk factors to determine the true extent of risk for a patient.30 The ACCP guidelines, in fact, point out that "specific knowledge about each patient's risk factors for VTE" is an essential component of the decision-making process when prescribing thromboprophylaxis. 19 Also, if many risk factors are present and a planned procedure is based on a quality-of-life decision rather than a critical medical need, the patient may come to a different decision about whether to proceed.30 A common misconception among physicians is that individual risk assessment takes longer and is more cumbersome than group risk assessment. However, individual assessment can be accomplished with, for example, a simple assessment form that merely captures information from the history and physical examination of the patient.

Among all patients with PE in the PIOPED II trial 94% had 1 or more of the following assessed risk factors: bed rest within the last month of 3 days or more, travel within the last month of 4 hours or more, surgery within 3 months, malignancy, past history of DVT or PE, trauma of lower extremities or pelvis, central venous instrumentation within 3 months, stroke, paresis or paralysis, heart failure or chronic obstructive pulmonary disease (COPD).31 Immobilization of only 1 or 2 days may predispose to PE, and 65% of those who were immobilized were immobilized for 2 weeks or less.[32]

2. Obesity and height

Investigations that reported an increased risk for VTE caused by obesity have been criticized because they failed to control for hospital confinement or other risk factors.33 High proportions of patients with VTE have been found to be obese,13,34 but the importance of the association is diminished because of the high proportion of obesity in the general population.35 Some investigations showed an increased risk ratio for DVT or PE in obese women,21,36,38 but data in men were less compelling. The Nurses' Health Study showed that the age-adjusted risk ratio for PE women with a body mass index (BMI, calculated as weight in kilograms divided by the square of height in meters) 29.0 kg/m2 or higher was 3.2 compared with the leanest category of less than 21.0 kg/m2.36 The Framingham Heart Study showed that metropolitan relative weight was significantly and independently associated with PE among women, but not men.39 However, the Study of Men Born in 1913 showed that men in the highest decile of waist circumference (>100 cm) had an adjusted relative risk for VTE of 3.92 compared with men with a waist circumference less than 100 cm.40 Among 1272 outpatients (men and women), the odds ratio for DVT, comparing obese (BMI> 30 kg/m2) with nonobese patients, was 2.39.41 Others showed a similar odds ratio for DVT of 2.26 compared with nonobese patients.37 BMI correlated linearly with the development of PE in women.42 On the other hand, the Olmsted County, Minnesota case-control study found no evidence that current BMI was an independent risk factor for VTE in men or women.33,43 Others did not show obesity to be a risk for VTE in men.21,38 Analysis of the huge database of the National Hospital Discharge Survey44 showed compelling evidence that obesity is a risk factor for VTE.45 Among patients hospitalized in short-term hospitals throughout the United States, in whom obesity was coded among the discharge diagnoses but not defined, 91,000 of 12,015,000 (0.8%) had PE.45 Among hospitalized patients who were not diagnosed with obesity, PE was diagnosed in 2,366,000 of 691,000,000 (0.3%). DVT was diagnosed in 243,000 of 12,015,000 (2.0%) of patients diagnosed with obesity, and in 5,524,000 of 691,000,000 (0.8%) who were not diagnosed with obesity. The relative risk of PE, comparing obese patients with nonobese patients, was 2.18 and for DVT it was 2.50.45 The relative risks for PE and DVT were age dependent. Obesity had the greatest effect on patients less than 40 years of age, in whom the relative risk for PE in obese patients was 5.19 and the relative risk for DVT was 5.20.45 The higher relative risk of obesity in younger patients may have reflected that younger patients uncommonly have multiple confounding- associated risk factors, which make the risk of obesity inapparent. Previous investigators used several indices of obesity including a BMI greater than 35 kg/m2 as well as BMI 30 to 35 kg/m2,46 BMI 29 kg/m2 or greater,36 weight more than 20% of median recommended weight for height,13 and for men, waist circumference 100 cm or greater.40 It is likely that all patients diagnosed with obesity in the National Hospital Discharge Survey database were obese, irrespective of the criteria used. However, some obese patients may not have had a listed discharge diagnosis of obesity, and they would have been included in the nonobese group. This situation would have tended to reduce the relative risk of obesity in VTE. Various abnormalities of hemostasis have been described in obesity, in particular increased plasminogen activator inhibitor-1 (PAI-1).47,48 Other abnormalities of coagulation have been reported as well,48 including increased platelet activation,39 increased levels of plasma fibrinogen, factor VII, factor VIII, and von Willebrand factor.49 Fibrinogen, factor VIIc, and PAI-1 correlated with BMI.50 Regarding height, in the study of Swedish men, those taller than 179 cm (5′ 10″) had a 1.5 times higher risk of VTE than men shorter than 172 cm.51 The Physicians' Health Study of male physicians also showed that taller men had a significantly increased risk of VTE.52

3. Air travel

The possibility of VTE after travel is not unique to air travel.53,54 Prolonged periods in cramped quarters, irrespective of travel, can lead to PE.55 The term economy class syndrome was introduced in 1988,56 but has since been replaced with flight-related DVT in recognition that all travelers are at risk, irrespective of the class of travel[57] Rates of development of PE with air travel lasting 12 to 18 hours have been calculated as 2.6 PE/million travelers.58 With air travel of 8 hours or longer, 1.65/million passengers had acute PE on arrival.59 With 6 to 8 hours of air travel the rate of acute PE on arrival was 0.25/million and among those who traveled for 6 hours or less none developed acute PE on arrival.59 The trend showing increasing rates of PE with duration of travel is compelling, but the incidence of DVT was about 3000 times higher in a prospective investigation.60 In a prospective investigation of travelers who traveled for 10 hours or longer, 4 of 878 (0.5%) developed PE and 5 of 878 (0.6%) developed DVT.60

4. Varicose veins

Varicose veins were found by some to be an agedependent risk factor for VTE.43 Among patients aged 45 years the odds ratio for VTE was 4.2.43 In patients aged 60 years the odds ratio was 1.9 and at aged 75 years, varicose veins were not associated with an increased risk of VTE.43 However, others did not find varicose veins to be a risk factor for DVT61 or PE found at autopsy.21

5. Oral contraceptives

Although the risk of VTE is higher among users of oral estrogen-containing contraceptives than nonusers, 62,63 the absolute risk is low.64 An absolute risk of VTE of less than 1/10,000 patients/y increased to only 3 to 4/10,000 patients/y during the time oral contraceptives were used.64 The relative risk for VTE in women using oral contraceptives containing 50 mg of estrogen, compared with users of oral contraceptives that contained less than 50 mg was 1.5.65 The relative risk for VTE in women using oral contraceptives containing more than 50 mg of estrogen, compared with users of oral contraceptives that contained less than 50 mg was 1.7.65 No difference in the risk of VTE was found with various levels of low doses of 20, 30, 40, and 50 mg/ d.66 With doses of estrogen of 50 mg/ d, the rate of VTE was 7.0/ 10,000 contraceptive users/ y and with more than 50 mg/ d, the rate of VTE was 10.0/10,000 oral contraceptive users/ y.65 However, some found no appreciable difference in the relative risk of VTE in relation to low or higher estrogen doses.67 Reports of the risk of VTE in relation to the duration of use of oral contraceptives are inconsistent. Some showed relative risks increased as the duration of use of estrogen-containing oral contraceptives increased.68 The relative risks were 0.7 in women who used oral contraceptives for less than 1 year, 1.4 for those who used oral contraceptives for 1 to 4 years and 1.8 in those who used it for 5 years or longer.68 Others showed the opposite effect, with a decreasing relative risk with duration of use.66 The relative risk for DVT or PE was 5.1 with use for less than 1 year, 2.5 with use for 1 to 5 years, and 2.1 with use for longer than 5 years.66 Some showed the risk to be unaffected by the duration of use.67 A synergistic effect of oral contraceptives with obesity has been shown.69,71 The odds ratio of DVT in obese women (BMI _30 kg/ m2) who were users of oral contraceptives ranged from 5.2 to 7.8 compared with obese women who did not use oral contraceptives37,69,71 and among women with a BMI 35 kg/ m2 or higher, the odds ratio was 3.1 compared with similarly obese nonusers of oral contraceptives.71

6. Tamoxifen

Tamoxifen is a selective estrogen-receptor modulator used for treatment of breast cancer and for prevention of breast cancer in high-risk patients.72,74 Among women with breast cancer currently being treated with tamoxifen, compared with previous users or those who never used it, the odds ratio was 7.1.74 Others found a lower odds ratio of 2.7.43 The odds ratio for VTE in women at high risk of breast cancer who received tamoxifen to prevent breast cancer was 2.1.73 Others found a hazard ratio of 1.63.72

7. Hormonal replacement therapy

There is a 2- to 3-fold increased risk of VTE with the use of hormone replacement therapy in postmenopausal women.75,76 Among postmenopausal women who had coronary artery disease and received estrogen plus progestin, the relative hazard of VTE was 2.7 compared with nonusers.77 Review showed that the risk of VTE is highest in the first year of hormone replacement therapy.78 The risk of VTE is increased for oral estrogen alone, oral estrogen combined with progestin, and probably for transdermal hormone replacement therapy.78

8. Congenital hypercoagulable disorders

8.1 Antithrombin deficiency

Antithrombin is a serine protease inhibitor of thrombin and also inhibits factors IXa, Xa, XIa, and XIIa. Thrombin is irreversibly bound by antithrombin and prevents thrombin's action on fi brinogen, on factors V, VIII, and XIII, and on platelets.[79] This anticoagulant is synthesized in the liver and endothelial cells, and has a half-life of 2.8 days.[80] Antithrombin deficiency has a prevalence of 1 : 5000 with more than 100 genetic mutations and an autosomal dominant inheritance pattern.[81] Homozygotes typically die *in utero* whereas heterozygotes typically have an antithrombin level that is 40 to 70% of normal.

Antithrombin deficiency is associated with lower extremity venous thrombosis as well as mesenteric venous thrombosis. The most common presentation in those with antithrombin deficiency is deep venous thrombosis with or without pulmonary embolism.[82]

8.2 Protein C and protein S deficiency

Protein C is a vitamin K dependent anticoagulant protein that, once activated by thrombin, will inactivate factors Va and VIIIa, thereby inhibiting the generation of thrombin.[83] Additionally, activated protein C stimulates the release of t-PA. It is produced in the liver and is the dominant endogenous anticoagulant with an eight-hour half-life. Protein C deficiency has a prevalence of 1 in 200–300 with more than 150 mutations and an autosomal dominant inheritance.[83,84]

Protein S is also a vitamin K dependent anticoagulant protein that is a cofactor to activated protein C. The actions of protein S are regulated by complement C4b binding protein and only the free form of protein S serves as an activated protein C cofactor.[85] Additionally, protein S appears to have independent anticoagulant function by directly inhibiting procoagulant enzyme complexes.[84,86] The prevalence of protein S defi ciency is about 1 : 500 with an autosomal dominant inheritance.

Clinically, protein C and S deficiencies are essentially identical. With homozygous protein C and S defi ciencies, infants typically will succumb to purpura fulminans, a state of unrestricted clotting and fi brinolysis. In heterozygotes, venous thromboses may occur at an early age especially in the lower extremity.[87] Thrombosis may also occur in mesenteric, renal, and cerebral veins.

8.3 Factor V Leiden mutation and activated protein C resistance

Factor V is a glycoprotein synthesized in the liver. With Factor V Leiden, a point mutation occurs when arginine is substituted by glutamine at position 506. This point mutation causes the activated Factor V to be resistant to inactivation by activated protein C thus causing a procoagulant state.

Clinically, patients may present with deep venous thrombosis in the lower extremities, or less commonly in the portal vein, cerebral vein, or superfi cial venous system.

8.4 Prothrombin G20210 polymorphism

Prothrombin (Factor II) is a zymogen synthesized in the liver and dependent on vitamin K. When prothrombin is activated, it forms thrombin (Factor IIa). A single mutation where adenine is substituted for guanine occurs at the 20210 position. The mechanism for increased thrombotic risk is not well understood, but individuals with this genetic variant have supranormal levels of prothrombin. The mutation is inherited as an autosomal dominant trait and is associated with both arterial and venous thrombosis.

Clinically, patients may present with deep venous thrombosis of the lower extremity, cerebral venous thrombosis, as well as arterial thrombosis. The risk of thrombosis increases in the presence of other genetic coagulation defects and with acquired risk factors.[88,84]

8.5 Hyperhomocysteinemia

Homocysteine is an amino acid formed during the metabolism of methionine and may be elevated secondary to inherited defects in two enzymes that are part of the conversion of homocysteine to cysteine. The two enzymes involved are N5,N10–methylene tetrahydrofolate reductase (MTHFR) or cystathionine beta-synthase. Hyperhomocysteinemia has been shown to increase the risk of atherosclerosis, atherothrombosis, and venous thrombosis. Elevated plasma homocysteine levels cause various dysfunctions of endothelial cells leading to a prothrombotic state.

Hypercoagulable syndromes include inherited and acquired thrombophilias. The former is discussed in detail in the article by Weitz in this issue. The latter includes the antiphospholipid syndrome, heparin-induced thrombocytopenia, acquired dysfibrinogenemia, myeloproliferative disorders, and malignancy. Myeloproliferative disorders and malignancy are described elsewhere in this article. Regarding the antiphospholipid syndrome, antiphospholipid antibodies are associated with both arterial and venous thrombosis.89 The most commonly detected subgroups of antiphospholipid antibodies are lupus anticoagulant antibodies, anticardiolipin antibodies and anti-b2-glycoprotein I antibodies.90 DVT, the most common manifestation of the antiphospholipid syndrome, occurs in 29% to 55% of patients with the syndrome, and about half of these patients have pulmonary emboli.91,92 The risk of heparin-associated thrombocytopenia is more duration related than dose related. Heparin-associated thrombocytopenia occurs more frequently with unfractionated heparin when used for an extended duration than with LMWH used for an extended duration.93 When used for prophylaxis, there was a higher prevalence of heparin-associated thrombocytopenia inthose receiving unfractionated heparin (1.6%, 57 of 3463) than in those receiving LMWH (0.6%, 23 of 3714).93 However, treatment resulted in only a small difference in the prevalence of heparinassociated thrombocytopenia comparing unfractionated heparin (0.9%, 22 of 2321) with LMWH (0.6%, 18 of 3126).93 Acquired dysfibrinogenemia occurs most often in patients with severe liver disease.94 The impairment of the fibrinogen is a structural defect caused by an increased carbohydrate content impairing the polymerization of the fibrin, depending on the degree of abnormality of the fibrinogen molecule.94

9. Heart failure

Congestive heart failure (CHF) is considered amajor risk factor for VTE.[13,41,61,95,96] Among patients with established CHF, those with lower ejection fractions had a higher risk of thromboembolic event.[97,98] However, some investigators did not evaluate CHF among the risk factors for VTE.[99] The reported frequency of PE in patients with heart failure has ranged widely from 0.9% to 39% of patients. [13,97,98,100,101] The reported frequency of DVT in patients with CHF also ranged widely from 10% to 59%.[13,41,61] The largest investigation was from the National Hospital Discharge Survey.[102] Among 58,873,000 patients hospitalized with heart failure in short-stay hospitals from 1979 to 2003, 1.63% had VTE (relative risk 5 1.47).[102] The relative risk for VTE was highest in patients less than 40 years old (relative risk 5 6.91). Some showed the lower the ejection fraction, the greater the risk of VTE.[103] Among 755,807 adults older than 20 years with heart failure who died from 1980 to 1998, PE was listed as the cause of death in 20,387 (2.7%).[104] Assuming that the accuracy of death certificates was only 26.7%,[105] the rate of death from PE in these patients may have been as high as 10.1%.

Therefore, the estimated death rate from PE in patients who died with heart failure was 3% to 10%. CHF seems to be a stronger risk factor in women. Dries and colleagues[97] reported a higher proportion of PE in women (24%) compared with men (14%). We too showed a higher relative risk of PE and of DVT in women with CHF than in men.[102] Although these data seemcompelling, multivariate logistic analysis failed to identify CHF as an independent risk factor for DVT or PE.[43] However, it was a risk factor for postmortem VTE that was not a cause of death.[43] In one study of pediatric patients with dilated cardiomyopathy awaiting transplant the incidence of pulmonary embolism was 13.9% [106].

Heart failure is the second most common risk factor for VTE in hospitalized patients, as shown in ENDORSE.[107]

10. COPD

Hospitalized patients with exacerbations of COPD, when routinely evaluated, showed PE in 25% to 29%.108,109From 1979 to 2003, 58,392,000 adults older than 20 years were hospitalized with COPD in short-stay hospitals in the United States.110 PE was diagnosed in 381,000 (0.65%) and DVT in 632,000 (1.08%).110 The relative risk for PE in adults hospitalized with COPD was 1.92 and for DVT it was 1.30. Among those aged 20 to 39 years with COPD, the relative risk for PE was 5.34. Among patients with COPD aged 40 to 59 years, the relative risk for PE decreased to 2.02, and among patients aged 60 to 79 years the relative risk for PE was 1.23.110 The relative risk for DVT was also higher in patients with COPD aged 20 to 39 years (relative risk 5 2.58) than in patients aged 40 years or older (relative risk 0.92-1.17, depending on age).110 In young adults, other risk factors in combination with COPD are uncommon, so the contribution of COPD to the risk of PE becomes more apparent than in older patients. Although these data strongly suggest that COPD is a risk factor for PE and DVT, multivariate logistic analysis did not identify it as an independent risk factor.43 Others, with univariate analysis, did not identify COPD as a risk factor.61

Neuhaus et al. [111] found pulmonary emboli in 27% of 66 autopsies performed in patients who had respiratory failure (not only as a decompensation of COPD) and died after admission to a Respiratory Intensive Care Unit.

The largest study was conducted by Schonhofer and Kohler [112] on a population of 196 patients admitted to a respiratory intensive care unit. The authors found a DVT rate of 10.7% as assessed by US. The majority (86%) of cases were asymptomatic and, interestingly, almost all major clinical variables (such as age, weight, severity of dyspnea, lung function, situation of blood gases) failed to predict patients who were more likely to develop DVT.

11. Stroke

There is considerable evidence that in spinal cord injury patients interruption of neurologic impulses and the ensuing paralysis cause profound metabolic changes in blood vessels accountable for venous thrombosis.

Vascular adaptations to inactivity and muscle atrophy, rather than the effect of a nonworking leg-muscle pump and sympathetic denervation, cause thrombosis, indicating that thrombosis established through venous incompetence cannot be reversed by anticoagulation alone.

Spinal cord injuries with paralysis result in an immobile state with retardation of the blood flow caused by the relaxation of muscle and the atony of blood vessels. It is not surprising that spinal cord injuries are frequently complicated by the development of venous thrombosis, which is inevitably linked to hospitalization, immobilization, vein wall damage, stasis, and hypercoagulability. Deep vein thrombosis and pulmonary emboli remain the major complications in spinal cord injuries below the C2 through T12 vertebrae associated with motor complete or motor nonfunctional paralysis. [113,114,115,116,117,118,119] Two surprising findings set spinal cord injury apart from other risk factors for venous thrombosis: incidence of leg DVT and pulmonary embolism in spinal cord injury is three times higher than in the general population.

Patients with stroke are at particular risk of developing DVT and PE because of limb paralysis, prolonged bed rest, and increased prothrombotic activity.120 Among 14,109,000 patients with ischemic stroke hospitalized in short-stay hospitals from 1979 to 2003, VTE was diagnosed in 165,000 (1.17%).121 Among 1,606,000 patients with hemorrhagic stroke, the incidence of VTE was higher (1.93%).

Among patients with ischemic stroke who died from 1980 to 1998, PE was the listed cause of death in 11,101 of 2,000,963 (0.55%).122 Based on an assumed sensitivity of death certificates for fatal PE of 26.7% to 37.2%,105,123 the corrected rate of fatal PE was 1.5% to 2.1%. Death rates from PE among patients with ischemic stroke decreased from 1980 to 1998, suggesting effective use of antithrombotic prophylaxis.

12. Cancer

Cancer is a major risk factor of venous thromboembolism (VTE) [124,125] as defined by deep-vein thrombosis (DVT) - including central venous catheter (CVC) related thrombosis - or pulmonaryembolism (PE), which occur in 4 to 20% of cancer patients [126,127].

12.1 Cancer-related factors

12.1.1 Site of cancer

In studies looking at pooled groups of patients with different types of malignancy, the rate of VTE is consistently highest in patients with cancer of the pancreas, stomach, brain, kidney, uterus, lung or ovary [128,129,130,131].

Both large retrospective studies by Stein et al and Chew et al based on discharge claims databases reported the highest rates of VTE in patients with pancreatic cancer (4.3% and 5.3%, respectively). Patients with stomach cancer had the second and third highest risk of developing VTE in these studies [128,132]. In patients with testicular and lung cancer, those with metastases to the liver and brain were shown to have higher rates of VTE compared with patients with other sites of metastases [133,134]. The rates of VTE for specific types of cancer have been reported in many studies.

12.1.2 Cancer stage

Multiple studies have shown an increased risk of VTE in patients with advanced-stage cancer. In a retrospective study of over 500 000 patients from the California Cancer Registry, patients with metastatic cancer stage were twice as likely to have developed VTE in the year prior to diagnosis of cancer [135]. In a population-based case–control study of patients with newly diagnosed VTE, including 389 patients with cancer, those with distant metastases had a higher risk of VTE (OR 19.8, CI 2.6–149) [136].

A multicentre retrospective study of VTE in hospitalized cancer patients reported an incidence of 10.3% in patients with advanced-stage cancer compared with 5.6% in patients with localized disease ($P < 0.0005$, OR 1.92, CI 1.21–3.04) [137], and these findings have been supported by other large studies in hospitalized cancer patients [138]. Other studies in ovarian, colorectal, pancreatic, lung and breast cancer support the finding that advanced-stage disease increases the risk of cancer- associated VTE [139,140,141,142,143,144].

12.2 Histology

In certain types of cancer, higher rates of VTE are found in some histological subtypes compared with others. For example, in patients with non-small-cell lung cancer, 9.9% of those with adenocarcinoma subtype develop VTE in the first 6 months after diagnosis compared with 7.7% with squamous cell carcinoma (HR 1.9, CI 1.7–2.1) [141].Inbreast and colon cancer patients, the type of histology does not predict for the incidence of cancer-associated VTE, but VTE-associated mortality rates are higher in patients with certain histological subtypes [141,143].

12.3 Time after diagnosis

Several studies have demonstrated that the risk of VTE is highest in the initial time period following cancer diagnosis. In a population-based study of patients with thrombosis, the risk of developing VTE was highest in the first few months following the initial diagnosis of malignancy. A retrospective analysis of over 200 000 cancer patients from the California Cancer Registry revealed that the rate of VTE per patient-year in the first year after diagnosis of cancer was 3.3, compared with 0.8 in the second year after diagnosis [145]. The rate of VTE in patients with colon cancer during the first 6 months after diagnosis is 5.0/100 patient-years, but this drops off dramatically to 1.4/100 patient-years in the next 6- month period [143].

12.4 Chemotherapy

Chemotherapy is one of the most important factors in VTE risk stratification of cancer patients. Large population-based studies in groups of pooled cancer patients have demonstrated a significantly increased risk in patients receiving chemotherapy. Heit et al used a population-based study of patients with a new diagnosis of VTE, 23% of which had a diagnosis of active malignancy, to demonstrate a significantly increased risk of VTE in those on chemotherapy (OR 6.5, CI 2.11–20) [146].

Studies in specific types of cancer and with specific antineoplastic agents have also supported the role of chemotherapy in predicting the risk of cancer-associated VTE. Two prospective studies of breast cancer patients demonstrated that the risk of VTE in patients receiving chemotherapy in addition to tamoxifen or surgery increased two- to seven-fold [147,148]. A recent meta-analysis of breast cancer patients revealed that use of adjuvant hormonal therapy was associated with a 1.5–7-fold increased risk of VTE [149].

12.5 Surgery

Surgery is a well-known risk factor for development of VTE in patients without cancer. The incidence of DVT in cancer patients undergoing general surgery is estimated at 37% compared with 20% in patients without cancer [150]. Factors related to immobility, tissue destruction and venous stasis are likely to be related to the increased risk of VTE after surgery.

12.6 Indwelling catheters

Indwelling central venous catheters (CVC) greatly facilitate treatment in cancer patients, but they are also associated with complications including a significant risk of catheter-associated thrombosis. The incidence of symptomatic catheter-related DVT in adult patients ranges from 0.3% to 28%, while the rate of catheter-related DVT assessed by venography is 27-66%[151].

Studies have not consistently demonstrated an association between use of haematopoietic growth factors and risk of cancer-associated VTE. İn a prospective study of ambulatory patients receiving chemotherapy, both the use of white cell growth factors and the use of red cell growth factors or decreased haemoglobin were independent predictors of VTE in multivariate analysis [152]. This association was only significant in types of cancer already known to have high rates of thrombosis, and it is possible that these agents are used more frequently in patients with other markers of poor prognosis or more aggressive disease.

12.7 Platelet and leukocyte counts

The authors' group was the first to identify an elevated prechemotherapy platelet count as a significant risk factor for cancer-associated thrombosis [152]. In a prospective study of outpatients receiving chemotherapy, 21.9% had a platelet count of 350 000/mm3 or more prior to starting chemotherapy. The incidence of VTE was 3.98% (1.66% per month) for these patients, which was significantly higher than the rate of 1.25% (0.52% per month) for patients with a prechemotherapy platelet count of less than 200 000/mm3 (P for trend¼ 0.0003). The distribution of rechemotherapy platelet counts in patients who subsequently developed VTE was significantly higher than that for patients who did not develop VTE (t-test P ¼0.002, Wilcoxon rank sum test P ¼0.0002).

12.8 Tissue factor

Tissue factor (TF), a transmembrane glycoprotein present on subendothelial tissue, platelets and leukocytes, is a key component in the initiation of coagulation and may play a role in cancer- associated thrombosis [153-155]. The authors recently demonstrated a correlation between the level of TF expression in pancreatic tumours and subsequent development of VTE [156]. VTE was four-fold more common (P ¼ 0.04) among patients with high TF-expressing carcinomas (26.5%) than among patients with low TF-expressing carcinomas (5.5%).

From 1979 to 1999, among 40,787,000 patients hospitalized in short-stay hospitals with any of 19 malignancies studied, 827,000 (2.0%) had VTE.157 This was twice the incidence in patients without these malignancies.157 The highest incidence of VTE was in patients with carcinoma of the pancreas (4.3%) and the lowest incidences were in patients with carcinoma of the bladder and carcinoma of the lip, oral cavity, or pharynx (<0.6% to 1.0%). Incidences with cancer were not age dependent.157 Myeloproliferative diseaseand lymphoma were associated with relative risks for VTE of 2.9 and 2.5, respectively157 Leukemia was associated with a lower relative risk (1.7). Based on death certificates from 1980 to 1998 among patients who died with cancer, PE was the listed cause of death in 0.21%.158 Adjustment of the data for the frailty of the diagnosis of fatal PE based on death certificates indicated a likely range of 0.31% to 1.97%.158

13. Pregnancy

Pregnancy-associated DVT based on data from the National Hospital Discharge Survey was diagnosed in 93,000 of 80,798,000 women (0.12%) from 1979 to 1999.151 The rate of pregnancyassociated DVT (vaginal delivery and cesarean section) increased from 1982 to 1999, although the rate of nonpregnancy-associated DVT decreased for most of this period. Some showed the rate of pregnancy-associated DVT was twice the rate of nonpregnancy-associated DVT.159 A 6-fold increase in the rate of thromboembolism during pregnancy and the puerperium compared with nonpregnant women has been reported by others.160 Although the rate of pregnancy-associated DVT was higher than the rate of nonpregnancyassociated DVT, the rate of pregnancyassociated PE was lower than

Pathophysiology of venous thromboembolism during Pregnancy:

Increased venous distensibility and capacity, with a resultant reduction in the velocity of blood flow in the lower limbs, are demonstrable from the first trimester of pregnancy[162,163]. These changes are compounded by a 20–25% increase in the overall circulatory volume during pregnancy[164]. Obstruction of the inferior vena cava by the enlarging gravid uterus may also result in increased stasis[165]. Compression of the left iliac vein by the right iliac artery as they cross [166] may explain the preponderance of left leg DVT during pregnancy [161,167].

Altered levels of coagulation factors have been described both during pregnancy and postpartum. Hypercoagulability is thought to be promoted by increases in coagulation factors such as fibrinogen, von Willebrand factor, and factor VIII:C [168,169-171], as well as by decreases in natural inhibitors of coagulation such as protein S [172] and the development of an acquired resistance to the endogenous anticoagulant, activated protein C [173]. In addition, a reduction in global fibrinolytic activity has been described during pregnancy [174], perhaps as a consequence of increases in the levels of plasminogen activator inhibitor 1 (PAI 1) and plasminogen activator inhibitor 2 (PAI 2) [174-176], the latter being produced by the placenta.

Exogenous risk factors also appear to determine the thrombotic risk associated with pregnancy. In a retrospective cohort study of unselected consecutive patients with confirmed pregnancy-related venous thromboembolism, approximately two-thirds of patients had an identifiable acquired risk factor (for example, age over 35 years, intercurrent illness, immobility, increased parity or caesarean section) [177].

The reason for this difference is unknown and could reflect difference of the natural history of DVT in pregnancy. It also could reflect a reluctance to expose pregnant women to ionizing radiation associated with imaging for PE, resulting in a decreased frequency of diagnosis of PE. The rate of pregnancy-associated DVT was higher among women aged 35 to 44 years than in younger women. The rate of pregnancyassociated DVT among black women was higher than among white women.159,178,179 DVT was more frequent among women who underwent cesarean section (104/100,000/y) than those who underwent vaginal delivery (47/ 100,000/y).159 VTE in pregnancy is discussed in detail in the article by Marik elsewhere in this issue.

14. Surgery and trauma

In PIOPED, trauma of the lower extremities was a predisposing factor in 10% of patients with PE, and in PIOPED II trauma of the lower extremities or pelvis was a predisposing factor in 14%.180,181 Surgery within 3 months of the acute PE was a predisposing factor in 54% in PIOPED and in 23% in PIOPED II.180,181 The prevalence of VTE following various categories of surgery and trauma has been reviewed in detail by Geerts and colleagues182.

15. Central venous access

The use of long-term venous access is now an integral component of treatment for patients receiving long-term antibiotic administration or hyperalimentation or undergoing chemotherapy. Externalized tunneled catheters were introduced almost 30 years ago, but required daily cleaning and frequent flushing[190,191]. On average, deep venous thrombosis (DVT) can complicate approximately 2%–6.7% of such port placements[192 - 194], although literature reports have ranged from 0% to 26%[195-198]. In 1991, Monreal et al.[199] observed that 4 of 30 consecutive patients with upper extremity deep venous thrombosis (DVT) had PE (13.3%), but more importantly, all these 4 occurred in 20 catheter related DVT patients (20%), while none of 10 patients with primary upper extremity DVT had PE.

16. Medical illnesses

16.1 Inflammatory bowel disease

The incidence of VTE among hospitalized medical patients with ulcerative colitis was 1.9% and the incidence with Crohn disease was lower (1.2%).200 Among medical patients who had neither ulcerative colitis nor Crohn disease the incidence was 1.1%.200 The relative risk of VTE among patients with ulcerative colitis compared with patients who did not have inflammatory bowel disease was 1.9 and with Crohn disease it was 1.2. Among patients younger than 40 years with ulcerative colitis, the relative risk of VTE compared with patients who did not haveinflammatory bowel disease was 2.96 and in patients younger than 40 years with Crohn disease the relative risk was 2.23.200

16.2 Liver disease

Patients with chronic liver disease (both alcoholic and nonalcoholic) seem to have a lower risk of PE than patients without liver disease,43,201 but data are inconsistent.202 Chronic liver disease may result in impaired production of vitamin-K dependent procoagulant factors.203 However, decreased production of vitamin-K dependent endogenous anticoagulants, such as protein C, protein S, and antithrombin III, may counter the hypocoagulability in such patients.203 Other prothrombotic factors may counteract the impaired production of vitamin Kdependent procoagulant factors including lupus anticoagulant, activated protein C resistance, PT20210A mutation, Factor V Leiden, MTHFR mutation, and increased levels of factor VIII.204 Based on data from the National Hospital Discharge Survey, among 4,927,000 hospitalized patients with chronic alcoholic liver disease from 1979 to 2006, the prevalence of VTE was 0.6% and among 4,565,000 hospitalized patients with chronic nonalcoholic liver disease it was 0.9%.201 The prevalence of VTE was higher in those with chronic alcoholic liver disease than with nonalcoholic liver disease, but the difference was small and of no clinical consequence.201

Both showed a lower prevalence of VTE than in hospitalized patients with most other medical diseases. It may be that both chronic alcoholic liver disease and chronic nonalcoholic liver disease have protective antithrombotic mechanisms although the mechanisms differ.

16.3 Hypothyroidism

Among 19,519,000 hospitalized patients with a diagnosis of hypothyroidism from 1979 to 2005, 119,000 (0.61%) had PE (relative risk 5 1.64).205 DVT was diagnosed in 1.36% of hypothyroid patients (relative risk 5 1.62).205 The relative risk for PE in patients with hypothyroidism was highest in patients younger than 40 years (relative risk 5 3.99) and the relative risk for DVT was also highest in patients younger than 40 years (relative risk 5 2.25). Hyperthyroidism was not associated with an increased risk for VTE (relative risk 5 0.98).

16.4 Rheumatoid arthritis

Rheumatoid arthritis is not generally considered a risk factor for VTE, although abnormalities of coagulation factors have been found in patients with rheumatoid arthritis.206,207 Among 4,818,000 patients hospitalized in short-stay hospitals from 1979 to 2005 with rheumatoid arthritis who did not have joint surgery, the incidence of PE was 2.3%, and the relative risk of VTE compared with those who did not have rheumatoid arthritis was 1.99.208 Among patients younger than 50 years the relative risk was higher (2.13).208

16.5 Diabetes mellitus

Among 92,240,000 patients with diabetes mellitus hospitalized from 1979 to 2005, 1,267,000 (1.4%) had VTE.209 The relative risk for VTE was increased only in patients younger than 50 years and was highest in patients aged 20 to 29 years (relative risk 5 1.73). In patients with diabetes mellitus who did not have obesity, stroke, heart failure, or cancer, compared with those who did not have diabetes mellitus and did not have any of these comorbid conditions, the relative risk for VTE was 1.52 in patients aged 20 to 29 years and 1.19 in patients 30 to 39 years. In older patients, the relative risk of VTE in patients with diabetes mellitus was not increased.209 Among all adults with diabetes mellitus, the relative risk of VTE was 1.05.209

16.6 Human immunodeficiency virus

Among 2,429,000 patients older than 18 years hospitalized in short-stay hospitals from 1990 through 2005 with human immunodeficiency virus (HIV) infection; the prevalence of VTE was 1.7% (relative risk 5 1.21).210 The prevalence of VTE in patients aged 30 to 49 years was also 1.7%, but the relative risk compared with patients who did not have HIV infection was higher (1.65).210

16.7 Nephrotic syndrome

From 1979 to 2005, 925,000 patients were discharged from short-stay hospitals with nephrotic syndrome and 14,000 (1.5%) had DVT (relative risk 5 1.72).211 In patients aged 18 to 39 years the relative risk for DVT was 6.81.211 Renal vein thrombosis was so uncommon that too few were reported to calculate its prevalence. Therefore, PE, if it occurs, is likely to be due to emboli from the lower extremities and not the renal vein.

16.8 Sickle cell disease

Sickle cell disease does not seem to be a risk factor for DVT.212 Among 1,804,000 patients hospitalized in short-stay hospitals with sickle cell disease from 1979 to 2003, 11,000 (0.61%) had a discharge diagnosis of DVT, which was not more than in African Americans without sickle cell disease (0.81%).212 Among patients with sickle cell disease, a discharge diagnosis of PE was made in 0.50% compared with 0.33% who did not have sickle cell disease. Regarding patients younger than 40 years, 0.44% had PE, whereas among patients who did not have sickle cell disease, 0.12% had PE.212 The higher prevalence of apparent PE in patients with sickle cell disease compared with African American patients the same age who did not have sickle cell disease, and the comparable prevalence of DVT in both groups, is compatible with the concept that thrombosis in situ may be present in many.

16.9 Systemic lupus erythematosus

Systemic lupus erythematosus is believed to be independently associated with the risk of developing DVT.61 The odds ratio for DVT in patients with systemic lupus erythematosus, compared with those without it, was 4.3.61

16.10 Behçet disease

Behcet disease is a rare multisystem inflammatory disorder of unknown cause.213 VTE occurs in about one-fifth of patients with Behc¸ et disease.213

16.11 Paroxysmal nocturnal hemoglobinuria

Review of 13 retrospective studies of patients with paroxysmal nocturnal hemoglobinuria showed a 30% prevalence of venous thrombotic events in patients from Western nations.214 The majority was within the hepatic and mesenteric veins.214

16.12 Buerger disease

PE associated with thromboangiitis obliterans (Buerger disease) is rare, and to our knowledge, limited to a case report.215

17. Sepsis

Initiation of coagulation takes place when TF is exposed, such as by fibroblasts, when there is tissue damage or by cytokine-stimulated monocytes and endothelial cells[216], as in sepsis. While TF is the major initiator of coagulation, endotoxin, foreign bodies, and negatively charged particles may initiate coagulation via contact system activation. TF binds to factor

VIIa, and this complex (TF:VIIa) may then activate factor X and factor IX[217]. Factor Xa, associated with factor Va, forms the prothrombinase complex, which subsequently turns prothrombin into thrombin.

The relationship between coagulation and inflammation is complex and, as yet, not completely understood. It is known that blood clotting not only leads to fibrin deposition and platelet activation, but it also results in vascular cell activation, which contributes to leukocyte activation[218]. On the other hand, inflammation can induce TF expression in monocytes, via nuclear factor kappa-B (NF-kB) activation, thus initiating coagulation[216].

Examples of this interaction are readily seen. First, leukocytes are found at relatively high concentrations in venous thrombi, and leukocytes and activated platelets can form rosettes mediated by P-selectin expression on the surface of the activated platelet [219,220].

These microscopic observations are probably elicited from the actions of thrombin, which can activate platelets and endothelium, increasing the surface expression of P-selectin[221,222]. P- electin is the primary initial mediator of leukocyte-endothelial cell rolling and is critical for leukocyte adhesion. Second, TF:VIIa and factor Xa have been shown to activate cells and generate responses similar to those mediated by thrombin[218]. Third, GAG and TM expression on cell surfaces are inhibited by inflammatory cytokines [223,224,225,226] and lipopolysaccharide (LPS)[227], thus blocking the augmentation of AT action by GAG, and APC formation by TM.

18. References

[1] Fowkes FJI, Price JF, Fowkes FGR. Incidence of diagnosed deep vein thrombosis in the general population: systematic review. *Eur J Vasc Endovasc Surg* 2003; 25: 1–5.

[2] Heit JA, Silverstein MD, Mohr DN, et al. The epidemiology of venous thromboembolism in the community. *Thromb Haemost* 2001; 86: 452–63.

[3] Stein PD, Patel KC, Kalra NK, et al. Deep venous thrombosis in a general hospital. *Chest* 2002; 122: 960–62.

[4] Kniffin WD, Baron JA, Barrett J, Birkmeyer JD, Anderson FA Jr. The epidemiology of diagnosed pulmonary embolism and deep venous thrombosis in the elderly. *Arch Intern Med* 1994; 154: 861–66.

[5] Heit JA, O'Fallon WM, Petterson TM, et al. Relative impact of risk factors for deep vein thrombosis and pulmonary embolism: a population-based study. *Arch Intern Med* 2002; 162: 1245–48.

[6] Cushman M, Tsai AW, White RH, et al. Deep vein thrombosis and pulmonary embolism in two cohorts: the longitudinal investigation of thromboembolism etiology. *Am J Med* 2004; 117: 19–25.

[7] Patel RK, Lambie J, Bonner L, Arya R. Venous thromboembolism in the black population. *Arch Intern Med* 2004; 164: 1348–49.

[8] Klatsky AL, Armstrong MA, Poggi J. Risk of pulmonary embolism and/or deep venous thrombosis in Asian-Americans. *Am J Cardiol* 2000; 85: 1334–37.

[9] Anderson FA, Wheeler HB, Goldberg RJ, et al. A population-based perspective of the hospital incidence and case-fatality rates of deep vein thrombosis and pulmonary embolism: the Worcester DVT Study. *Arch Intern Med* 1991; 151: 933–38.

[10] Kyrle PA, Minar E, Bialonczyk C, Hirschl M, Weltermann A, Eichinger S. The risk of recurrent venous thromboembolism in men and women. *N Engl J Med* 2004; 350: 2558–63.
[11] Anderson FA Jr, Spencer FA. Risk factors for venous thromboembolism. Circulation 2003;107:I9 -I16.
[12] Coleridge-Smith PD, Hasty JH, Scurr JH. Venous stasis and vein lumen changes during surgery. Br J Surg 1990;77:1055–9.
[13] Coleridge Smith PD, Hasty JH, Scurr JH. Deep vein thrombosis: effect of graduated compression stockings on distension of the deep veins of the calf. Br J Surg 1991;78:724–6.
[14] Comerota AJ, Stewart GJ, Alburger PD, et al. Operative venodilation: a previously unsuspected factor in the cause of postoperative deep vein thrombosis. Surgery 1989;106:301–9.
[15] Comerota AJ, Stewart GJ, White JV. Combined dihydroergotamine and heparin prophylaxis of postoperative deep vein thrombosis: proposed mechanism of action. Am J Surg 1985;150:39–44.
[16] Stamatakis JD, Kakkar VV, Sagar S, et al. Femoral vein thrombosis and total hip replacement. BMJ 1977;2:223–5.
[17] Mammen EF. Pathogenesis of venous thrombosis. Chest 1992;102:640S–4S.
[18] Mackman N. Role of tissue factor in hemostasis, thrombosis, and vascular development. Arterioscler Thromb Vasc Biol 2004;24:1015–22.
[19] Geerts WH, Bergqvist D, Pineo GF, et al. Prevention of venous thromboembolism: American College of Chest Physicians Evidence-Based Clinical Practice Guidelines. Chest 2008;133:381S- 453S.
[20] Thromboembolic Risk Factors (THRIFT) Consensus Group. Risk of and prophylaxis for venous thromboembolism in hospital patients. BMJ 1992;305:567–74.
[21] Wheeler HB. Diagnosis of deep vein thrombosis. Review of clinical evaluation and impedance plethysmography. Am J Surg 1985;150:7–13.
[22] Nguyen GC, Sam J. Rising prevalence of venous thromboembolism and its impact on mortality among hospitalized inflammatory bowel disease patients. Am J Gastroenterol 2008;103:2272- 80.
[23] Kröger K, Weiland D, Ose C, et al. Risk factors for venous thromboembolic events in cancer patients. Ann Oncol 2006;17:297–303.
[24] Kovacevich GJ, Gaich SA, Lavin JP, et al. The prevalence of thromboembolic events among women with extended bed rest prescribed as part of the treatment for premature labor or preterm premature rupture of membranes. Am J Obstet Gynecol 2000;182:1089 -92.
[25] Anderson FA Jr, Wheeler HB, Goldberg RJ, et al. A population-based perspective of the hospital incidence and case-fatality rates of deep vein thrombosis and pulmonary embolism. The Worcester DVT Study. Arch Intern Med 1991;151:933- 8.
[26] Borow M, Goldson H. Postoperative venous thrombosis. Evaluation of five methods of treatment. Am J Surg 1981;141:245–51.
[27] Borow M, Goldson HJ. Prevention of postoperative deep venous thrombosis and pulmonary emboli with combined modalities. Am Surg 1983;49:599–605.

[28] Sugerman HJ, Sugerman EL, Wolfe L, et al. Risks and benefits of gastric bypass in morbidly obese patients with severe venous stasis disease. Ann Surg 2001;234:41–6.
[29] Geerts WH, Heit JA, Clagett GP, et al. Prevention of venous thromboembolism. Chest 2001;119:132S–75S.
[30] Caprini JA. Thrombosis risk assessment as a guide to quality patient care. Dis Mon 2005;51:70–8.
[31] Stein PD, Beemath A, Matta F, et al. Clinical characteristics of patient with acute pulmonary embolism: data from PIOPED II. Am J Med 2007;120:871e9.
[32] Stein PD, Terrin ML, Hales CA, et al. Clinical, laboratory, roentgenographic and electrocardiographic findings in patients with acute pulmonary embolism and no pre-existing cardiac or pulmonary disease. Chest 1991;100:598e603
[33] Heit JA, Silverstein MD, Mohr DN, et al. The epidemiology of venous thromboembolism in the community. Thromb Haemost 2001;86:452e63.
[34] Anderson FA Jr, Wheeler HB, Goldberg RJ, et al. The prevalence of risk factors for venous thromboembolism among hospital patients. Arch Intern Med 1992;152:1660e4.
[35] Hedley AA, Ogden CL, Johnson CL, et al. Prevalence of overweight and obesity among US children, adolescents, and adults, 1999e2002. JAMA 2004;291:2847e50.
[36] Goldhaber SZ, Grodstein F, Stampfer MJ, et al. A prospective study of risk factors for pulmonary embolism in women. JAMA 1997;277:642e5.
[37] Abdollahi M, Cushman M, Rosendaal FR. Obesity: risk of venous thrombosis and the interaction with coagulation factor levels and oral contraceptive use. Thromb Haemost 2003;89:493e8.
[38] Coon WW, Coller FA. Some epidemiologic considerations of thromboembolism. Surg Gynecol Obstet 1959;109:487e501.
[39] Basili S, Pacini G, Guagnano MT, et al. Insulin resistance as a determinant of platelet activation in obese women. J Am Coll Cardiol 2006;48:2531e8.
[40] Hansson PO, Eriksson H, Welin L, et al. Smoking and abdominal obesity: risk factors for venous thromboembolism among middle-aged men: "the study of men born in 1913". Arch Intern Med 1999;159:1886e90.
[41] Samama MM. An epidemiologic study of risk factors for deep vein thrombosis in medical outpatients: the Sirius study. Arch Intern Med 2000;160: 3415e20.
[42] Kabrhel C, Varraso R, Goldhaber SZ, et al. Prospective study of BMI and the risk of pulmonary embolism in women. Obesity (Silver Spring) 2009; 17:2040e6.
[43] Heit JA, Silverstein MD, Mohr DN, et al. Risk factors for deep vein thrombosis and pulmonary embolism: a population-based case-control study. Arch Intern Med 2000;160:809e15.
[44] US Department of Health and Human Services. Public Health Service, National Center for Health Statistics National Hospital Discharge Survey 1979-2006 Multi-year Public-Use Data File Documentation. Available at: http://www.cdc.gov/nchs/about/major/hdasd/nhds.htm. Accessed April 28, 2010.
[45] Stein PD, Beemath A, Olson RE. Obesity as a risk factor in venous thromboembolism. Am J Med 2005;118:978e80.

[46] Farmer RD, Lawrenson RA, Todd JC, et al. A comparison of the risks of venous thromboembolic disease in association with different combined oral contraceptives. Br J Clin Pharmacol 2000;49:580e90.
[47] Pannaciulli N, De Mitrio V, Marino R, et al. Effect of glucose tolerance status on PAI-1 plasma levels in overweight and obese subjects. Obes Res 2002; 10:717e25.
[48] De Pergola G, Pannacciulli N. Coagulation and fibrinolysis abnormalities in obesity. J Endocrinol Invest 2002;25:899e904.
[49] Mertens I, Van Gaal LF. Obesity, haemostasis and the fibrinolytic system. Obes Rev 2002;3:85e101.
[50] Bara L, Nicaud V, Tiret L, et al. Expression of a paternal history of premature myocardial infarction on fibrinogen, factor VIIC and PAI-1 in European offspringethe EARS study. European Atherosclerosis Research Study Group. Thromb Haemost 1994;71:434e40.
[51] Rosengren A, Frede´n M, Hansson PO, et al. Psychosocial factors and venous thromboembolism: a long-term follow-up study of Swedish men. J Thromb Haemost 2008;6:558e64.
[52] Glynn RJ, Rosner B. Comparison of risk factors for the competing risks of coronary heart disease, stroke, and venous thromboembolism. Am J Epidemiol 2005;162:975e82.
[53] Homans J. Thrombosis of the deep leg veins due to prolonged sitting. N Engl J Med 1954;250:148e9.
[54] Tardy B, Page Y, Zeni F, et al. Phlebitis following travel. Presse Med 1993;22:811e4.
[55] Simpson K. Shelter deaths from pulmonary embolism. Lancet 1940;2:744.
[56] Cruickshank JM, Gorlin R, Jennett B. Air travel and thrombotic episodes: the economy class syndrome. Lancet 1988;2:497e8.
[57] Collins J. Thromboembolic disease related to air travel: what you need to know. Semin Roentgenol 2005;40:1e2.
[58] Hertzberg SR, Roy S, Hollis G, et al. Acute symptomatic pulmonary embolism associated with long haul air travel to Sydney. Vasc Med 2003;8:21e3.
[59] Perez-Rodriguez E, Jimenez D, Diaz G, et al. Incidence of air travel-related pulmonary embolism at the Madrid-Barajas airport. Arch Intern Med 2003; 163:2766e70.
[60] Hughes RJ, Hopkins RJ, Hill S, et al. Frequency of venous thromboembolism in low to moderate risk long distance air travellers: the New Zealand Air Traveller's Thrombosis (NZATT) study. Lancet 2003;362:2039e44.
[61] Cogo A, Bernardi E, Prandoni P, et al. Acquired risk factors for deep-vein thrombosis in symptomatic outpatients. Arch Intern Med 1994;154:164e8.
[62] Lewis MA. The epidemiology of oral contraceptive use: a critical review of the studies on oral contraceptives and the health of young women. Am J Obstet Gynecol 1998;179:1086e97.
[63] Realini JP, Goldzieher JW. Oral contraceptives and cardiovascular disease: a critique of the epidemiologic studies. Am J Obstet Gynecol 1985;152:729e98.
[64] Vandenbroucke JP, Rosing J, BloemenkampK W, et al. Oral contraceptives and the risk of venous thrombosis. N Engl J Med 2001;344:1527e35.
[65] Gerstman BB, Piper JM, Tomita DK, et al. Oral contraceptive estrogen dose and the risk of deep venous thromboembolic disease. Am J Epidemiol 1991;133:32e7.

[66] Lidegaard O, Edstrom B, Kreiner S. Oral contraceptives and venous thromboembolism. A casecontrol study. Contraception 1998;57:291e301.
[67] World Health Organization Collaborative Study of Cardiovascular Disease and Steroid Hormone Contraception. Venous thromboembolic disease and combined oral contraceptives: results of international multicentre case-control study. Lancet 1995;346:1575e82.
[68] Helmrich SP, Rosenberg L, Kaufman DW, et al. Venous thromboembolism in relation to oral contraceptive use. Obstet Gynecol 1987;69:91e5.
[69] Pomp ER, le Cessie S, Rosendaal FR, et al. Risk of venous thrombosis: obesity and its joint effect with oral contraceptive use and prothrombotic mutations. Br J Haemotol 2007;139:289e96.
[70] Lidegaard O, Edstrom B, Kreiner S. Oral contraceptives and venous thromboembolism: a fiveyear national case-control study. Contraception 2002;65:187e96.
[71] Nightingale AL, Lawrenson RA, Simpson EL, et al. The effects of age, body mass index, smoking and general health on the risk of venous thromboembolism in users of combined oral contraceptives. Eur J Contracept Reprod Healthcare 2000;5:265e74.
[72] Decensi A, Maisonneuve P, Rotmensz N, et al. Italian Tamoxifen Study Group. Effect of tamoxifen on venous thromboembolic events in a breast cancer prevention trial. Circulation 2005;111:650e6.
[73] Duggan C, Marriott K, Edwards R, et al. Inherited and acquired risk factors for venous thromboembolic disease among women taking tamoxifen to prevent breast cancer. J Clin Oncol 2003;21:3588e93.
[74] Meier CR, Jick H. Tamoxifen and risk of idiopathic venous thromboembolism. Br J Clin Pharmacol 1998;45:608e12.
[75] Daly E, Vessey MP, Hawkins MM, et al. Risk of venous thromboembolism in users of hormone replacement therapy. Lancet 1996;348:977e80.
[76] Varas-Lorenzo C, Garcı´a-Rodriguez L, Cattaruzzi C, et al. Hormone replacement therapy and the risk of hospitalization for venous thromboembolism: a population-based study in southern Europe. Am J Epidemiol 1998;147:387e90.
[77] Grady D, Wenger NK, Herrington D, et al. Postmenopausal hormone therapy increases risk for venous thromboembolic disease. The Heart and Estrogen/progestin Replacement Study. Ann Intern Med 2000;132:689e96.
[78] Peverill RE. Hormone therapy and venous thromboembolism. Best Pract Res Clin Endocrinol Metab 2003;17:149e64.
[79] Whiteman T, Hassouna HI. Hypercoagulable States, Hem/Onc Clin N Am. 2000. 14: 2.
[80] Bick RL. Prothrombin G20210A mutation, antithrombin, heparin cofactor II, protein C, and protein S defects, Hematol Oncol Clin N Am. 2003. 17: 9–36.
[81] Johnson CM, Mureebe L, Silver D. Hypercoagulable states: A review, Vasc Endovasc Surg. 2005. 39: 123–133.
[82] Bick RL. Clinical relevance of antithrombin III, Semin Thromb Hemost. 1982. 8: 276.
[83] Seligsohn U, Lubetsky A. Genetic susceptibility to venous thrombosis, N Engl J Med. 2001. 344: 1222–1231.
[84] Bick RL. Prothrombin G20210A mutation, antithrombin, heparin cofactor II, protein C, and protein S defects, Hematol Oncol Clin N Am. 2003. 17: 9–36.

[85] Nicolaes GAF, Dahlback B. Activated protein C resistance (FVLeiden) and thrombosis: Factor V mutations causing hypercoagulable states, Hematol Oncol Clin N Am. 2003. 17: 37–61.
[86] Koppelman SJ, Hackeng TM, Sixma JJ et al. Inhibition of the intrinsic factor X activating complex by protein S: Evidence for specifi c binding of protein S to factor VIII, Blood. 1995. 86:1062–1071.
[87] Allaart CF, Poort SR, Rosendaal FR et al. Increased risk of venous thrombosis in carriers of hereditary protein C defi ciency defect, Lancet. 1993. 341: 134–138.
[88] Silver D, Vouyouka A. The caput medusae of hypercoagulability, J Vasc Surg. 2000. 31: 396–495.
[89] Greaves M. Antiphospholipid antibodies and thrombosis. Lancet 1999;353:1348e53.
[90] Levine JS, Branch DW, Rauch J. The antiphospholipid syndrome. N Engl J Med 2002;346: 752e63.
[91] Asherson RA, Khamashta MA, Ordi-Ros J, et al.The "primary" antiphospholipid syndrome: major clinical and serological features. Medicine (Baltimore) 1989;68:366e74.
[92] Vianna JL, Khamashta MA, Ordi-Ros J, et al. Comparison of the primary and secondary antiphospholipid syndrome: a European Multicenter Study of 114 patients. Am J Med 1994;96:3e9.
[93] Stein PD, Hull RD, Matta F, et al. Incidence of thrombocytopenia in hospitalized patients with venous thromboembolism. Am J Med 2009;122: 919e30.
[94] Brick W, Burgess R, Faguet GB. Dysfibrinogenemia. WebMD. Available at: www.webmd.com. Accessed March 19, 2010.
[95] Shively BK. Deep venous thrombosis prophylaxis in patients with heart disease. Curr Cardiol Rep 2001;3:56e62.
[96] Jafri SM, Ozawa T, Mammen E, et al. Platelet function, thrombin and fibrinolytic activity in patients with heart failure. Eur Heart J 1993;14:205e12.
[97] Dries DL, Rosenberg YD, Waclawiw MA, et al. Ejection fraction and risk of thromboembolic events in patients with systolic dysfunction and sinus rhythm: evidence for gender differences in the studies of left ventricular dysfunction trials. J Am Coll Cardiol 1997;29:1074e80.
[98] Kyrle PA, Korninger C, Gossinger H, et al. Prevention of arterial and pulmonary embolism by oral anticoagulants in patients with dilated cardiomyopathy. Thromb Haemost 1985;54:521e3.
[99] Nordstro¨m M, Lindblad B, Bergqvist D, et al. A prospective study of the incidence of deep-vein thrombosis within a defined urban population. J Intern Med 1992;232:155e60.
[100] Segal JP, Harvey WP, Gurel T. Diagnosis and treatment of primary myocardial disease. Circulation 1965;32:837e44.
[101] Roberts WC, Siegel RJ, McManus BM. Idiopathic dilated cardiomyopathy: analysis of 152 necropsy patients. Am J Cardiol 1987;60:1340e55.
[102] Beemath A, Stein PD, Skaf E, et al. Risk of venous thromboembolism in patients hospitalized with heart failure. Am J Cardiol 2006;98:793e5.
[103] Howell MD, Geraci JM, Knowlton AA. Congestive heart failure and outpatient risk of venous thromboembolism: a retrospective, case-control study. J Clin Epidemiol 2001;54:810e8166.

[104] Beemath A, Skaf E, Stein PD. Pulmonary embolism as a cause of death in adults who died with heart failure. Am J Cardiol 2006;98:1073e5.

[105] Attems J, Arbes S, Bohm G, et al. The clinical diagnostic accuracy rate regarding the immediate cause of death in a hospitalized geriatric population; an autopsy study of 1594 patients. Wien Med Wochenschr 2004;154:159e62.

[106] Hsu DT, Addonizio LJ, Hordof AJ, Gersony WM. Acute pulmonary embolism in pediatric patients awaiting heart transplantation. J Am Coll Cardiol 1991;17:1621–5.

[107] Cohen AT, Tapson VF, Bergmann JF, et al. Venous thromboembolism risk and prophylaxis in the acute hospital care setting (ENDORSE study): a multinational cross-sectional study. Lancet 2008;371: 387-94.

[108] Mispelaere D, Glerant JC, Audebert M, et al. Pulmonary embolism and sibilant types of chronic obstructive pulmonary disease decompensations. Rev Mal Respir 2002;19:415e23.

[109] Tillie-Leblond I, Marquette CH, Perez T, et al. Pulmonary embolism in patients with unexplained exacerbation of chronic obstructive pulmonary disease: prevalence and risk factors. Ann Intern Med 2006;144:390e6.

[110] Stein PD, Beemath A, Meyers FA, et al. Pulmonary embolism and deep venous thrombosis in patients hospitalized with chronic obstructive pulmonary disease. J Cardiovasc Med 2007;8:253e7.

[111] Neuhaus A, Bentz RR, Weg JG. Pulmonary embolism in respiratory failure. Chest 1978;73(4):460 –5.

[112] Schonhofer B, Kohler D. Prevalence of deep-vein thrombosis of the leg in patients with acute exacerbation of Chronic Obstructive Pulmonary Disease. Respiration 1998;65:173- 7.

[113] Gunduz S, Ogur E, Mohur H, et al: Deep vein thrombosis in spinal cord injured patients. Paraplegia 31:606410, 1993

[114] Hull R Venous thromboembolism in spinal cord injury patients Chest 102:658-662, 1992

[115] Merli GJ: Management of deep vein thrombosis in spinal cord injury. Chest 102652-657, 1992

[116] Myllynen P, Kammonen M, Rokkanen P, et al: Deep venous thrombosis and pulmonary embolism in patients with acute spinal cord injury: A comparison with non-paralyzed patients immobilized due to spinal fractures. J Trauma 25:541-543, 1985

[117] Prasad DK, Banerjee AK, Howard H Incidence of deep vein thrombosis and the effect of the pneumatic compression if the calf in elderly hemiplegics. Age Aging 11:424, 1982

[118] Waring WP, Karunas RS: Acute spinal cord injuries and the incidence of clinically occurring thromboembolic disease. Paraplegia 29:8-16, 1991

[119] Yao JST Deep vein thrombosis in spinal cord-injured patients. Evaluation and assessment. Chest 102:645-648, 1992

[120] Harvey RL. Prevention of venous thromboembolism after stroke. Topics Stroke Rehab 2003;10:61e9.

[121] Skaf E, Stein PD, Beemath A, et al. Venous thromboembolism in patients with ischemic and hemorrhagic stroke. Am J Cardiol 2005;96:1731e3.

[122] Skaf E, Stein PD, Beemath A, et al. Fatal pulmonary embolism and stroke. Am J Cardiol 2006;97:1776e7.
[123] Dismuke SE, VanderZwaag R. Accuracy and epidemiological implications of the death certificate diagnosis of pulmonary embolism. J Chronic Dis 1984;37:67e73.
[124] Heit JA, Silverstein MD, Mohr DN, Petterson TM, O'Fallon WM, Melton 3rd LJ. Risk factors for deep vein thrombosis and pulmonary embolism: a populationbased case-control study. Arch Intern Med 2000;160(6):809–15.
[125] Spencer FA, Lessard D, Emery C, Reed G, Goldberg RJ. Venous thromboembolism in the outpatient setting. Arch Intern Med 2007;167(14):1471-5.
[126] Levitan N, Dowlati A, Remick SC, Tahsildar HI, Sivinski LD, Beyth R, et al. Rates ofinitial and recurrent thromboembolic disease among patients with malignancy versus those without malignancy. Risk analysis using Medicare claims data. Medicine (Baltimore) 1999;78(5):285–91.
[127] Khorana AA, Francis CW, Culakova E, Kuderer NM, Lyman GH. Frequency, risk factors, and trends for venous thromboembolism among hospitalized cancer patients. Cancer 2007;110(10):2339–46.
[128] Stein PD, Beemath A, Meyers FA, et al. Incidence of venous thromboembolism in patients hospitalized with cancer. Am J Med 2006;119:60–8.
[129] Khorana AA, Francis CW, Culakova E, et al. Thromboembolism in hospitalized neutropenic cancer patients. J Clin Oncol 2006;24:484–90.
[130] Sallah S, Wan JY, Nguyen NP. Venous thrombosis in patients with solid tumors: determination of frequency and characteristics. Thromb Haemost 2002;87:575–9.
[131] Levitan N, Dowlati A, Remick SC, et al. Rates of initial and recurrent thromboembolic disease among patients with malignancy versus those without malignancy. Risk analysis using Medicare claims data. Medicine (Baltimore) 1999;78:285–91.
[132] Stein PD, Beemath A, Meyers FA, et al. Incidence of venous thromboembolism in patients hospitalized with cancer. Am J Med 2006;119:60–8.
[133] Chew HK, Wun T, Harvey D, et al. Incidence of venous thromboembolism and its effect on survival among patients with common cancers. Arch Intern Med 2006;166:458–64.
[134] Numico G, Garrone O, Dongiovanni V, et al. Prospective evaluation of major vascular events in patients with nonsmall cell lung carcinoma treated with cisplatin and gemcitabine. Cancer 2005;103:994–9.
[135] Weijl NI, Rutten MF, Zwinderman AH, et al. Thromboembolic events during chemotherapy for germ cell cancer: a cohort study and review of the literature. J Clin Oncol 2000;18:2169–78.
[136] White RH, Chew HK, Zhou H, et al. Incidence of venous thromboembolism in the year before the diagnosis of cancer in 528,693 adults. Arch Intern Med 2005;165:1782–7.
[137] Blom JW, Doggen CJ, Osanto S, et al. Malignancies, prothrombotic mutations, and the risk of venous thrombosis. JAMA 2005;293:715–22.
[138] Sallah S, Wan JY, Nguyen NP. Venous thrombosis in patients with solid tumors: determination of frequency and characteristics. Thromb Haemost 2002;87:575–9.
[139] Khorana AA, Francis CW, Culakova E, et al. Thromboembolism in hospitalized neutropenic cancer patients. J Clin Oncol 2006;24:484–90.
[140] Rodriguez AO, Wun T, Chew H, et al. Venous thromboembolism in ovarian cancer. Gynecol Oncol 2007;105:784–90.

[141] Tateo S, Mereu L, Salamano S, et al. Ovarian cancer and venous thromboembolic risk. Gynecol Oncol 2005;99:119–25.
[142] Chew HK, Wun T, Harvey DJ, et al. Incidence of venous thromboembolism and the impact on survival in breast cancer patients. J Clin Oncol 2007;25:70–6.
[143] Chew HK, Davies AM,Wun T, et al. The incidence of venous thromboembolism among patients with primary lung cancer. J Thromb Haemost 2008;6:601–8.
[144] Alcalay A, Wun T, Khatri V, et al. Venous thromboembolism in patients with colorectal cancer: incidence and effect on survival. J Clin Oncol 2006;24:1112–8.
[145] Mandala M, Reni M, Cascinu S, et al. Venous thromboembolism predicts poor prognosis in irresectable pancreatic cancer patients. Ann Oncol 2007;18:1660–5.
[146] Chew HK, Wun T, Harvey D, et al. Incidence of venous thromboembolism and its effect on survival among patients with common cancers. Arch Intern Med 2006;166:458–64.
[147] Heit JA, Silverstein MD, Mohr DN, et al. Risk factors for deep vein thrombosis and pulmonary embolism: a populationbased case-control study. Arch Intern Med 2000;160:809–15.
[148] Pritchard KI, Paterson AH, Paul NA, et al. Increased thromboembolic complications with concurrent tamoxifen and chemotherapy in a randomized trial of adjuvant therapy for women with breast cancer. National Cancer Institute of Canada Clinical Trials Group Breast Cancer Site Group. J Clin Oncol 1996;14:2731–7.
[149] Fisher B, Dignam J, Wolmark N, et al. Tamoxifen and chemotherapy for lymph node-negative, estrogen receptor-positive breast cancer. J Natl Cancer Inst 1997;89:1673–82.
[150] Deitcher SR, Gomes MP. The risk of venous thromboembolic disease associated with adjuvant hormone therapy for breast carcinoma: a systematic review. Cancer 2004;101:439–49.
[151] Agnelli G, Caprini JA. The prophylaxis of venous thrombosis in patients with cancer undergoing major abdominal surgery: emerging options. J Surg Oncol 2007;96:265–72.
[152] Verso M, Agnelli G. Venous thromboembolism associated with long-term use of central venous catheters in cancer patients. J Clin Oncol 2003;21:3665–75.
[153] Khorana AA, Francis CW, Culakova E, et al. Risk factors for chemotherapy-associated venous thromboembolism in a prospective observational study. Cancer 2005;104:2822–9.
[154] Edgington TS, Mackman N, Brand K, et al. The structural biology of expression and function of tissue factor. Thromb Haemost 1991;66:67–79.
[155] Nemerson Y. Tissue factor and hemostasis. Blood 1988;71:1–8.
[156] Nemerson Y. Tissue factor: then and now. Thromb Haemost 1995;74:180–4.
[157] Khorana AA, Ahrendt SA, Ryan CK, et al. Tissue factor expression, angiogenesis, and thrombosis in pancreatic cancer. Clin Cancer Res 2007;13:2870–5.
[158] Stein PD, Beemath A, Meyers FA, et al. Incidence of venous thromboembolism in patients hospitalized with cancer. Am J Med 2006;119:60e8.
[159] Stein PD, Beemath A, Meyers FA, et al. Pulmonary embolism as a cause of death in patients who died with cancer. Am J Med 2006;119:163e5.
[160] Stein PD, Hull RD, Kayali F, et al. Venous thromboembolism in pregnancy: 21 year trends. Am J Med 2004;117:121e5.

[161] Anonymous. Oral contraception and thromboembolic disease. J R Coll Gen Pract 1967;13: 267e79.
[162] Ginsberg JS, Brill-Edwards P, Burrows RF, Bona R, Prandoni P, Buller HR, et al. Venous thrombosis during pregnancy: leg and trimester of presentation. Thromb Haemost 1992;67:519- 20
[163] Ikard RW, Ueland K, Folse R. Lower limb venous dynamics in pregnant women. Surg Gynecol Obstet 1971;132:483- 8.
[164] Macklon NC, Greer IA, Bowman AW. An ultrasound study of gestational and postural changes in the deep venous system of the leg in pregnancy. Br J Obstet Gynaecol 1997;104:191–7.
[165] Metcalfe J, Ueland K. Maternal cardiovascular adjustments to pregnancy. Prog Cardiovasc Dis 1974;16:363–74.
[166] Kerr MG, Scott DB, Samuel E. Studies of the inferior vena cava in late pregnancy. Br Med J 1964;1:532- 3.
[167] Cockett FB, Thomas ML. The iliac compression syndrome. Br J Surg 1965;52:816- 21.
[168] Hull RD, Raskob GE, Carter CJ. Serial impedance plethysmography in pregnant patients with clinically suspected deep vein thrombosis. Ann Intern Med 1990;112:663- 7.
[169] Rutherford SE, Phelan JP. Thromboembolic disease in pregnancy. Clin Perinatol 1986;13:719- 39.
[170] Stirling Y, Woolf L, North WR, Seghatchian MJ, Meade TW. Haemostasis in normal pregnancy. Thromb Haemost 1984;52:176–82.
[171] Woodhams BJ, Candotti G, Shaw R, Kernoff PB. Changes in coagulation and fibrinolysis during pregnancy: evidence of activation of coagulation preceding spontaneous abortion. Thromb Res 1989;55:99- 107.
[172] Bonnar J. Blood coagulation and fibrinolysis in obstetrics. Clin Hematol 1973;12:58 - 63.
[173] Comp PC, Thurnau GR, Welsh J, Esmon CT. Functional and immunologic protein S levels are decreased during pregnancy. Blood 1986;68:881- 5.
[174] Clark P, Brennand J, Conkie JA, McCall F, Greer IA, Walker ID. Activated protein C sensitivity, protein C, protein S, and coagulation in normal pregnancy. Thromb Haemost 1998;79:1166- 70.
[175] Wright JG, Cooper P, Astedt B, Lecander I, Wilde JT, Preston FE, et al. Fibrinolysis during normal human pregnancy: complex interrelationships between plasma levels of tissue plasminogen activator and inhibitors and the euglobulin clot lysis time. Br J Haematol 1988; 69:253- 8.
[176] Bremme K, Ostlund E, Almqvist I, Heinonen K, Blomback M. Enhanced thrombin generation and fibrinolytic activity in normal pregnancy and the puerperium. Obstet Gynecol 1992;80:132- 7.
[177] Kruithof EK, Tran-Thang C, Gudinchet A, Hauert J, Nicoloso G, Genton C, et al. Fibrinolysis in pregnancy: a study of plasminogen activator inhibitors. Blood 1987;69:460–6.
[178] McColl MD, Ramsay JI, Tait RD, Walker ID, McCall F, Conkie JA, et al. Risk factors for pregnancy associated venous thromboembolism. Thromb Haemost 1997;78:1183–8.

[179] Geerts WH, Bergqvist D, Pineo GF, et al. Preventive of venous thromboembolism. American College of Chest physicians evidence-based clinical practice guidelines (8th edition). Chest 2008;133: 381Se453S.
[180] Kroger K, Schelo C, Gocke C, et al. Colour Doppler sonographic diagnosis of upper limb venous thromboses. Clin Sci 1998;94:657e61.
[181] Dollery CM, Sullivan ID, Bauraind O, et al. Thrombosis and embolism in long-term central venous access for parenteral nutrition. Lancet 1994;344: 1043e5.
[182] Mustafa S, Stein PD, Patel KC, et al. Upper extremity deep venous thrombosis. Chest 2003; 163:1213e9.
[183] Hingorani A, Ascher E, Lorenson E, et al. Upper extremity deep venous thrombosis and its impact on morbidity and mortality rates in a hospitalbased population. J Vasc Surg 1997;26:853e60.
[184] Monreal M, Lafoz E, Ruiz J, et al. Upperextremity deep venous thrombosis and pulmonary embolism. A prospective study. Chest 1991;99:280e3.
[185] Horattas MC, Wright DJ, Fenton AH, et al. Changing concepts of deep venous thrombosis of the upper extremityereport of a series and review of the literature. Surgery 1988;104:561e7.
[186] Joffe HV, Kucher N, Tapson VF, et al. Upper-extremity deep vein thrombosis: a prospective registry of 592 patients. Circulation 2004;110:1605e11.
[187] Broviac JW, Cole JJ, Scribner BH. A silicone rubber atrial catheter for prolonged parenteral alimentation. Surg Gynecol Obstet 1973; 136:602- 606.
[188] Hickman RO, Buckner CD, Clift RA, Sanders JE, Stewart P, Thomas ED. A modified right atrial catheter for access to the venous system in marrow trans-plant recipients. Surg Gynecol Obstet 1979; 148:871- 875.
[189] Foley MJ. Radiologic placement of long-term central venous peripheral access system ports (PAS Port): results in 150 patients. J Vasc Interv Radiol1995; 6:255–262.
[190] Rubenstein EB, Fender A, Rolston KV, et al. Vascular access by physician as-sistants: evaluation of an implantable peripheral port system in cancer patients. J Clin Oncol 1995; 13:1513–1519.
[191] Shetty PC, Mody MK, Kastan DJ, et al. Outcome of 350 implanted chest ports placed by interventional radiologists. J Vasc Interv Radiol 1997; 8:991–995.
[192] Schwarz RE, Groeger JS, Coit DG. Subcutaneously implanted central venous access devices in cancer patients: a prospective analysis. Cancer 1997; 79: 1635–1640.
[193] Struk DW, Bennett JD, Kozak RI. Insertion of subcutaneous central venous infusion ports by interventional radiologists. Can Assoc Radiol J 1995; 46:32–36.
[194] Hata Y, Morita S, Morita Y, et al. Peripheral insertion of a central venous access device under fluoroscopic guidance using a peripherally accessed system (PAS) port in the forearm. Cardiovasc Intervent Radiol 1998; 21:230 –233.
[195] Deppe G, Kahn ML, Malviya VK, Malone JM, Christensen CW. Experience with the P.A.S.-Port venous access device in patients with gynecologic malignancies. Gynecol Oncol 1996; 62:340 –343.
[196] Monreal M, Lafoz E, Ruiz J, Valls R, Alastrue A. Upper extremity deep venous thrombosis and pulmonary embolism; a prospective study. Chest 1991;99:280–3.
[197] Saleh T, Matta F, Yaekoub AY, et al. Risk of venous thromboembolism with inflammatory bowel disease. Clin Appl Thromb Hemost 2010. [Epub ahead of print].

[198] Saleh T, Matta F, Alali F, et al. Liver disease and risk of venous thromboembolism. Submitted for publication.
[199] Søgaard KK, Horva´th-Puho´ E, Grønbaek H, et al. Risk of venous thromboembolism in patients with liver disease: a nationwide population-based case-control study. Am J Gastroenterol 2009;104: 96e101.
[200] Northup PG, McMahon MM, Ruhl AP, et al. Coagulopathy does not fully protect hospitalized cirrhosis patients from peripheral venous thromboembolism. Am J Gastroenterol 2006;101:1524e8.
[201] Tripodi A, Primignani M, Chantarangkul V, et al. An imbalance of pro- vs anti-coagulation factors in plasma from patients with cirrhosis. Gastroenterology 2009;137:2105e11.
[202] Danescu L, Badshah A, Danescu SC, et al. Venous thromboembolism in patients hospitalized with thyroid dysfunction. Clin Appl Thromb Hemost 2009;15:676e80.
[203] Seriolo B, Accardo S, Garnero A, et al. Anticardiolipin antibodies, free protein S levels and thrombosis: a survey in a selected population of rheumatoid arthritis patients. Rheumatology 1999; 38:675e8.
[204] McEntegart A, Capell HA, Creran D, et al. Cardiovascular risk factors, including thrombotic variables, in a population with rheumatoid arthritis. Rheumatology 2001;40:640e4.
[205] Matta F, Singala R, Yaekoub AY, et al. Risk of venous thromboembolism with rheumatoid arthritis. Thromb Haemost 2009;101:134e8.
[206] Stein PD, Goldman J, Matta F, et al. Diabetes mellitus and risk of venous thromboembolism. Am J Med Sic 2009;337:259e64.
[207] Matta F, Yaekoub AY, Stein PD. Human immunodeficiency virus infection and risk of venous thromboembolism. Am J Med Sci 2008;336:402e6.
[208] Kayali F, Najjar R, Aswad F, et al. Venous thromboembolism in patients hospitalized with nephrotic syndrome. Am J Med 2008;121:226e30.
[209] Stein PD, Beemath A, Meyers FA, et al. Deep venous thrombosis and pulmonary embolism in patients hospitalized with sickle cell disease. Am J Med 2006;119:897e901.
[210] Navarro S, Ricart JM, Medina P, et al. Activated protein C levels in Behc¸ et's disease and risk of venous thrombosis. Br J Haematol 2004;126:550e6.
[211] Ray JG, Burows RF, Ginsberg JS, et al. Paroxysmal nocturnal hemoglobinuria and the risk of venous thrombosis: review and recommendations for management of the pregnant and nonpregnant patient. Haemostasis 2000;30:103e17.
[212] Fischer MD, Hopewell PC. Recurrent pulmonary emboli and Buerger's disease. West J Med 1981; 135:238e41.
[213] Osterud B (1998) Tissue factor expression by monocytes: regulation and pathophysiological roles. Blood Coagul Fibrinolysis 9[Suppl 1]:S9–14
[214] Osterud B, Rapaport SI (1977) Activation of factor IX by the reaction product of tissue factor and factor VII: additional pathway for initiating blood coagulation. Proc Natl Acad Sci USA 74:5260–5264
[215] Esmon CT (2001) Role of coagulation inhibitors in inflammation. Thromb Haemost 86:51–56

[216] Schaub RG, Simmons CA, Koets MH, Romano PJ, Stewart GJ (1984) Early events in the formation of a venous thrombus following local trauma and stasis. Lab Invest 51:218–224

[217] Yang J, Furie BC, Furie B (1999) The biology of P-selectin glycoprotein ligand-1: its role as a selectin counterreceptor in leukocyte-endothelial and leukocyte-platelet interaction. Thromb Haemost 81:1–7

[218] Coughlan AF, Hau H, Dunlop LC, Berndt MC, Hancock WW (1994) P-selectin and platelet-activating factor mediate initial endotoxin- induced neutropenia. J Exp Med 179:329–334

[219] Lim YC, Snapp K, Kansas GS, Camphausen R, Ding H, Luscinskas FW (1998) Important contributions of P-selectin glycoprotein ligand-1-mediated secondary capture to human monocyte adhesion to P-selectin, E-selectin, and TNF-alpha-activated endothelium under flow in vitro. J Immunol 161:2501–2508

[220] Ramasamy S, Lipke DW, McClain CJ, Hennig B (1995) Tumor necrosis factor reduces proteoglycan synthesis in cultured endothelial cells. J Cell Physiol 162:119–126

[221] Klein NJ, Shennan GI, Heyderman RS, Levin M (1992) Alteration in glycosaminoglycan metabolism and surface charge on human umbilical vein endothelial cells induced by cytokines, endotoxin and neutrophils. J Cell Sci 102[Pt 4]:821–832

[222] Conway EM, Rosenberg RD (1988) Tumor necrosis factor suppresses transcription of the thrombomodulin gene in endothelial cells. Mol Cell Biol 8:5588–5592

[223] Murugesan G, Rani MR, Ransohoff RM, Marchant RE, Kottke-Marchant K (2000) Endothelial cell expression of monocyte chemotactic protein-1, tissue factor, and thrombomodulin on hydrophilic plasma polymers. J Biomed Mater Res 49:396–408

[224] Moore KL, Andreoli SP, Esmon NL, Esmon CT, Bang NU (1987) Endotoxin enhances tissue factor and suppresses thrombomodulin expression of human vascular endothelium in vitro. J Clin Invest 79:124–130

2

Venous Stasis and Deep Vein Thrombosis Prevention in Laparoscopic Surgery

Mindaugas Kiudelis, Dalia Adukauskienė and Rolandas Gerbutavičius
Medical Academy of Lithuanian University of Health Sciences, Kaunas, Lithuania

1. Introduction

Laparoscopic surgery - is one of the most progressive minimal invasive surgery branches. About 25–40% of all abdominal operations are performed laparoscopicaly in our days and this rating is going in ascending order. Laparoscopic operations (cholecystectomy, fundoplication, appendectomy, bypass due to morbid obesity et at.) have rapidly become the operations of choice in abdominal surgery. Several authors reported that deep vein thrombosis (DVT) in the legs developed in 30% of postoperative patients and pulmonary embolism (PE) in 10% of these patients.

Many studies explored the frequency of deep leg vein thrombosis after various open abdominal surgery operations. Some studies (Geerts and al.,1994) determined that deep leg vein thrombosis develops in 55% of polytrauma patients. Clagett &Reisch, 1988; found 25% rate of DVT after open abdominal surgery. Literature data on the incidence of DVT after laparoscopic operations is limited. Patel MI and al., 1996; carried out the prospective clinical study, studying the frequency of DVT after laparoscopic cholecystectomy. The rate of DVT, diagnosed by ultrasound Doppler, was 55%. The incidence of DVT and PE after laparoscopic fundoplications was 1.8% in our prospective randomized study. Lord RV and al., 1998; performed the prospective clinical study and compared the incidence of DVT after laparoscopic or microlaparotomic (open) cholecystectomy. The incidence of DVT was 1.7% after laparoscopic and 2.4% after open cholecystectomy. Nevertheless, many authors states, that the incidence of DVT should be less after laparoscopic surgery when comparing with open one. Laparoscopic operations, in comparison with open ones, have few basic differences:

1. Laparoscopic operation involves a specific manipulation called abdominal insufflation in addition to the routine procedure of general anesthesia. The increased intra-abdominal pressure associated with pneumoperitoneum (12-14 mm Hg) during laparoscopic upper gastrointestinal surgery has the potential to compound any lower-limb venous stasis already present due to general anesthesia by compressing the retroperitoneal vena cava and iliac veins.
2. Most of laparoscopic operations often last more than 1.5 hours and often are performed with patient in the reverse Trendelenburg position. These differences also have the potential for an increased risk of significant venous stasis.

2. Venous stasis and deep vein thrombosis prevention in laparoscopic surgery

Lower – limb venous stasis is one of the major pathophysiological elements involved in the development of intraoperative DVT and postoperative PE. Factors influencing venous return in the healthy subject are left ventricular output, negative intrathoracic pressure during inspiration, the calf's soleal muscle pump, squeezing of the inferior vena cava by increased intra-abdominal pressure during diaphragmatic descent, and the suction effect of the right atrium during systole. Thus, in the anesthetized patient, venous return from the legs depends mainly on the pressure gradient between the venules (12-18 mm Hg) and the right atrium (4-5 mm Hg). It is expected that the introduction of a pressure barrier between legs venules and the right atrium impedes venous return. Venous thrombosis is major causes of morbidity and mortality. Venous thrombosis leads to pulmonary embolism, which can be fatal, and to postphlebitic syndrome. Venous thrombosis occurs when procoagulant stimuli overwhelm natural protective mechanisms. Procoagulant stimuli include the excessive activation of coagulation, particularly when protective pathways are copromised by thrombophilic abnormalities, vessel wall damage, or stasis. Although of less degree than open surgery, laparoscopic surgery may potentially predispose to thombosis since it salters venous flow and coagulability and cause endothelian injuries.

Little attention has been appointed by the scientists of venous intimal irregularity, as one of the pathogenesis factors of venous thrombosis. Schaub RG and al. 1978; performing experimental studies with dogs, noticed endothelium rupture of small veins, which occurred away from the surgical field and were caused by intra-abdominal surgery. These multiple micro tears often occur in the place of small and large vein (femoral, jugular) fusion sites. Histological studies found that these ruptures are infiltrated with leukocytes and platelets. Comerota AJ and al., 1990; have shown that venous endothelial micro tears occur in dilated veins, which normally are always present during laparoscopic surgery. When the micro tears of endothelium occurs, appeared subendothelial blood vessel collagen stimulates the release of coagulation predisposing factors - thromboplastin and Wilebrand factor.

General anesthesia has been shown to decrease profoundly lower-limb venous return. In one series, 50% of anesthetized patients developed same degree of venous stasis intraoperatively, similar to that produced by 10-14 days of bed rest. We performed a prospective randomized clinical study in which 72 patients undergoing elective laparoscopic fundoplications because of gastroesophagial reflux disease, caused by hiatal hernia were studied. One of our study aims was to evaluate the effect of general anesthesia and the effect of pneumoperitoneum (12 mm Hg) on a femoral venous outflow. Lower extremity venous blood velocity and the femoral vein diameter were evaluated using Doppler ultrasonography. Doppler ultrasound images of the longitudinal section of the femoral vein were obtained at its segment proximal to the bifurcation of the deep femoral artery from the femoral artery.

Our study results demonstrated that both factors - general anesthesia and abdominal insufflation reduced the blood velocity in the femoral vein (figure 1 and 2) and increased cross-sectional area of this vein (figure 3 and 4).

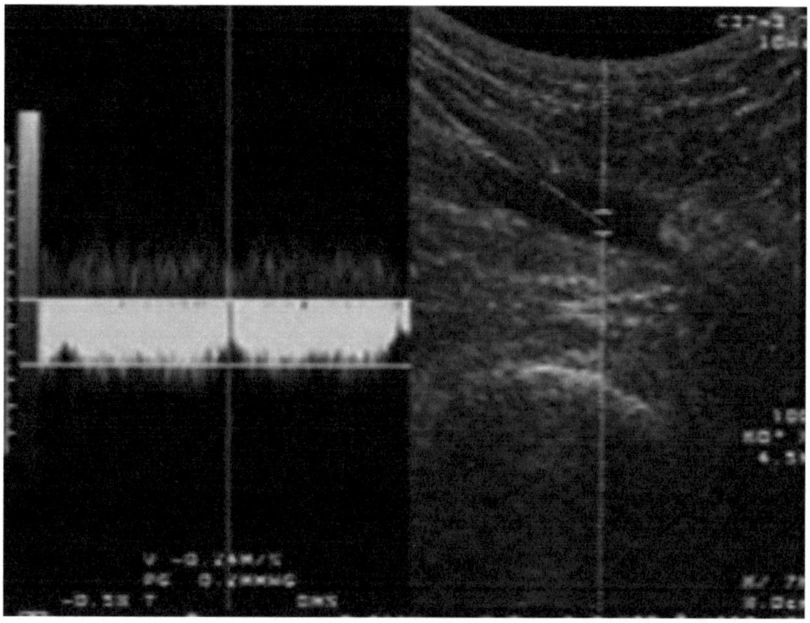

Fig. 1. Ultrasonography of the common femoral vein before the general anesthesia. Figure on the left side shows blood velocity in the femoral vein using doppler ultrasound; the right side shows longitudinal section of the femoral vein.

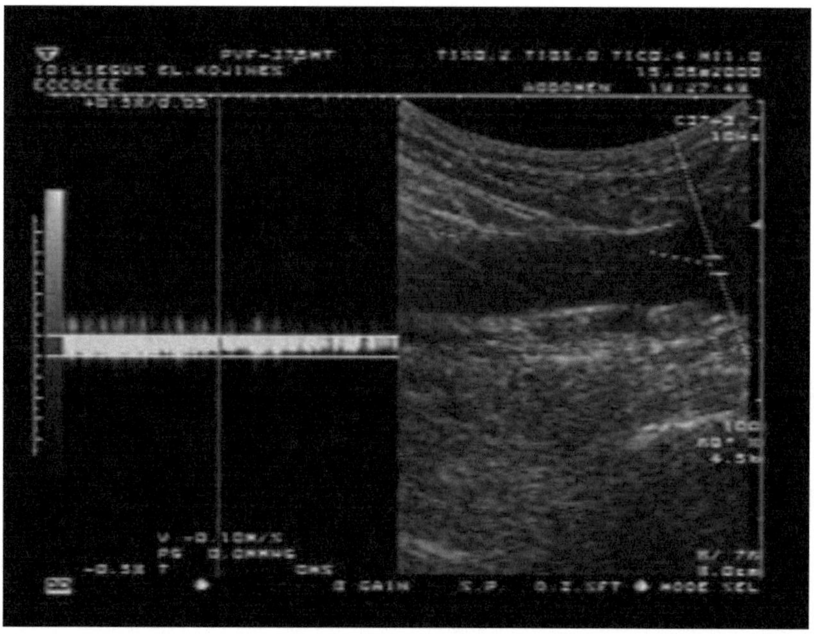

Fig. 2. Ultrasonography of the common femoral vein at the 12 mm Hg insufflation when the patient was placed in the reverse Trendelenburg position (angle 45°). Figure on the left side shows blood velocity in the femoral vein using doppler ultrasound; the right side shows longitudinal section of the femoral vein.

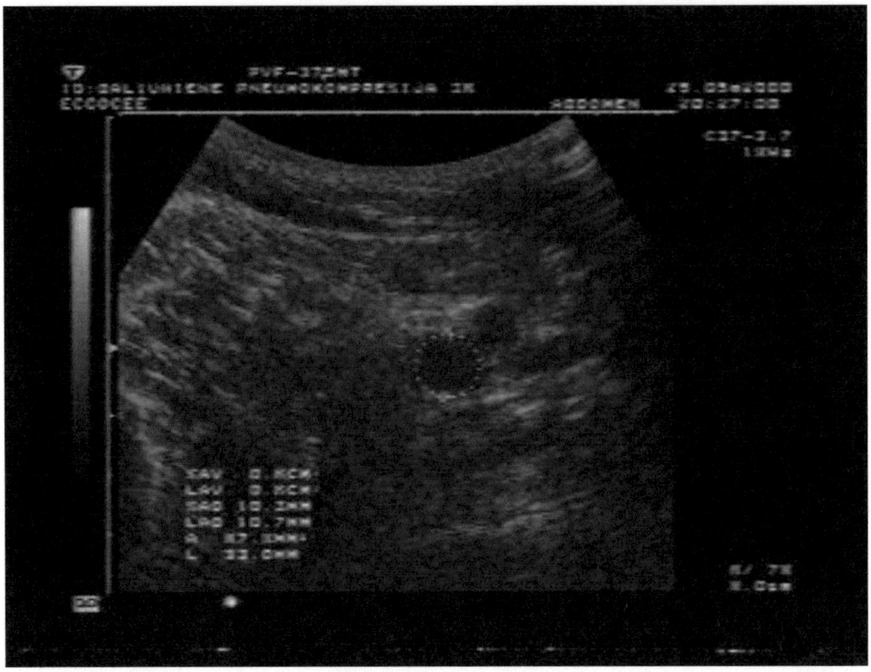

Fig. 3. Ultrasonography of the common femoral vein before the general anesthesia. Figure shows the cross-sectional area of the femoral vein.

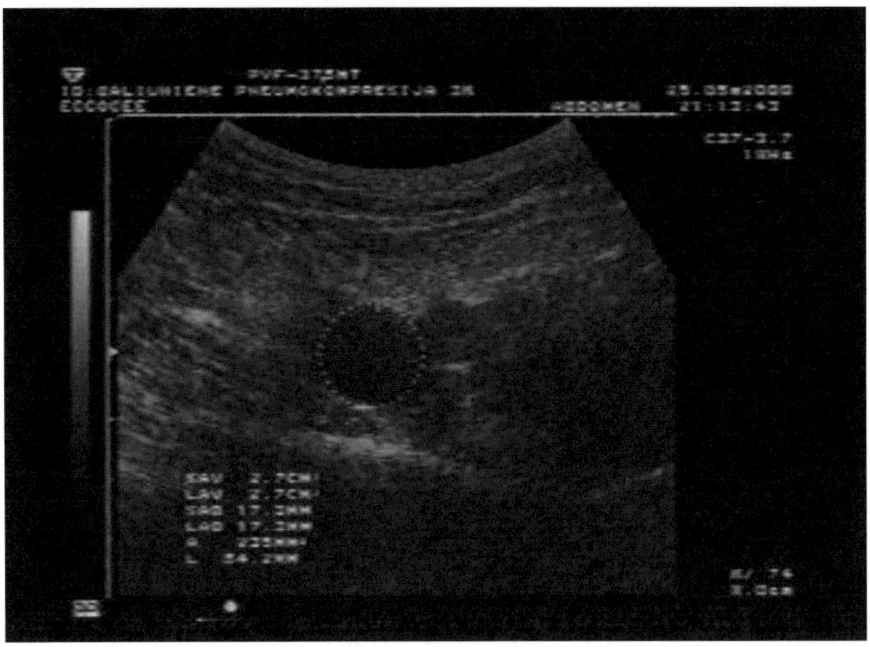

Fig. 4. Ultrasonography of the common femoral vein at the 12 mm Hg insufflation when the patient was placed in the reverse Trendelenburg position (angle 45°). Figure shows the cross-sectional area of the femoral vein.

The decrease in the blood velocity of the femoral vein and increase of the cross-sectional area differed significantly between 5-mm Hg insufflation, 10-mm Hg insufflation and 12-mm Hg insufflation. Futhermore, the blood velocity of the femoral vein decreased significantly and the femoral vein cross-sectional area increased significantly when the patient was placed in the reverse Trendelenburg position with the presence of 12 mm Hg pneumoperitoneum. These findings suggest that venous stasis, caused by abdominal insufflation during laparoscopic operations, can be reduced by using lower pressures. Postural changes during laparoscopic operation also greatly affect venous stasis. The large increase in femoral venous blood flow and large decrease in femoral vein cross-sectional area observed after release of the pneumoperitoneum in our study confirmed that venous stasis is present through all laparoscopic operation.

Several other scientists (Ido et al.,1995; Jorgensen et al., 1994; Beebe et al., 1993) also investigated femoral vein blood flow velocities during and after abdominal insufflation in patients, who underwent laparoscopic cholecystectomy, using color Doppler ultrasonography. They also found, that abdominal insufflation reduced the blood velocity in the femoral vein and suggested that abdominal insufflation during laparoscopic operation can cause femoral vein stasis. The femoral vein stasis, which appears in laparoscopic operations, can be minimized by reducing the intraabdominal pressure during operation, and avoiding reverse Trendelenburg position as much as possible.

2.1 Mechanical deep vein thrombosis prevention in laparoscopic surgery

A variety of mechanical techniques and devices has been used in an attempt to reduce the venous stasis, which appears during laparoscopic surgery. Compression bandages, passive exercise, electrical calf stimulation, intermittent pneumatic compression have been employed in reducing venous stasis and the incidence of postoperative DVT.

The other aim of our randomized clinical study was to evaluate the efficacy of mechanical antistasis devices: intermittent pneumatic compression (IPC), intermittent electric calf stimulation (IECS) and graded compression leg bandages (LB) in reducing venous stasis during laparoscopic fundoplication.

Of the physical methods, simple compression using elastic stockings has been reported to be ineffective. The effectiveness of the graded compression bandage, which we used in the present study, has been noted by several investigators. They found the incidence of deep vein thrombosis 7 % in the graded compression bandage groups and 19 % in the controls groups. In our study we found, that femoral venous blood velocity was significantly increased and cross-sectional area significantly decreased over control values (IPC and IECS groups) before the general anesthesia and after the induction of anesthesia in the supine position. However, after the start of abdominal insufflation (5 mmHg) in the supine position, the difference in venous blood flow velocity and cross-sectional area between LB group and IPC and IECS groups (at that time antistasis devices were not acting on the legs and these groups served as controls) was minimized. These our findings suggest that graded compression leg bandages is effective for patients, undergoing open surgery without abdominal insufflation or postural changes, but it is ineffective in patients undergoing laparoscopic surgery, which involves abdominal insufflation. Ido et al., 1995 also found that this type of bandage is ineffective in patients, undergoing laparoscopic cholecystectomy with abdominal insufflation.

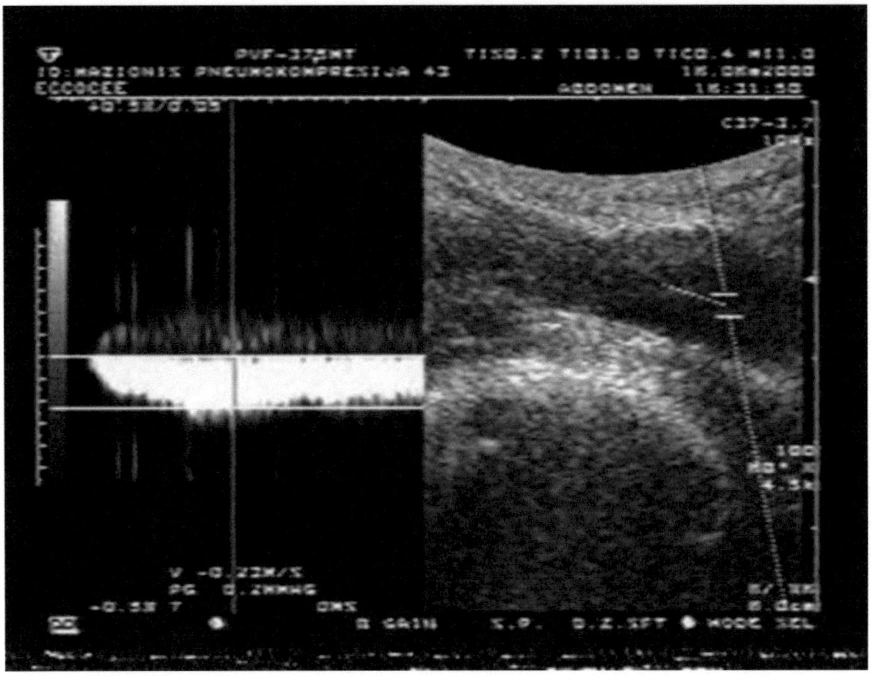

Fig. 5. Venous blood flow velocity at 12 mm Hg insufflation in the reverse Trendelenburg position when intermittent pneumatic compression is acting on the legs.

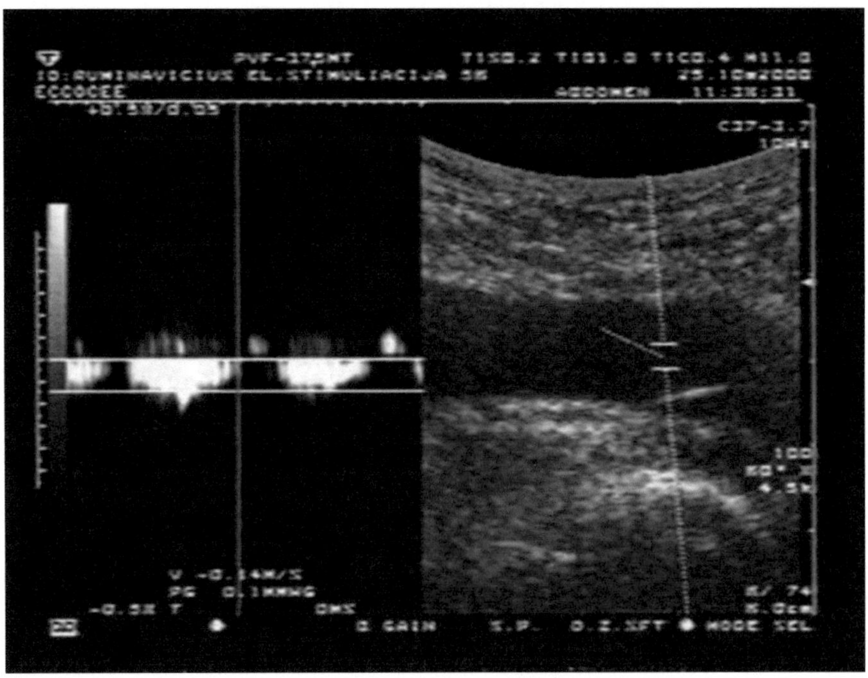

Fig. 6. Venous blood flow velocity at 12 mm Hg insufflation in the reverse Trendelenburg position when intermittent electric calf stimulation is acting on the legs.

The creation of pulsatile venous blood flow is thought to be crucial for the function of mechanical antistasis devices. This pulsatile blood flow episodically flushes activated clotting factors from stagnant soleal sinuses, thereby preventing thrombosis. Both IPC and IECS were able to achieve pulsatile blood flow with a pneumoperitoneum (figure 5 and 6).

The maximum blood velocity generated by the IPC when a pneumoperitoneum (12 mm Hg) was present and the patient was placed in the reverse Trendelenburg position was significantly greater than the maximum blood velocity generated by the IECS. The femoral vein cross-sectional area decreased 25 % when IPC was acting on the legs, when pneumoperitoneum (12 mmHg) was present and the patient was placed in the reverse Trendelenburg position, while the femoral vein cross-sectional area decreased only 3 % when IECS was acting on the legs during laparoscopic operation. The femoral vein cross-sectional area changes received by IPC were significantly greater than changes received by IECS when the pneumoperitoneum (12 mm Hg) was present. These findings show that IPC is more effective than IECS in reducing venous stasis induced by the pneumoperitoneum and the reverse Trendelenburg position. Graded compression leg bandages is totally ineffective in patients, undergoing laparoscopic operations (figure 7).

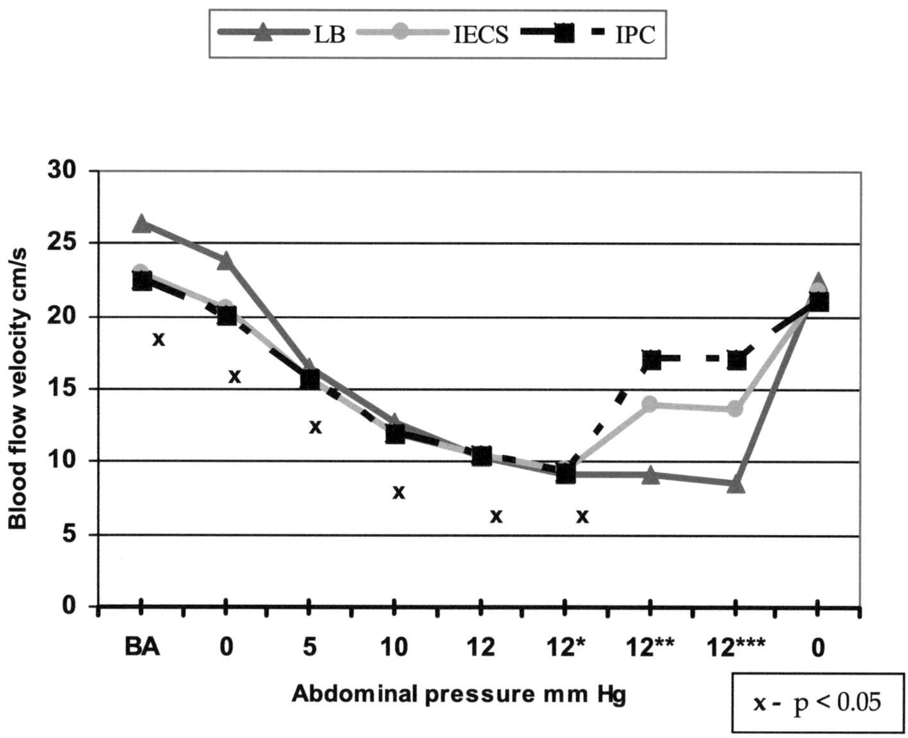

BA - Before the general anesthesia, * - the patient placed in the reverse Trendelenburg position (angle 45°), ** - the patient placed in the reverse Trendelenburg position, when the mechanical antistasis devices is acting on the legs, *** - the patient placed in the reverse Trendelenburg position, when the mechanical antistasis devices is acting on the legs and 1 h after the beginning of the operation

Fig. 7. Mean blood flow velocity changes in the relationship with pneumoperitoneum, reverse Trendelenburg position and antistasis devices.

With a pneumoperitoneum in place, neither device is able to return the depressed blood flow velocity to the values recorded without a pneumoperitoneum. The incidence of DVT and PE after laparoscopic fundoplications was 1.8% in our study.

2.2 Pharmaceutical deep vein thrombosis prevention in laparoscopic surgery

Methods that have conventionally been used to prevent postoperative deep vein thrombosis during laparoscopic surgery include not only mechanical techniques or devices (compression bandages, electrical calf stimulation, passive exercise, intermittent pneumatic compression), but also drug therapy (low-dose heparin, low-molecular-weight-heparin).

Stasis alone does not cause thrombosis, but the combination of stasis, hypercoagulability, and endothelial damage allows thrombus to develop. Some studies demonstrated that laparoscopic operations lead to postoperative activation of the coagulation system, which is one of the factors for postoperative thromboembolic complications.

We performed other prospective randomized clinical study and the aim of this study was to evaluate the hypocoagulation effect of intermittent pneumatic compression (IPC) or combination of low molecular weight heparin (LMWH) and IPC during and after laparoscopic fundoplication. The patients were randomized in to two groups - 10 patients in each group. The first group received IPC during laparoscopic fundoplications. The second group received 40mg LMWH enoxaparin subcutaneous 1h before operation and IPC during laparoscopic fundoplication.

A series of highly sensitive and specific immunochemical tools has been developed that can quantitate the levels and activities of various steps of the haemostatic mechanism in vivo at the sub abnormal level. These include prothrombin F1+2, which measures the cleavage of prothrombin molecule by factor Xa and thrombin –antithrombin complex (TAT) reflecting the in vivo thrombin generation process. The increases in plasma prothrombin fragment F1+2 and thrombin - antithrombin complex indicate increased formation of thrombin. In this study plasma prothrombin fragment F1+2 and TAT were used as markers of coagulation pathway activation. Our study results demonstrated that hypercoagulable state is present during and after laparoscopic fundoplication when using IPC alone for deep-vein thrombosis prevention (tables 1 and 2).

Variable	Before operation (Baseline)	1 h after introduction of laparoscope	10 min after extubation
IPC group (n = 10)	1.07 (0.89-1.23)	1.0 (0.73-1.26)	1.85 (1.31-5.36)[ab]
IPC + LMWH group (n = 10)	1.11 (0.83-1.94)	1.01 (0.77-1.93)	1.44 (0.89-2.17)

Values are expressed as median (range)
[a] $p < 0.0001$ vs baseline
[b] $p < 0.0001$ vs 1h after introduction of laparoscope

Table 1. Changes of prothrombin fragment F1+2 plasma levels (nmol/L) in the IPC and IPC + LMWH groups.

Variable	Before operation (Baseline)	1 h after introduction of laparoscope	10 min after extubation
IPC group (n = 10)	1.5 (1.2-2.5)	6.5 (2.7-9.5)[a]	9.1 (1.4-45.2)[bc]
IPC + LMWH group (n = 10)	2.5 (1.2-7.3)	4.8 (1.3-20.1)	4.7 (1.3-7.1)

Values are expressed as median (range)

[a] $p < 0.0001$ vs baseline
[b] $p < 0.0001$ vs baseline
[c] $p < 0.0001$ vs 1h after introduction of laparoscope

Table 2. Changes of thrombin - antithrombin complex plasma levels (μg/L) in the IPC and IPC + LMWH groups.

Coagulation is regulated at several levels. Key inhibitors include tissue factor pathway inhibitor, antithrombin, and the protein C pathway. The inhibition of the factor VIIa/tissue factor complex (extrinsic coagulation pathway) is effected by TFPI. TFPI acts in a two-step manner. In the first step, TFPI complexes and inactivates factor Xa to form a TFPI/factor Xa complex. The TFPI within this complex then inactivates tissue factor-bound VIIa as the second step. Because the formation of the TFPI/factor Xa complex is a prerequisite for the efficient inactivation of factor VIIa, the system ensures that some factor Xa generation occurs before factor VIIa-mediated initiation of the coagulation system is shut down. In this study plasma free tissue factor pathway inhibitor as marker of hypocoagulation effect was used. Our study results demonstrated that a combination of LMWH and IPC generates hypocoagulation effect and are more effective than IPC alone to prevent deep-vein thrombosis after laparoscopic fundoplication (table 3).

Variable	Before operation (Baseline)	1 h after introduction of laparoscope	10 min after extubation
IPC group (n = 10)	13.7 (7.2-22.3)	13.7 (7.3-20.1)	11.3 (7.9-15.2)
IPC + LMWH group (n = 10)	13.4 (8.3-20.4)	27.9 (20.6-43.6)[a]	21.3 (11.5-32.3)[b]

Values are expressed as median (range)
[a] $p < 0.001$ vs baseline
[b] $p < 0.05$ vs baseline

Table 3. Changes of free tissue pathway factor inhibitor plasma levels (ng/ml) in the IPC and IPC + LMWH groups.

The antithrombotic effect of IPC is thought to be the result of increased venous velocity and stimulation of endogenous fibrinolysis. However, the results of several studies on the enhancement of hypocoagulation effect by an IPC have been controversial. Cahan et al., 2000; showed that external pneumatic compression devices did not enhance systemic fibrinolysis or prevent postoperative shutdown either by decreasing plasminogen activator inhibitor-1 activity or by increasing tissue plasminogen activator activity. Their data suggest that external pneumatic compression devices do not prevent deep venous thrombosis by fibrinolytic enhancement; effective prophylaxis is achieved only when the devices are used in a manner that reduces lower extremity venous stasis. Jacobs et al., 1996; reported that sequential gradient intermittent pneumatic compression induces prompt, but short-lived, alterations in both fibrinolytic function, and the values quickly reverted to baseline on termination of compression. Okuda et al., 2002; reported that intermittent compression boot did not prevent increased intravascular thrombogenesis and platelet activation through significant increases of plasma D-dimmer and β-thromboglobulin after laparoscopic cholecystectomy. Killewich et al., 2002; also reported that enhanced regional fibrinolysis in the lower extremities could not be detected with the use of external pneumatic compression devices, as measured with tissue plasminogen activator and plasminogen activator inhibitor-1 activity in common femoral venous blood samples in patients undergoing abdominal surgery. On the other hand, Comerota et al., 1997; reported that external pneumatic compression devices induced a significant decrease in plasminogen activator inhibitor-1 activity in normal volunteers.

In our study, the IPC used alone during laparoscopic fundoplication, did not prevent increased intravascular thrombogenesis through significant increases of plasma F1+2 and TAT during and after laparoscopic fundoplication.

Giddings et al.,1999; reported that IPC led to highly significant falls in factor VIIa, associated with increased levels of tissue factor pathway inhibitor in non-smoking volunteers. Chouhan et al., 1999; investigated the effect of IPC on the tissue factor pathway in 6 normal subjects and 6 patients with postthrombotic venous disease. Their study results demonstrated that IPC results in an increase in plasma TFPI and decline in FVIIa in both groups. Authors speculated that inhibition of tissue factor pathway, the initiating mechanism of blood coagulation, is a possible mechanism for the antithrombotic effect of IPC. Our study results demonstrate that IPC used alone did not increase TFPI in plasma and didn't produce hypocoagulation effect during laparoscopic fundoplication.

Most circulating TFPI is bound to lipoproteins. TFPI is also found in platelet α-granules and on the endothelium cell surface. TFPI bound to the endothelium is released with therapeutic doses of heparin or low molecular weight heparin, suggesting that TFPI binds to endogenous glycosaminoglycans on the endothelium wall surface.

Our clinical data suggest that LMWH, administered 1 h before operation, together with IPC induce more favorable hypocoagulation profile compared with LMWH alone. However, clinical data, comparing the rate of DVT between these two prophylactic methods are still lacking. On the other hand, alone LMWHs have been evaluated in a large number of randomized clinical trials and have been shown to be safe and effective for the prevention and treatment of venous thrombosis in laparoscopic or in open surgery.

Our recommendation is LMWH, administered 1 h before operation, together with IPC against postoperative venous tromboembolism in laparoscopic operations. Of course, this recommendation has to be proved in future prospective randomized clinical trials, comparing the incidence of DVT between these two prophylactic methods.

3. Conclusions

1. Venous stasis, which appears in laparoscopic operations, can be minimized by reducing the intraabdominal pressure during operation and avoiding reverse Trendelenburg possition as much as possible.
2. IPC is more effective than IECS in reducing venous stasis induced by the pneumoperitoneum and the reverse Trendelenburg position.
3. Graded compression leg bandages is ineffective in patients, undergoing laparoscopic operations with pneumoperitoneum.
4. With a pneumoperitoneum in place, neither mechanical device is able to return the depressed blood flow velocity to the values recorded without a pneumoperitoneum.
5. Hypercoagulable state is present during and after laparoscopic fundoplications when using IPC alone for deep-vein thrombosis prevention: the IPC, used alone, did not prevent increased intravascular thrombogenesis through significant increases of plasma F1+2 and TAT during operation.
6. A combination of LMWH and IPC generates hypocoagulation effect and can be more effective than IPC alone to prevent deep-vein thrombosis after laparoscopic operations.
7. Our recommendation is LMWH, administered 1 h before operation, together with IPC against postoperative venous tromboembolism in laparoscopic operations.

4. References

Allan, A.; Williams, JT & Bolton J.P. (1983). The use of graduated compression stockings in the prevention of postoperative deep vein thrombosis. Br J Surg 70:172-4.

Beebe, D.S.; Mc Nevin, M.P.; Crain, J.M. & al. (1993). Evidence of venous stasis after abdominal insufflation for laparoscopic cholecystectomy. Surg Gynec Obstet 176:443-7.

Borow, M., & Goldson, H.J. (1981). Postoperative venous thrombosis: Evaluation of five methods of prophylaxis. Am J Surg 141:245-51.

Broze, G.J.J. (1995). Tissue factor pathway inhibitor. Thromb Haemost 95:90-3.

Browse, N.L. & Negus, D. (1970). Prevention of postoperative leg vein thrombosis by electrical muscle stimulation. An evaluation with I-labeled fibrinogen. Br Med J 3:615-8.

Cahan, M.A.; Hanna, D.J.; Wiley, L.A.; Cox , D.K. & Killewich, L.A. (2000). External pneumatic compression and fibrinolysis in abdominal surgery. J Vasc Surg 32(3):537-43.

Caprini, J.A.; Arcelus, J.I.; Laubach, M.; Size, G.; Hoffman, K.N. & Coats, R.W. (1995). Postoperative hypercoagulability and deep-vein thrombosis after laparoscopic cholecystectomy. Surg Endosc 9(3):304-9.

Chouhan, V.D.; Comerota, A.J.; Sun, L.; Harada, R.; Gaughan, J.P. & Rao, A.K. (1999). Inhibition of tissue factor pathway during intermittent pneumatic compression: A possible mechanism for antithrombotic effect. Arterioscler Thromb Vasc Biol 19(11):2812-7.

Comerota ,A.J.; Gwendolyn, J. & Stewart, J. (1990). Operative venodilatation: a previously unsuspected factor in the cause of postoperative deep vein thrombosis. Surgery 106:301-9.

Comerota, A.J.; Chouhan, V.; Harada, R.N.; Sun, L.; Hosking, J. & Veermansunemi R. (1997). The fibrinolytic effects of intermittent pneumatic compression: mechanism of enhanced fibrinolysis. Ann Surg 226:306-13.

Dexter, S.P.; Griffith, J.P.; Grant, P.J. & McMahon, M.J. (1996). Activation of coagulation and fibrinolysis in open and laparoscopic cholecystectomy. Surg Endosc 10(11):1069-1074.

Di, V.G.; Frazzetta, M.; Sciume, C.; Lauria, L.G.; Patti, R. & Leo P. (2000). Changes in the hemostatic system after laparoscopic cholecystectomy. G Chir 21(5):213-8.

Ido, K. ; Suzuki, T. & Taniguchi Y. (1995). Femoral vein stasis during laparoscopic cholecystectomy: effects of graded elastic compression leg bandages in preventing thrombus formation. Gastrointestinal Endoscopy 42:151-5.

Ido, K.; Suzuki, T. & Kimura K. (1995). Lower-extremity venous stasis during laparoscopic cholecystectomy as assessed using color Doppler ultrasound. Surg Endosc 9:310-3.

Jacobs, D.G.; Piotrowski, J.J.; Hoppensteadt, D.A.; Salvator, A.E. & Fareed, J. (1996). Hemodinamic and fibrinolytic consequences of intermittent pneumatic compression: preliminary results. J Trauma 40:710-7.

Jorgensen, J.O.; Lalak, N.J. & North L. (1994). Venous stasis during laparoscopic cholecystectomy. Surgical laparoscopy and Endoscopy 4:128-33.

Killewich, L.A.; Cahan, M.A.; Hanna, D.J.; Murakami, M.; Uchida, T. & Wiley, L.A. (2002). The effect of external pneumatic compression on regional fibrinolysis in a prospective randomized trial. J Vasc Surg 36(5):953-8.

Kiudelis, M.; Endzinas, Z.; Mickevicius, A. & Pundzius, J. (2002). Venous stasis and deep vein thrombosis prophylaxis during laparoscopic fundoplication. Zentrallbl Chir (127):944-9.

Lindberg, F.; Rasmussen, I.; Siegbahn, A. & Bergqvist, D. (2000). Coagulation activation after laparoscopic cholecystectomy in spite of thromboembolism prophylaxis. Surg Endosc 14(9):858-61.

Lord, R.V.; Ling, J.J.; Hugh, T.B.; Coleman, M.J.; Doust, B.D. & Nivison-Smith, I. (1998). Incidence of deep vein thrombosis after laparoscopic vs minilaparotomy cholecystectomy. Arch Surg 133(9):967-73.

Okuda, Y.; Kitajima, T.; Egawa, H.; Hamaguchi, S.; Yamaguchi, S. & Yamazaki, H. (2002). A combination of heparin and an intermittent pneumatic compression device may be more effective to prevent deep-vein thrombosis in the lower extremities after laparoscopic cholecystectomy. Surg Endosc 16:781-4.

Patel, M.I.; Hardman, D.T.; Nicholls, D.; Fisher; C.M. & Appleberg, M. (1996). The incidence of deep venous thrombosis after laparoscopic cholecystectomy. Med J Aust 164(11):652-4, 656.

Risberg, B. (1988). Pathophysiological mechanisms of thromboembolism. Acta Chir Scand Suppl (550):104-14.

Rosengarten, D.S.; Laird, J. & Jeyasingh K. (1970). The failure of compression stockings (Tubigrip) to prevent deep venous thrombosis after operation. Br J Surg 57:296-9.

Schaub, R.G.; Lynch, P.R. & Stewart, G.J. (1978). The response of canine veins to three abdominal surgery; a scanning and transmission electron microscopic study. Surgery 83:411-24.

Vecchio, R.; Cacciola, E.; Martino, M.; Cacciola, R.R. & MacFadyen, B.V. (2003). Modifications of coagulation and fibrinolytic parameters in laparoscopic cholecystectomy. Surg Endosc 17(3):428-433.

3

Vena Cava Malformations as an Emerging Etiologic Factor for Deep Vein Thrombosis in Young Patients

Massimiliano Bianchi[1], Lorenzo Faggioni[1], Virna Zampa[1], Gina D'Errico[1], Paolo Marraccini[2] and Carlo Bartolozzi[1]
[1]*Azienda Ospedaliero-Universitaria Pisana,*
[2]*Istituto di Fisiologia Clinica del CNR*
[1,2]*Italia*

1. Introduction

Deep venous thrombosis (DVT) is an illness of clinical interest, due to the associated morbidity and mortality and its social and health care consequences. The etiology in young patients has shown it frequently associated with congenital coagulation abnormalities and acquired/inherited risk factors (table I) [(a,b)].

Inherited
Common
G169A mutation in the factor V gene (factor V Leiden)
G20219A mutation in the protrombin (factor II) gene
Homozygous C677T mutation in the methylenetetrahydrofolate reductase gene
Rare
Antitrombin deficiency
Protein C deficiency
Protein S deficiency
Very rare
Dysfibrinogenemia
Homozygous homocystinuria
Probably inherited
Increased levels of factor VII, IX, XI or fibrinogen
Acquired
Surgery and trauma
Prolonged immobilization
Older age
Cancer
Myeloproliferative disorders
Previous thrombosis
Pregnancy and the puerperium
Use of contraceptives or hormone-replacement therapy

Resistence to activated protein C (not due alterations in the factor V gene
Antiphospholipid antibodies)
Mild to moderate hyperomocysteinemia

Table 1. inherited and acquired risk factors for DVT.

However, recent radiological advances derived from multislice computerized tomography (CT) and magnetic resonance imaging (MRI) have identified vena cava malformations as a new etiologic factor to be considered.[c-g]

The objectives of the present chapter are to describe the embryogenesis and the spectrum of congenital anomalies of the inferior vena cava (IVC) as a risk factor in DVT in young patients. Anomalies of the inferior vena cava (IVC) and its tributaries have been known to anatomists since 1793, when Abernethy[h] described a congenital meso-caval shunt and azygos continuation of the IVC in a 10-month-old infant with polysplenia and dextrocardia. Since the development of cross-sectional imaging, congenital anomalies of the IVC and its tributaries have become more frequently encountered in asymptomatic patients[c]. The imaging study with CT and MRI of the abdominal vein structures require a specific thecnique of acquisition in relation with contrast medium injection. During the usual vascular study, that are acquired in arterial phase, the visualization of veins is not adequate for the recognition of the vein system. This may are usually readily identified on CT and magnetic resonance (MR) imaging scans of the abdomen and pelvis obtained with intravenously administered contrast medium. In addition, with helical acquisition, the venous structures may be imaged during the arterial phase, when little or no contrast material is present in the veins. Therefore, in these cases the diagnostic request is essential for correct interpretation of vein vasculature and to avoid erroneous diagnosis (retroperitoneal and mediastinal masses or adenopathy) and to alert the surgeon and angiographer about the characteristics of vascular anatomy.

1.1 The embryogenesis of the IVC

The embryogenesis and the anatomic variations of the IVC become more clear with the development of the CT and magnetic resonance (MR) imaging in clinical practice. In the past Phillips[i] has published a comprehensive review of the embryogenesis of the IVC. In brief, the infrahepatic IVC develops between the 6th and 8th weeks of embryonic life as a composite structure formed from the continuous appearance and regression of three paired embryonic veins. In order of appearance, they are the posterior cardinal, the subcardinal, and the supracardinal veins (Fig 1).

Under ordinary circumstances, the prerenal division is formed from union of the hepatic segment (green area), a vitelline vein derivative, and the right subcardinal vein (magenta area). The renal segment is formed from the suprasubcardinal anastomosis (yellow area) and the postsubcardinal anastomosis (light violet area). The infrarenal segment derives from the right supracardinal vein (goldenrod area). The posterior cardinal veins (dark violet area) form the iliac veins (Adapted and reprinted, with permission, from reference d). Initially, all blood return from the body wall caudal to the heart proceeds through the posterior cardinal veins (dark violet in Fig 1). Blood return from the viscera is conveyed by the vitelline veins (green in Fig 1), which drain the yolk sac. Subsequently, the subcardinal veins (magenta in

Fig 1) develop ventromedial to the posterior cardinal veins and ventrolateral to the aorta. The intersubcardinal anastomosis forms between the paired subcardinal veins, anterior to the aorta, and caudal to the superior mesenteric artery.

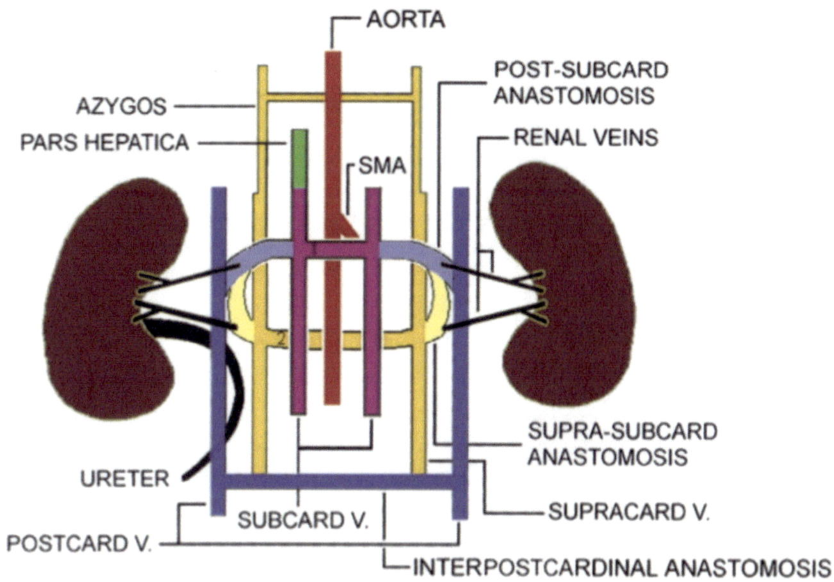

Fig. 1. Conceptual framework for development of the IVC. Composite schematic shows the relative positions and interrelationships of the three paired embryonic vessels that contribute to development of the IVC. The pictured veins are not all present simultaneously. card= cardinal, post= posterior, SMA= superior mesenteric artery, v= vein, 1= intersubcardinal anastomosis, 2 = intersupracardinal anastomosis.

Anastomosis between the posterior cardinal and subcardinal veins (light violet in Fig 1) develop on each side at approximately the level of the intersubcardinal anastomosis. At the same time, union occurs between the right subcardinal vein and the hepatic segment of the IVC, which forms from the vitelline vein. As the cranial portions of the posterior cardinal veins begin to atrophy, blood return from the lower extremities is shunted through the postsubcardinal anastomosis, then through the subcardinal-hepatic anastomosis to the hepatic segment of the IVC. This process establishes the pre-renal division of the IVC. The next major development is the appearance of the paired supra-cardinal veins (goldenrod in Fig 1), which lie dorso-medial to the posterior cardinal veins and dorso-lateral to the aorta. Initially, multiple anastomosis form between the posterior and supracardinal veins. On each side, a suprasubcardinal anastomosis (yellow in Fig 1) develops from union of the postsupracardinal and the postsubcardinal anastomosis. In addition, intersupracardinal anastomosis develop dorsal to the aorta. The supracardinal veins then separate into cranial (azygos) and caudal (lumbar) ends. Meanwhile, inferiorly, anastomosis develop between the two posterior cardinal veins and between the posterior and lumbar supracardinal veins. With further atrophy of the posterior cardinal veins, blood return from the lower extremities is shunted through the supracardinal system to the suprasubcardinal anastomosis, then to the pre-renal division of the IVC. In addition, blood return from the left side of the body is shunted to the right across the intersupracardinal and interpostcardinal anastomosis.

Finally, the left supracardinal vein is one of the last veins to disappear, although Huntington and McLure[j] state that the vessel does not so much atrophy as become incorporated into the right supracardinal vein by coalescence of the multiple anastomosis. In summary, the normal IVC is composed of four segments: hepatic, suprarenal, renal, and infrarenal. The hepatic segment is derived from the vitelline vein. The right subcardinal vein develops into the suprarenal segment by formation of the subcardinal-hepatic anastomosis. The renal segment develops from the right suprasubcardinal and postsubcardinal anastomosis. It is generally accepted that the infra-renal segment derives from the right supracardinal vein, although this idea is somewhat controversial[i]. In the thoracic region, the supracardinal veins give rise to the azygos and hemiazygos veins. In the abdomen, the postcardinal veins are progressively replaced by the subcardinal and supracardinal veins but persist in the pelvis as the common iliac veins.

2. Variations in IVC anatomy

In a study of the development of the IVC in the domestic cat (Felis domestica), Huntington and McLure[j] proposed a classification system for IVC anomalies based on abnormal regression or abnormal persistence of various embryonic veins. These investigators suggested that there could be up to 14 theoretical variations in the anatomy of the infra-renal IVC. They noted that 11 of the 14 variants had been observed in the domestic cat or in humans. In addition, these authors observed that other anomalies seen in humans, such as abnormal development of the pre-renal division of the IVC and persistence of the renal collar in the adult, could be explained on a similar basis.

2.1 Left IVC

A left IVC results from regression of the right supra-cardinal vein with persistence of the left supra-cardinal vein. The prevalence is 0.2%–0.5%[i]. Typically, the left IVC joins the left renal vein, which crosses anterior to the aorta in the normal fashion, uniting with the right renal vein to form a normal right-sided prerenal IVC (Fig 2).

2.2 Double IVC

Duplication of the IVC results from persistence of both supracardinal veins. The prevalence is 0.2%–3%[i]. The left IVC typically ends at the left renal vein, which crosses anterior to the aorta in the normal fashion to join the right IVC (Fig 3).

2.3 Azygos continuation of the IVC

Azygos continuation of the IVC has also been termed absence of the hepatic segment of the IVC with azygos continuation[k]. The embryonic event is theorized to be failure to form the right sub-cardinal–hepatic anastomosis, with resulting atrophy of the right sub-cardinal vein. Consequently, blood is shunted from the supra-sub-cardinal anastomosis through the retro-crural azygos vein, which is partially derived from the thoracic segment of the right supra-cardinal vein. The prevalence is 0.6%[k]. The renal portion of the IVC receives blood return from both kidneys and passes posterior to the diaphragmatic crura to enter the thorax as the azygos vein (Fig 4).

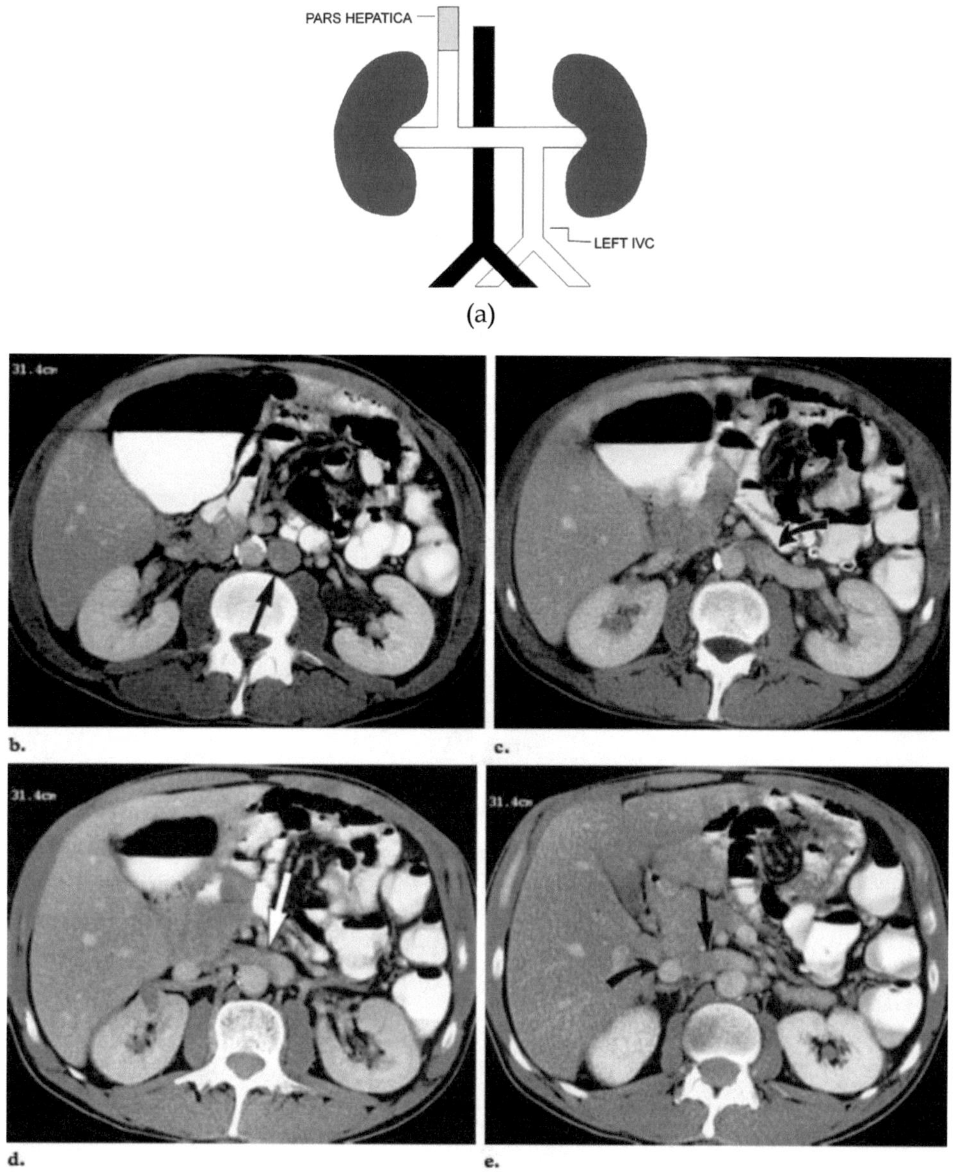

Fig. 2. Partial malrotation and left IVC in a 49-year-old man. (a) Schematic shows a left IVC terminating at the left renal vein. (b-e) CT scans presented from caudal to cranial show the anomaly. (b) Note the left IVC (arrow) inferior to the renal veins. (c) The left IVC joins the left renal vein (arrow). (d) The left renal vein (arrow) crosses anterior to the aorta in the normal fashion. (e) A normal right-sided prerenal IVC is formed from the confluence of the left (straight arrow) and right (curved arrow) renal veins. Note the increased attenuation of the right renal vein relative to that of the left due to absence of dilution from relatively unenhanced lower-extremity venous return. The major clinical significance of this anomaly is the potential for misdiagnosis as left-sided paraaortic adenopathy[k].

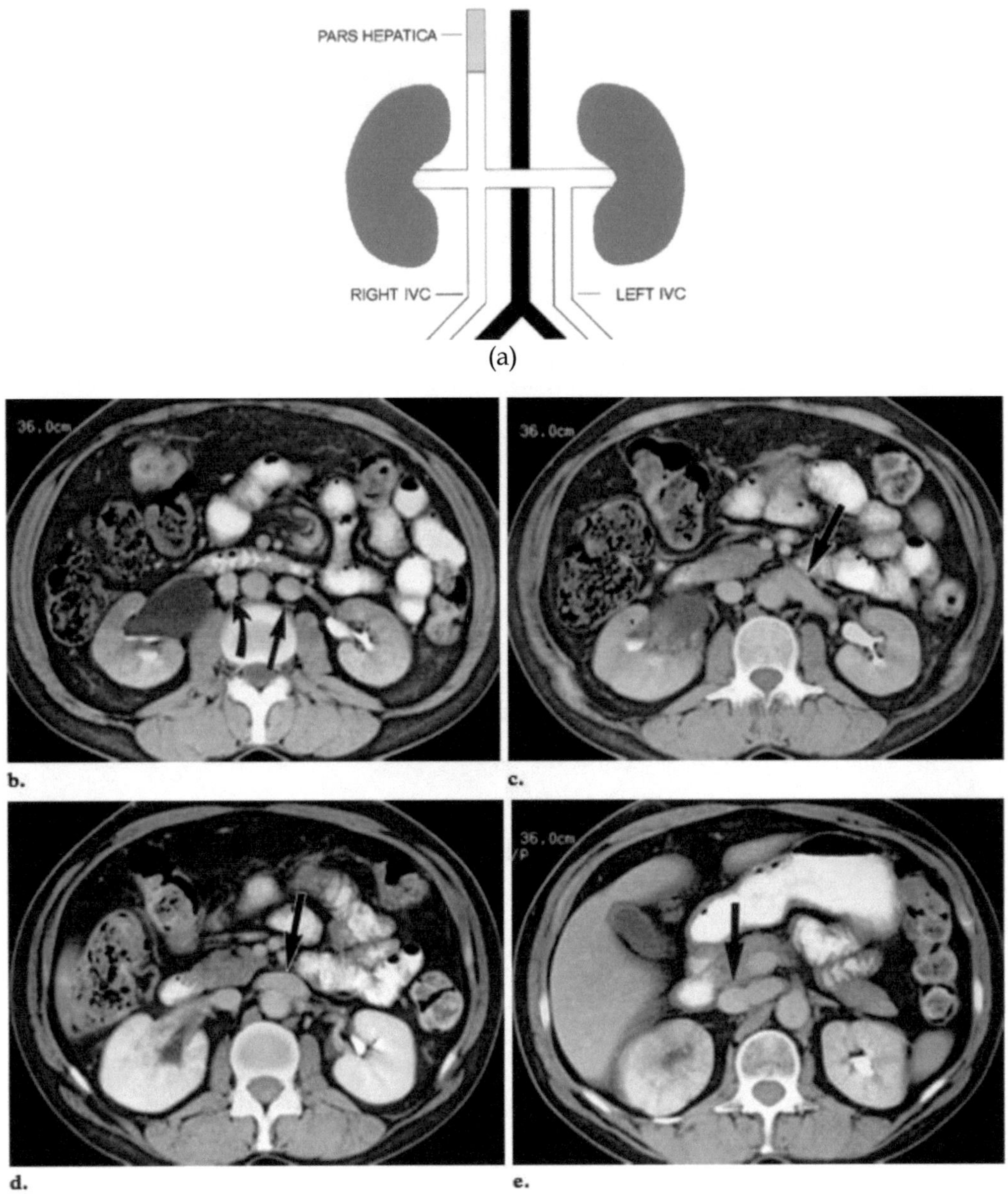

Fig. 3. Double IVC in a 53-year-old woman with lymphoma. (a) Schematic shows left and right infrarenal IVCs. The left IVC terminates at the left renal vein. (b) CT scan obtained inferior to the renal veins shows left (straight arrow) and right (curved arrow) IVCs. (c-e) CT scans show the left IVC ending at the confluence with the left renal vein (arrow in c), which crosses anterior to the aorta in the normal fashion (arrow in d) to join a normal pre-renal IVC (arrow in e). There may be morphological variation and asymmetry of the left and right veins. Double IVC should be suspected in cases of recurrent pulmonary embolism following placement of an IVC filter(i).

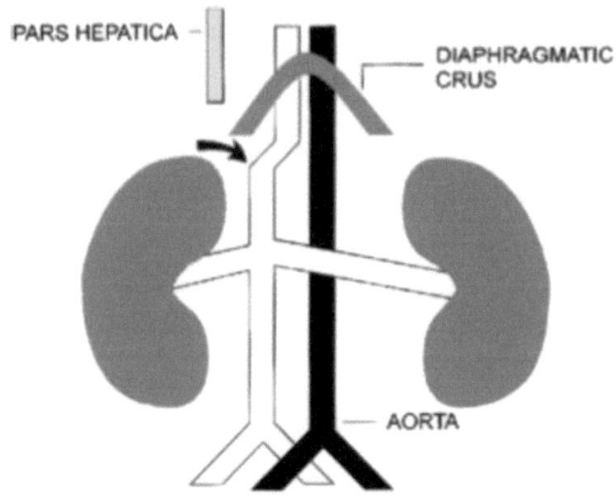

(a)

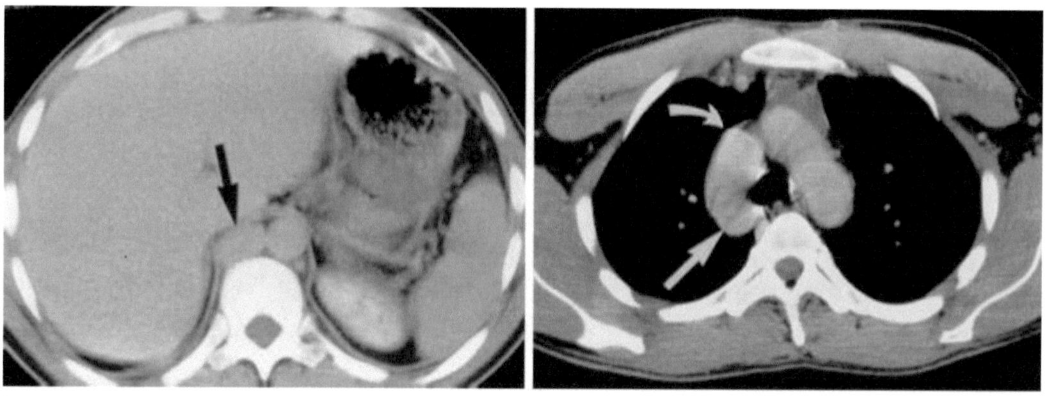

b. c.

Fig. 4. CT images of azygos continuation of the IVC in a 48-year-old man. (a) Schematic shows lack of contiguity between the pre-renal segment of the IVC (arrow) and the hepatic segment. The vessel parallel to the aorta under the crus is the azygos vein. (b, c) CT scans obtained at the level of the diaphragmatic crus (b) and the level of the azygos vein arch (c) show the enlarged azygos vein (straight arrow) draining into the superior vena cava (curved arrow in c).

The azygos vein joins the superior vena cava at the normal location in the right para-tracheal space. The hepatic segment (often termed the post-hepatic segment) is ordinarily not truly absent; rather, it drains directly into the right atrium. Since the post-sub-cardinal anastomosis does not contribute to formation of the IVC, each gonadal vein drains to the ipsi-lateral renal vein[j]. Formerly thought to be predominantly associated with severe congenital heart disease and a-splenia or poly-splenia syndromes, azygos continuation of the IVC has become increasingly recognized in otherwise asymptomatic patients since the advent of cross-sectional imaging. It is important to recognize the enlarged azygos vein at the confluence with the superior vena cava and in the retrocrural space to avoid misdiagnosis as a right-sided para-tracheal mass or retro-crural adenopathy[k,l]. Preoperative knowledge of the anatomy may be important in planning cardiopulmonary bypass and to avoid difficulties in catheterizing the heart[m].

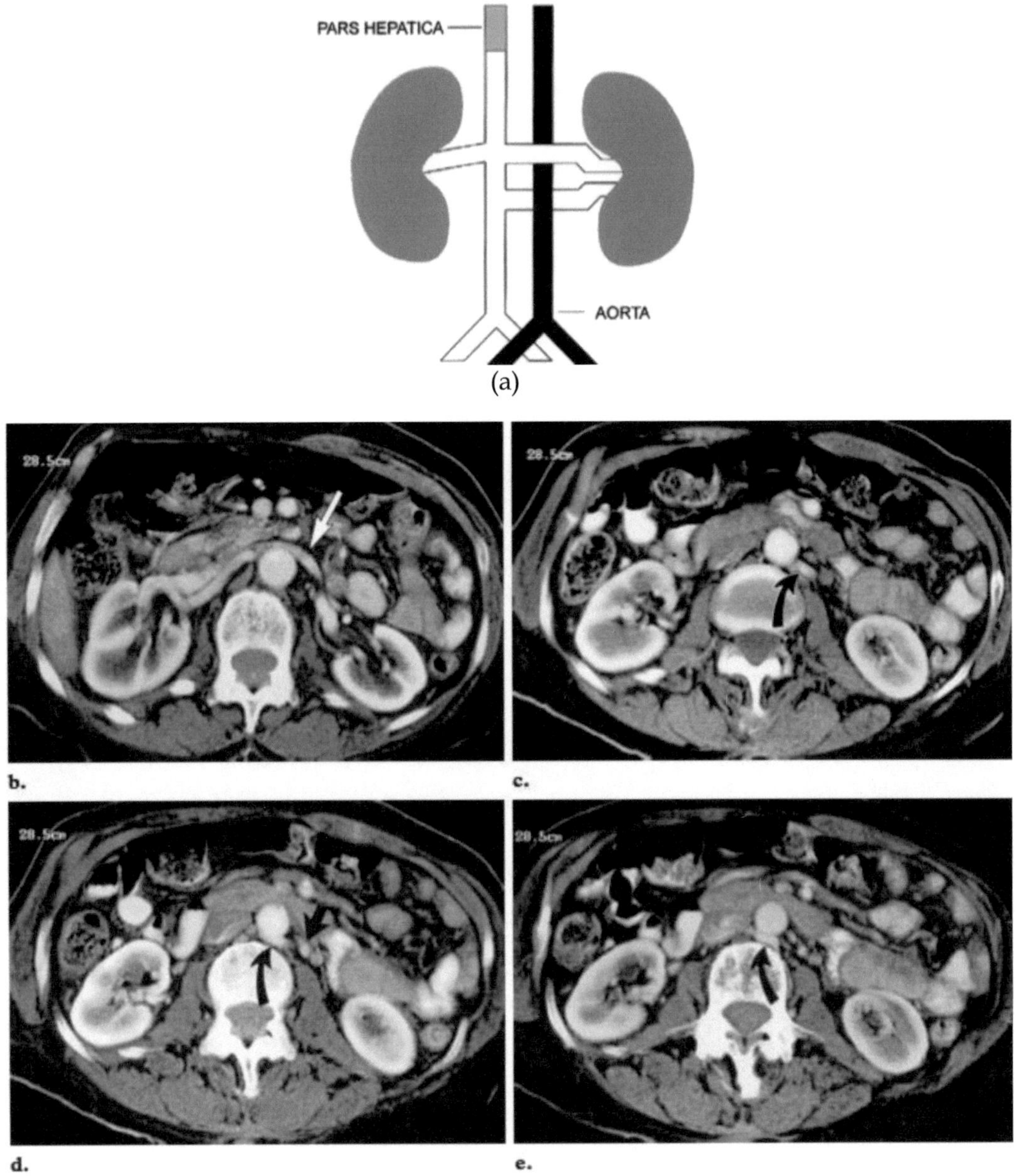

Fig. 5. Circumaortic left renal vein in a 73-year-old woman. (a) Schematic shows two left renal veins, with the inferior vein crossing posterior to the aorta. (b-e) Contiguous 5-mm-thick CT sections presented from cranial to caudal show the anomaly. (b) The superior left renal vein (arrow) crosses anterior to the aorta. (c-e) The inferior vein (curved arrow) descends approximately 2 cm and receives the left gonadal vein (straight arrow in d) before crossing posterior to the aorta. The major clinical significance is in preoperative planning prior to nephrectomy and in renal vein catheterization for venous sampling. Misdiagnosis as retroperitoneal adenopathy should be avoided.

2.4 Circum-aortic left renal vein

A circum-aortic left renal vein results from persistence of the dorsal limb of the embryonic left renal vein and of the dorsal arch of the renal collar (inter-supra-cardinal anastomosis). The prevalence may be as high as 8.7%(i). Two left renal veins are present. The superior renal vein receives the left adrenal vein and crosses the aorta anteriorly. The inferior renal vein receives the left gonadal vein and crosses posterior to the aorta approximately 1–2 cm inferior to the normal anterior vein (Fig 5).

2.5 Retro-aortic left renal vein

As with circum-aortic left renal vein, a retro-aortic left renal vein results from persistence of the dorsal arch of the renal collar. However, in this variation the ventral arch (inter-subcardinal anastomosis) regresses so that a single renal vein passes posterior to the aorta (Fig 6). The prevalence is 2.1%(i). The clinical significance is preoperative recognition of the anomaly.

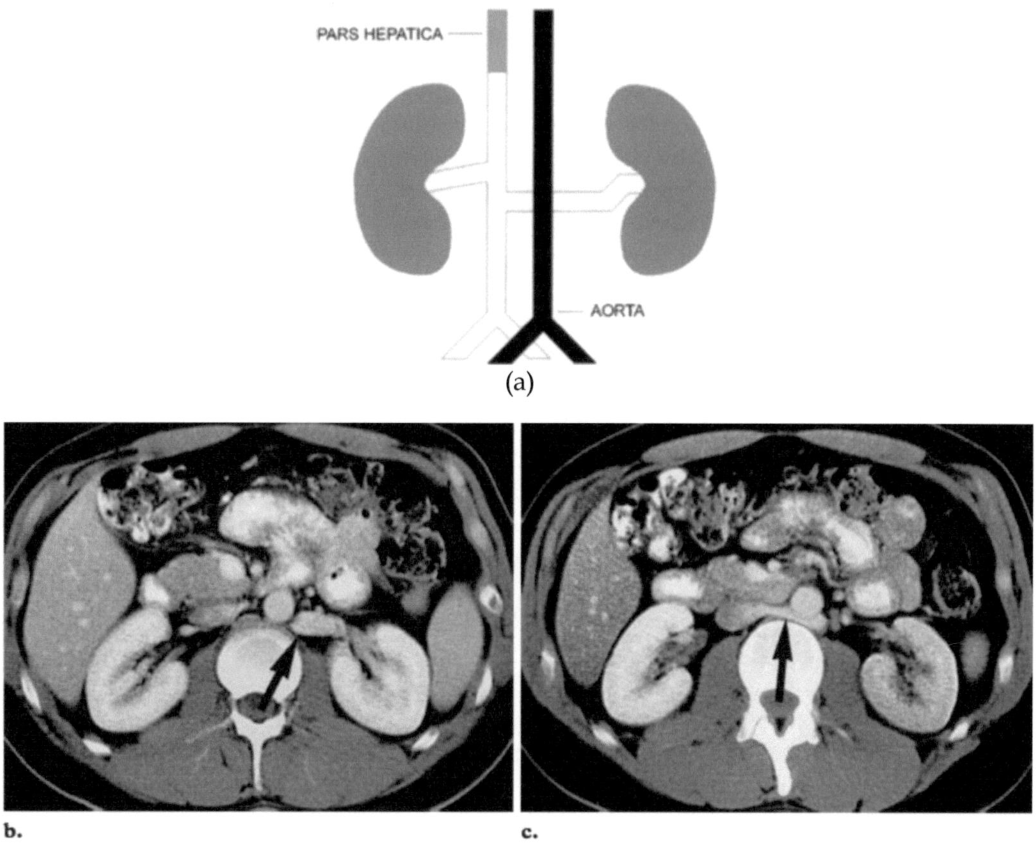

Fig. 6. Retroaortic left renal vein in a 27-year-old man. (a) Schematic shows a single left renal vein, which crosses posterior to the aorta. (b, c) CT scans show the left renal vein (arrow) descending to cross posterior to the aorta.

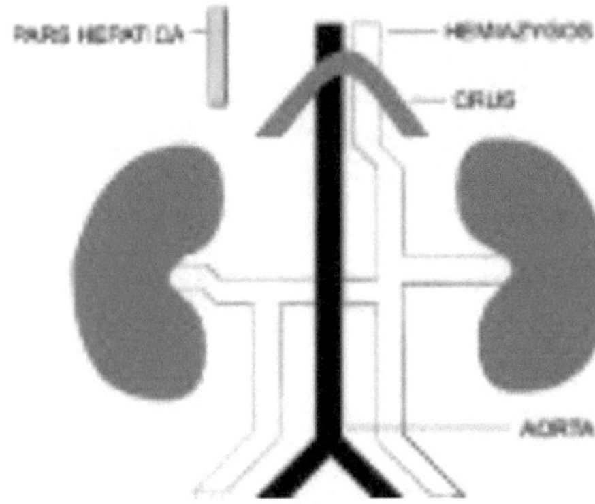

(a)

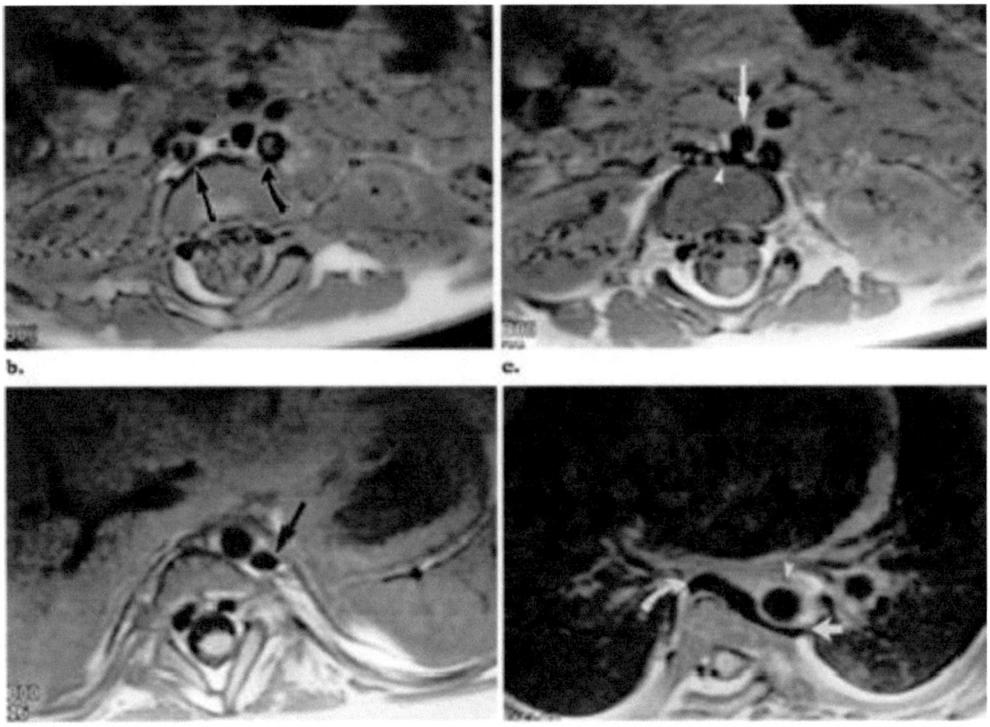

Fig. 7. Spinal dysraphism and double IVC with hemiazygos continuation in a 2-year-old boy. (a) Schematic shows failed development of the right pre-renal IVC and hemi-azygos continuation of the left IVC. (b-e) MR images presented from caudal to cranial show the anomaly. (b) Note the right (straight arrow) and left (curved arrow) IVCs. (c) The right renal vein (arrowhead) descends to receive the right IVC and crosses posterior to the aorta (arrow) to join the left IVC. (d) The left IVC continues cephalad left of the aorta under the diaphragmatic crus as the hemi-azygos vein (arrow). (e) In the thorax, the hemi-azygos vein (straight arrow) crosses posterior to the aorta (arrowhead) to join a rudimentary azygos vein (curved arrow) approximately 1-2 cm below the carina.

2.6 Double IVC with retro-aortic right renal vein and hemi-azygos continuation of the IVC

More than one anomaly can coexist in a patient. In the case of a double IVC with a retro-aortic right renal vein and hemi-azygos continuation of the IVC, the embryologic basis is persistence of the left lumbar and thoracic supra-cardinal vein and the left supra-sub-cardinal anastomosis, together with failure of formation of the right sub-cardinal–hepatic anastomosis. In addition, the right renal vein and right IVC meet and cross posterior to the aorta to join the left IVC and continue cephalad as the hemi-azygos vein (Fig 7). Thus, there is also persistence of the dorsal limb of the renal collar and regression of the ventral limb. In the thorax, the hemi-azygos vein crosses posterior to the aorta at approximately T8 or T9 to join the rudimentary azygos vein. Alternate collateral pathways for the hemi-azygos vein include cephalad continuation to join the coronary vein of the heart via a persistent left superior vena cava and an accessory hemi-azygos continuation to the left brachio-cephalic vein[n].

2.7 Double IVC with retro-aortic left renal vein and hemiazygos continuation of the IVCA

Double IVC with a retro-aortic left renal vein and azygos continuation of the IVC is an interesting combination. It results from persistence of the left supracardinal vein and the dorsal limb of the renal collar with regression of the ventral limb. In addition, the sub-cardinal-hepatic anastomosis fails to form (Fig 7). A recent study demonstrated that azygos continuation of the IVC can be predicted with ultrasonography by identifying the right renal artery crossing abnormally anterior to the IVC [15].

2.8 Circum-caval ureter

A circum-caval ureter is also termed a retro-caval ureter. The right supra-cardinal system fails to develop, whereas the right posterior cardinal vein persists. The anomaly always occurs on the right side. The proximal ureter courses posterior to the IVC, then emerges to the right of the aorta, coming to lie anterior to the right iliac vessels (Fig 8). Patients with this anomaly may develop partial right ureteral obstruction or recurrent urinary tract infections. Therapeutic options include surgical relocation of the ureter anterior to the cava[i].

2.9 Absent Infra-renal IVC with preservation of the supra-renal segment

Several reports have described absence of the entire IVC [o–r] or absence of the infra-renal IVC with preservation of the supra-renal segment (Fig 9) [s,t]. Absence of the entire posthepatic IVC suggests that all three paired venous systems failed to develop properly.

Absence of the infrarenal IVC implies failure of development of the posterior cardinal and supracardinal veins. Since it is difficult to identify a single embryonic event that can lead to either of these scenarios, there is controversy as to whether these conditions are true embryonic anomalies or the result of perinatal IVC thrombosis [p,s,t].

3. Implications for treatment of DVT and prevention of recurrences

The therapy of acute DVT in this kind of patients is similar of the currently recommended strategies and includes un-fractioned heparin, low-molecular weight heparin, fondaparinux

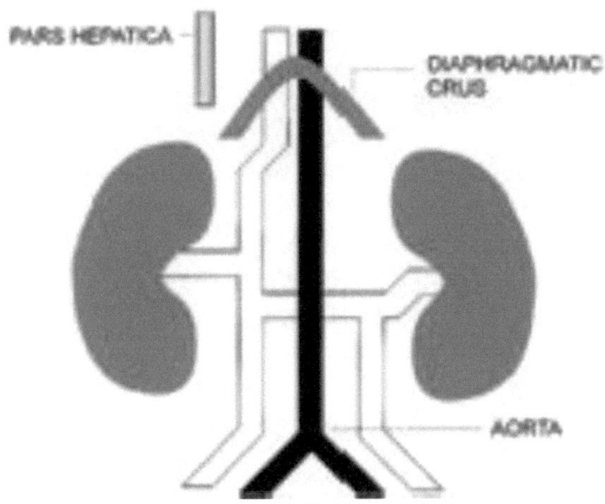

(a)

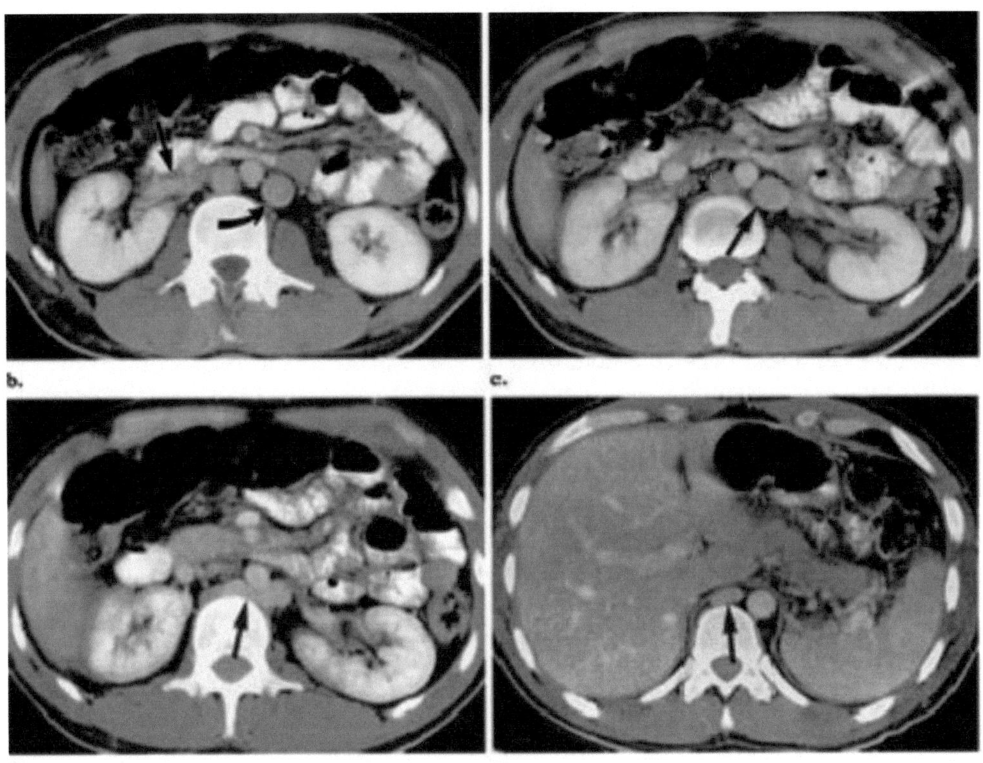

Fig. 8. Circumcaval ureter in a 65-year-old man. (a) Schematic shows the right ureter encircling the IVC. (b-d) CT scans presented from cranial to caudal show the anomaly. (b) The right ureter (arrow) is positioned posterior to the IVC. (c) The ureter (arrow) then courses to the left of the IVC. (d) Finally, the ureter (arrow) crosses anterior to the IVC. (Courtesy of Akira Kawashima, MD, Lyndon B. Johnson General Hospital, Houston, Tex.)

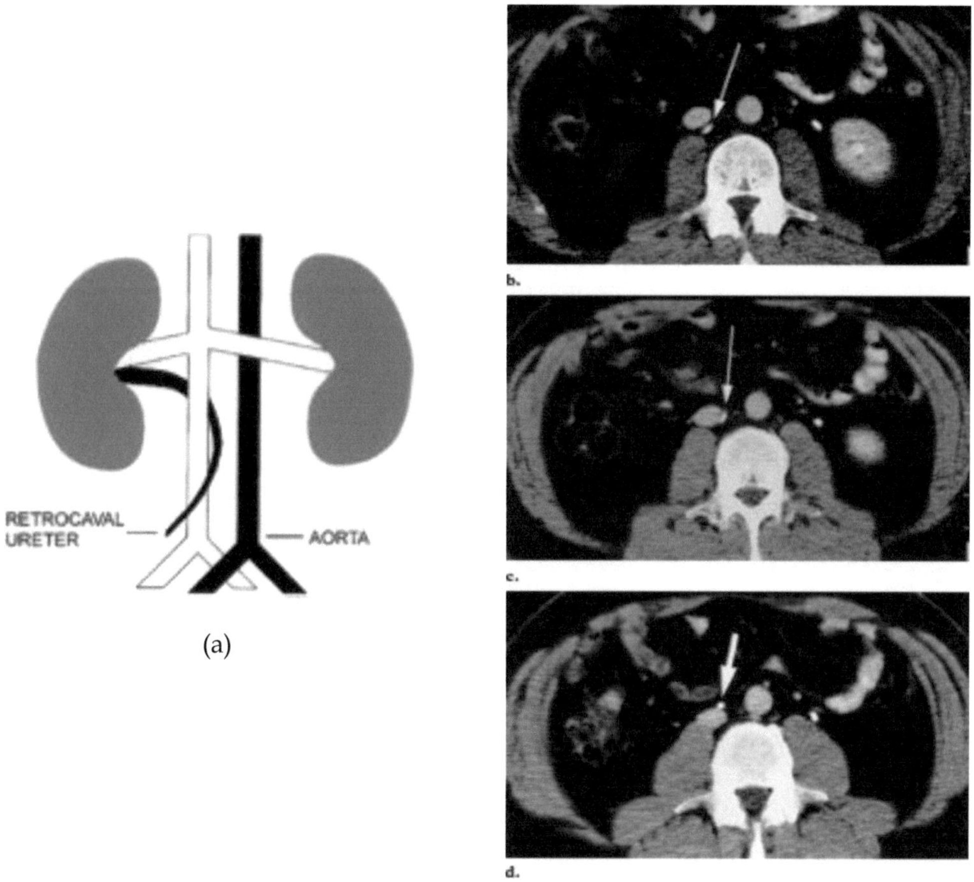

Fig. 9. Absent infra-renal IVC. (a) Schematic shows absence of the IVC below the renal veins. Collateral flow from the lower extremities reaches the azygos vein via para-vertebral collateral veins. (b) CT scan obtained inferior to the aortic bifurcation shows absence of the common iliac veins. Enlarged ascending lumbar veins are present (black arrow). Note the iliac arteries (white arrow). (c) CT scan obtained inferior to the kidneys shows absence of the IVC (white arrow). Enlarged ascending lumbar veins are present (black arrow). (d) CT scan obtained at the level of the renal veins shows a normal pre-renal IVC formed at the confluence of the renal veins (arrow). (e) CT scan obtained at the level of the pre-renal IVC (white arrow) shows prominent para-vertebral collateral veins (black arrow), which lead to a prominent azygos vein (arrowhead). (f) Coronal T1-weighted MR image shows the enlarged ascending lumbar veins (arrow). (g) Lateral maximum-intensity projection reconstruction of two-dimensional time-of-flight MR images shows formation of enlarged ascending lumbar veins at the confluence of the internal and external iliac veins (solid straight arrow). Note the anastomosis between the ascending lumbar veins and the azygos vein (open straight arrow) via prominent anterior para-vertebral veins (white curved arrow). Also note the pre-renal IVC (black arrowhead) posterior to the portal vein (black curved arrow), as well as prominent anterior abdominal wall collateral veins (white arrowheads). (Figs 10b, 10c, and 10g reprinted, with permission, from references).

and vitamin-K antagonists(u). The diagnosis of anomalies in the inferior vena cava influences the strategy for prevention the pulmonary embolism and long them maintenance treatment.

The use of mechanical device as caval filter is clearly limited by the anomalous anatomy of the inferior vena cava and, generally, is-not indicated. On the other hand the use of oral anti-coagulant (commonly warfarin) should be adjusted to maintain a target international normalized ratio of 2.5 (range 2-3) and extended indefinitely in absence of main contra-indications(d).

At present the introduction of new drugs as the factor Xa antagonists (rivarixaban, apixaban, edoxaban, ect) and the direct thrombin inhibitors as dabigatran etexilate could improve the therapeutic options. The promising results of the recent clinical studies in terms of efficacy and safety, suggest that these new drugs may allow a reduction of the length of hospital stay after an acute DVT, and a better adherence to guidelines in the long term treatment. The principal advantages of these drugs are the absence of the need of a routine coagulation monitoring and a therapeutic activity not influenced by dietary regimen and by drugs as NSADIs and statins(u). Potential limitations are the lack of specific antidotes (however the hal-life of these drugs is relative short) and the absence of a simple assay for quantification of activity or plasma level.

In conclusion these interesting pharmacological characteristics could improve the benefit-risk balance of long-term anti-coagulant therapy and the overall clinical outcome.

4. Conclusions

The complexity of the ontogeny of the IVC, with numerous anastomosis formed between the three primitive paired veins, can lead to a wide array of variations in the basic plan of venous return from the abdomen and lower extremity. Some of these anomalies have significant clinical implications. Although vascular structures can usually be readily identified on contrast-enhanced CT scans, identification of unusual venous arrangements may be difficult in those cases in which intravenous contrast material is contraindicated. In such patients, MR imaging may be used to distinguish aberrant vessels from masses by demonstrating flow voids or flow-related enhancement. The echo-scanning may suggest the presence of venous anomalies but usually it insufficient for a detailed diagnosis. A knowledge of IVC and renal vein anomalies is essential to avoid diagnostic pitfalls.

5. References

[1] Rosendaal F. Thrombosis in the young: epidemiology and risk factors. A focus on venous thrombosis. *Thromb Haemost.* 1997;78:1-6.

[2] García-Fuster MJ, Fernández C, Forner MJ, & Vayá A. Estudio prospectivo de los factores de riesgo y las características clíni- cas de la enfermedad tromboembólica en pacientes jóvenes. *Med Clin (Barc).* 2004;123:217-9.

[3] Ruggeri M, Tosseto A, Castaman G & Rodeghiero F. Congenital absence of the inferior vena cava: a rare risk factor for idiopathic deep vein thrombosis. *Lancet.* 2001;357:441.

[4] M. Bianchi, D. Giannini, A. Balbarini, M.G. & Castiglioni. Congenital hypoplasia of inferior vena cava and inherited thrombophilia: rare associated risk factor for

idiopathic deep vein thrombosis. A case report. *J Cardiovasc Med* (Hagerstown). 2008 Jan;9(1):101-4.

[5] Obernosterer A, Aschauer M, Schnedl W & Lipp RW. Anomalies of the inferior vena cava in patients with iliac venous thrombosis. *Ann Intern Med.* 2002;136:37-41.

[6] Chee YL, Culligan DJ & Watson HG. Inferior vena cava malformation as a risk factor for deep venous thrombosis in the young. *Br J Haematol.* 2001;114:878-80.

[7] Gayer G, Luboshitz J, Hertz M, Zissen R, Thaler M, Lubetsky A & et al. Congenital anomalies of the inferior vena cava revealed on CT in patients with deep vein thrombosis. *AJR.* 2003;180:729-32.

[8] Abernethy J. Account of two instances of uncommon formation in the viscera of the human body. *Philos Trans R Soc* 1793; 83:59

[9] Phillips E. Embryology, normal anatomy, and anomalies. In: Ferris EJ, Hipona FA, Kahn PC, Phillips E, Shapiro JH, eds. Venography of the inferior vena cava and its branches. Baltimore, Md: *Williams & Wilkins*, 1969; 1-32.

[10] Huntington GS, McLure CFW. The development of the veins in the domestic cat (felis domestica) with especial reference, 1) to the share taken by the supracardinal vein in the development of the postcava and azygous vein and 2) to the interpretation of the variant conditions of the postcava and its tributaries, as found in the adult. *Anat Rec* 1920; 20:1-29.

[11] Ginaldi S, Chuang VP & Wallace S. Absence of hepatic segment of the inferior vena cava with azygous continuation. *J Comput Assist Tomogr* 1980; 4:112-114.

[12] Schultz CL, Morrison S & Bryan PJ. Azygous continuation of the inferior vena cava: demonstration by NMR imaging. *J Comput Assist Tomogr* 1984; 8:774-776.

[13] Mazzucco A, Bortolotti U, Stellin G & Galucci V. Anomalies of the systemic venous return: a review. *J Card Surg* 1990; 5:122-133.

[14] Haswell DM, Berrigan TJ, Jr. Anomalous inferior vena cava with accessory hemiazygos continuation. *Radiology* 1976; 119:51-54.

[15] Geley TE, Unsinn KM, Auckenthaller TM, Fink CJ & Gassner I. Azygos continuation of the inferior vena cava in pediatric patients: sonographic demonstration of the renal artery ventral to the azygos vein as a clue to diagnosis. *Am J Roentgenol* 1999; 172:1659-1662.

[16] Milner LB, Marchan R. Complete absence of the inferior vena cava presenting as a paraspinous mass. *Thorax* 1980; 35:798

[17] Dougherty MJ, Calligaro KD, DeLaurentis DA. Congenitally absent inferior vena cava presenting in adulthood with venous stasis and ulceration: a surgically treated case. *J Vasc Surg* 1996; 23:141

[18] Debing E, Tielemans Y, Jolie E & Van den Brande P. Congenital absence of inferior vena cava. *Eur J Vasc Surg* 1993; 7:201-203.

[19] D'Archambeau O, Verguts L & Myle J. Congenital absence of the inferior vena cava. *J Belge Radiol* 1990; 73:516-517.

[20] Bass JE, Redwine MD, Kramer LA & Harris JH, Jr. Absence of the infrarenal inferior vena cava with preservation of the suprarenal segment as revealed by CT and MR venography. *Am J Roentgenol* 1999; 172:1610-1612.

[21] Mavrakanas T, Bounameaux H. The potential role of new oral anticoagulants in the prevention and treatment of thromboembolism. *Pharmacology & Therapeutics* 130 (2011) 46–58

4

Endovascular Therapies in Acute DVT

Jeff Tam and Jim Koukounaras
The Alfred Hospital
Australia

1. Introduction

Deep venous thrombosis of the lower limb is a common disease with an incidence of 80 per 10000 (Patel et al 2011) and has potential fatal consequences in the form of pulmonary embolism.

It is usually seen in patients undergoing major surgery particularly orthopaedic surgery, trauma, prolonged immobilisation or hypercoagulable states (such as in the context of malignancy). There are associations with drugs such as the oral contraceptive pill and hormone replacement therapy (tamoxifen) that predispose to hypercoagulability.

2. Pathology and clinical presentation

Deep venous thrombosis of the lower extremity can occur anywhere from the ankle to the IVC, however it is those that occur between the IVC and femoral veins that most often lead to venous hypertension, resulting in the more severe symptoms. They are also more likely to recur (Vendatham 2006).

The clinical spectrum can range from being completely asymptomatic to post thrombotic syndrome: ulceration, pain, and intractable oedema.

Traditionally, DVTs have been treated with the use of oral anticoagulation medication (such as warfarin) for a period of 6 months. However, this is associated with a high risk for recurrent thrombosis, and approximately one third will develop post thrombotic syndrome despite treatment (Prandoni et al 1996). The recurrence of DVT is thought to be related to damage to the venous valves during an episode of thrombosis and the low rate of recanalisation particularly in caval/iliac/femoral venous thrombosis, which leads to obstruction and venous hypertension. It has been suggested that anticoagulation therapy alone may be inadequate to prevent the damage to the venous valves in the setting of caval/iliac/femoral DVT. Moreover, it has been shown that early thrombus removal is associated with a lower incidence of symptoms related to post thrombotic syndrome (Sharafuddin 2003). These factors have prompted use of invasive techniques such as catheter directed thrombolysis and mechanical thrombectomy, particularly in the acute setting, for thrombus removal.

There are currently two large randomised controlled trials (TORPEDO and ATTRACT) underway investigating the efficacy of these invasive techniques and early results suggest that early intervention in the setting of acute DVT is associated with lower recurrence rates, lower incidence of post thrombotic syndrome and lower rates of fatal PE.

Pending the results of these trials however, clinicians should assess the need for invasive measures on a case by case basis, based on the timing of the DVT, associated risk factors for development of DVT, risk factors for thrombolysis related bleeding, age and prognosis of the patient.

3. Endovascular techniques

The goals of endovascular treatment of acute DVT include: prevention of PE, early symptom relief, and prevention of post thrombotic syndrome (Vendatham 2006).

The endovascular techniques available to achieve these goals include catheter directed thrombolysis, mechanical/rheolytic thrombectomy and stent placement. IVC filters can theoretically be used in conjunction with these techniques to reduce the rate of PE during therapy, although this is controversial.

These techniques require knowledge of, and skills in, ultrasound guided needle punctures, wire and catheter manipulation, thrombolysis drug administration, placement of endovascular stents, and familiarity with the use of various mechanical/rheolytic thrombectomy devices. The specific equipment will vary according to their availability and preference.

3.1 Catheter directed thrombolysis

Thrombolytic agents activate plasminogen which leads to the breakdown of clot. Systemic thrombolysis results in better short and long term clinical results (Comerota & Aldridge 1993; Gallus AS 1998; Schweizer J, et al 2000; Wells PS 2001) when compared with anticoagulation, but this is at the expense of an increase in serious bleeding and PEs.

Catheter directed thrombolysis (CDT) has developed in response, in an effort to reduce the dose of systemic thrombolytic by delivering the agent at the site of thrombosis, allowing a relative higher concentration to reach the thrombus with a lower systemic dose. This also reduces the duration of the therapy and complication rates. In addition, this technique allows the simultaneous treatment of underlying lesions that are often the cause of the thrombosis itself.

Indications for CDT should focus on patients who ideally are young and active and have a normal life expectancy. In older patients, CDT should be performed in cases of an acutely threatened limb. Both these groups should have acute symptomatic DVT or severe clot burden that involves the IVC. Threshold for thrombolysis in iliofemoral DVT should be lower than that for femoro-popliteal DVT, due to the higher risk of developing post thrombotic syndrome in the former group (discussed in previous sections). Patients who have propagation of clot despite anticoagulation should also be considered for treatment. CDT is most effective when instituted within 4 weeks of thrombosis.

Contraindications are similar to thrombolysis of any site, and include recent major surgery, recent cerebrovascular bleed, recent CPR, pregnancy or coagulopathy. In cases of phlegmasia cerulea dolens with contraindications to thrombolysis, surgical thrombectomy may be considered (Sharafuddin 2003).

In order to effectively deliver the thrombolytic agent, the location and extent of the affected vessels must be elucidated, and this can be performed with ultrasound in the lower extremity. For the central venous system or the peripheral system, a venogram using CT, MRI or angiography can be used, which give a better appreciation of the extent and location of the clot.

Once the inflow and outflow of the occluded segment is elucidated, the access site can be selected. Early experience with access sites centred on the internal jugular vein (Grosman & Macpherson 1999). However this has technical disadvantages such as the longer route of access causing catheter migration, catheters stimulating cardiac arrhythmias, and difficulty crossing venous valves. In the past, some authors also used the brachial vein and contralateral common femoral vein, which have also fallen out of favour. The ipsilateral popliteal access later became the route of choice for most authors, being easily punctured with ultrasound guidance, having less problems with venous valves, and providing direct access to the thrombosed segment (Grossman, 1998; Sharafuddin 2003). Other common access routes include the common femoral vein (used in iliocaval disease) and posterior tibial vein (for infrapopliteal disease). Occasionally, antegrade and retrograde access is simultaneously used, with the catheters crossed, to treat both up and downstream disease (Molina et al 1992, Raju et al 1998, Tarry et al 1994). In extensive and severe disease, particularly in the calf, selection of the smaller veins with the catheter is extremely difficult, and sometimes impossible, which leads to poor inflow and higher rates of rethrombosis. Comerota (1993) described infusion through the ipsilateral femoral artery to push the thrombolytic agent through the capillary bed and into the small veins of the calf, and potentially improving clearance of thrombosis in those very small veins.

The equipment required in CDT includes:

- Ultrasound machine and sterile probe cover
- Local anaesthesia
- Micropuncture set
- 0.035in J-wire
- Vascular sheath (usually 6 Fr or larger to accommodate infusion catheters, stents and mechanical thrombectomy devices)
- 0.035in glidewire
- Angiographic catheters (according to clinician's preference such as Davis, Angled tapered, Bern)
- Infusion catheters
- Thombolytic agent
- Heparin
- IV Infusion sets

Once access is achieved, usually via ultrasound guided micropuncture (Cook Inc, Bloomington, IN) of the popliteal vein, a vascular sheath is inserted (6Fr or larger to allow passage of an infusion catheter), and a diagnostic venogram performed either via the sheath or via a catheter. This may or may not be sufficient to visualise the extent of thrombosis. In either case, this is followed by a wire and angiographic catheter (usually 0.035in system, such as glidewire (Terumo, Somerset NJ) and a 5Fr angled tapered glidecatheter), which traverses the occluded segment. A venogram past the level of the occlusion is performed, usually in the IVC, to confirm intraluminal position, and absence of more centrally located clot.

The thrombolytic agent is usually injected at this point, and a number of different thrombolytic strategies have been described. At our institution, we would lace the length of the thrombosed segment using 200,000IU of Urokinase as the diagnostic catheter is being retracted. An infusion catheter with an infusion length that covers the occluded segment is then selected, and is inserted over a wire. The active infusion segment of the catheter is placed over the thrombosed segment of vein, which allows direct delivery of thrombolytic agent throughout the length of the thrombus. An infusion of Urokinase would then be commenced, at a rate of between 100,000-150,000 IU per hour. A Heparin infusion through the vascular sheath side arm is also commenced. The infusion is continued overnight, and patient nursed in a High Dependency Unit or Intensive Care Unit with one to one nursing. If the case arrives early in the morning, the infusion is left running until the mid afternoon. The patient will then return to the angiography suite for a venogram to reassess the degree of thrombosis and treat any underlying lesions.

If significant thrombus remains after the initial infusion, the infusion can be continued if it is felt that the clot will continue to disintegrate. However, this increases the dose and the duration of therapy with the associated increased risks of thrombolysis. It also increases the length of hospital stay and potentially increases the costs of treatment. Currently, CDT combined with mechanical thrombectomy is the preferred treatment (Sharaffudin 2003).

3.2 Mechanical thrombectomy

Mechanical thrombectomy devices disturb and break up the thrombus and allow rapid clearance of a large clot burden without the risks of pharmacological thrombolysis. They can be used alone, in situations where rapid debulking of thrombus is crucial, without the need for pharmacological therapy. However, adjunctive use of mechanical thrombectomy with thrombolysis is the preferred option. They can be used before, after or both before and after thrombolytic therapy.

The mechanism employed in the device can be divided into rotational devices and rheolytic devices.

Rotational devices include the Amplatz Thrombectomy Device (Microvena, White Bear Lake, MN), and Trerotola Percutaneous Thrombectomy Device (Arrow International, Reading, PA). These employ a high-velocity rotating helix or nitinol cage to macerate thrombus. The Trellis device (Trellis-8; Bacchus Vascular, Santa Clara, California, USA) employs a sinusoidal nitinol wire to disintegrate thrombus and with thrombolytic agent between proximal and distal balloons for control and to prevent PE. Rotational devices have direct contact with the endothelium and subsequently have the potential for endothelial damage. However there have been no studies to analyse their efficacy compared with rheolytic devices.

Rheolytic devices include the Angiojet (Possis, Minneapolis,MN). The device uses high-pressure saline jets to fragment the thrombus. The jets also create a negative pressure zone which draws the fragmented thrombus toward the catheter where it is aspirated and removed. A possible advantage of the Angiojet device is that there is no contact of the maceration component of the device with the vessel wall. However, its use of high-pressure saline jets carries a theoretical risk of haemolysis and the release of adenosine and potassium. (Zhu, 2008) This has been linked to the incidence of bradyarrhythmia in cardiac applications of the device (Lee et al, 2005) or haemoglobinuria.

Ultrasound enhanced devices include the EKOS Endowave (EKOS Corporation, Bothell, WA, USA) and Omniwave (Omnisonics Medical Technologies, Wilmington, MA, USA). These are catheters that contain multiple ultrasound transducers, which radially emit high-frequency, low-energy ultrasound energy. The ultrasonic energy expands and thins the fibrin component of thrombus, exposing plasminogen receptor sites, and the ultrasound forces thrombolytic into the clot and keeps it there (Francis et al, 1995). This technique may be associated with fewer haemolytic effects than rheolytic thrombectomy (Lang et al, 2008) and has a lower potential for endothelial damage than rotational thrombectomy devices.

We prefer the use of the Angiojet system at our institution, as an adjunctive modality to CDT. The timing of its use is dependent on the case, and preference of the interventionist. However, the method is the same in either situation. The Angiojet catheters come in a range of sizes and lengths, we prefer the 5 and 6Fr systems. The device is passed several times across the thrombosed segment over a wire and under fluoroscopic visualisation. In order to minimise the risk of haemolysis, each pass is limited to 30 seconds with 10 second rests in between.

The potential added benefit of the Angiojet system is the ability of the catheters to 'pulse spray' thrombolytic agent using high pressure jets into the thrombus itself, improving delivery.

4. Results

4.1 Catheter directed thrombolysis

To date, the largest DVT thrombolytic database is the venous registry (Mewissen 1999), which is a prospective registry of patients with a DVT who underwent CDT with urokinase. 473 patients were enrolled with 287 patients followed up at 1 year. 83% of patients had thrombolysis >50%. There were also a strong relationship between early thrombus removal and 1- year patency (primary patency rate of 60%). Major bleeding complications occurred in 11%, most often at the puncture site. 1% of patients developed a PE. Two patients (<1%) died (one from PE and one from intracranial haemorrhage).

Grunwald and Hofmann (2004) retrospectively analysed 74 patients who underwent CDT for DVT and compared Urokinase, Alteplase and Reteplase. They found that there was no statistical difference between infusion times, success rates and complication rates between the three agents. However, they did find that the new recombinant agents are significantly less expensive than Urokinase in the United States.

No RCTs have been published looking at CDT in acute DVT. However, currently the TORPEDO trial is underway which is a large scale RCT looking at the efficacy of CDT vs anticoagulation in treatment of DVT. Mid term results show that CDT is superior to anticoagulation therapy alone in the prevention of recurrence of DVT, reduction in PTS, and reduction of hospital stays.

Similarly the ATTRACT Trial is currently underway looking at the efficacy of CDT.

4.2 Mechanical thrombectomy

No large randomised control studies have been published looking at mechanical thrombectomy in DVT.

An analysis by Karthikesalingam et al (2011) on 16 retrospective case series on the use of mechanical thrombectomy in DVT, with a total of 481 patients, looked at its efficacy. They found successful thrombolysis (>50% lysis) in 83-100% of patients. Bleeding complications requiring transfusion were seen in 7.5%. Symptomatic PE was seen in <1%. No procedure related deaths or strokes were seen. Of the studies that did look at mid term follow up, 75-98% of patients demonstrated significant improvement of symptoms and similar improvement in radiological findings.

5. Adjunctive procedures

DVT, particularly in the iliocaval system, can be associated with chronic venous obstruction, which can lead to valvular insufficiency and consequently venous hypertension. This in turn is associated with a higher incidence of post thrombotic syndrome (PTS). There are multiple other causes of venous obstruction, which include May Thurner syndrome, external compression (e.g. cancer, lymphocoeles) and retroperitoneal fibrosis. Very frequently, thrombolysis and thrombectomy can uncover the underlying lesion which precipitated the venous thrombosis. Failure to identify and treat these lesions, despite successful thrombolysis, can result in higher rates of recurrence, and the development of PTS.

The advantage of CDT as compared with anticoagulation therapy alone in the treatment of acute DVT, is that it allows the opportunity to treat the underlying lesion and restore flow in most cases. Obviously, non mechanical underlying issues must also be addressed, such as underlying prothrombotic syndromes.

The objective is to restore flow and the measures employed usually involve angioplasty and stenting of the lesion. Angioplasty and stenting in the setting of obstruction has been shown to improve quality of life and improve symptoms (Hartung et al 2005, Neglen P et al 2005, Raju S et al 2002;). The lesions treated usually lie within the IVC, iliac and femoral veins. It has not been shown that angioplasty and stenting of lesions below this level is of any benefit. However, chronic lesions do benefit as well as acute obstructions (Titus 2011).

The procedure is similar to angioplasty of the arterial system. Once access is achieved, heparin is given if anticoagulation has not been already instituted. A wire is passed across the lesion, followed by a catheter. Any wire can be used however 0.035in wires are preferred. This is usually not too difficult in an acute thrombus, which is soft, and has not had time to organise. Contrast is injected beyond the lesion to ensure intraluminal position. The catheter is then exchanged for a balloon which is usually sized approximately 20% greater than the expected calibre of the vein. Angioplasty of the venous system is different from the arterial system, in that the balloons can be oversized to a greater extent than in the arteries. There is also a greater propensity for veins to have elastic recoil, such that even with aggressive angioplasty using high pressure balloons, the veins collapse back to their obstructed state. In other cases there is persistent stenosis in the vein post angioplasty. When this is the case, stenting is performed. These are also oversized in relation to the vein.

6. Use of IVC filters

The use of CDT and mechanical thrombectomy devices carry the theoretical increased risk of pulmonary embolisation. This has not been proven in any large scale study, and it is unclear based on current data whether this is true. In a review study by Grossman 1998, 2 out of 263 (0.7%) patients developed a PE post CDT. This is compared to the incidence of PE in patients treated with heparin alone for DVT ranging from 0-56% for symptomatic emboli, and 0-8% for asymptomatic emboli (Leizorovicz et al 1994, Sirgusa et al 1996, Levine et al 1995, Piccioli et al 1996).

In addition, no large studies are available that looks at whether IVC filters reduce the incidence of PE following CDT or mechanical thrombectomy. Given the lack of data on their use, prophylactic IVC filters prior to commencement of CDT and/or mechanical thrombectomy has been debated.

In a systematic review (Karthikesalingam et al 2011) of mechanical thrombectomy between 1999 and 2009, the use of prophylactic IVC filters was variable between the various authors. Almost all authors report 0% PE on follow up CTPA whether IVC filters were inserted or not. One author (Arko et al 2007) reports a 17% PE rate, all asymptomatic, in patients where no IVC filter was placed. In those that had a filter, Arko found no PE. All deaths were unrelated to the thrombectomy (either myocardial infarct or cancer) and no patients died of PE.

The role IVC filters therefore is not known and there are no current recommendations regarding their use. However they are not without risk, albeit small. Filter migration, filter fracture, break through PE have all been described, as well as complications associated with their retrieval.

Placement of IVC filters remain at the discretion of the interventionist. In the presence of free-floating IVC thrombus or in patients with limited cardiopulmonary reserve who are unlikely to tolerate minor embolic events, IVC filtration may be appropriate with use of permanent (Tarry WC Ann Vasc Surg 1994) or temporary filters (Lorch et al 2000).

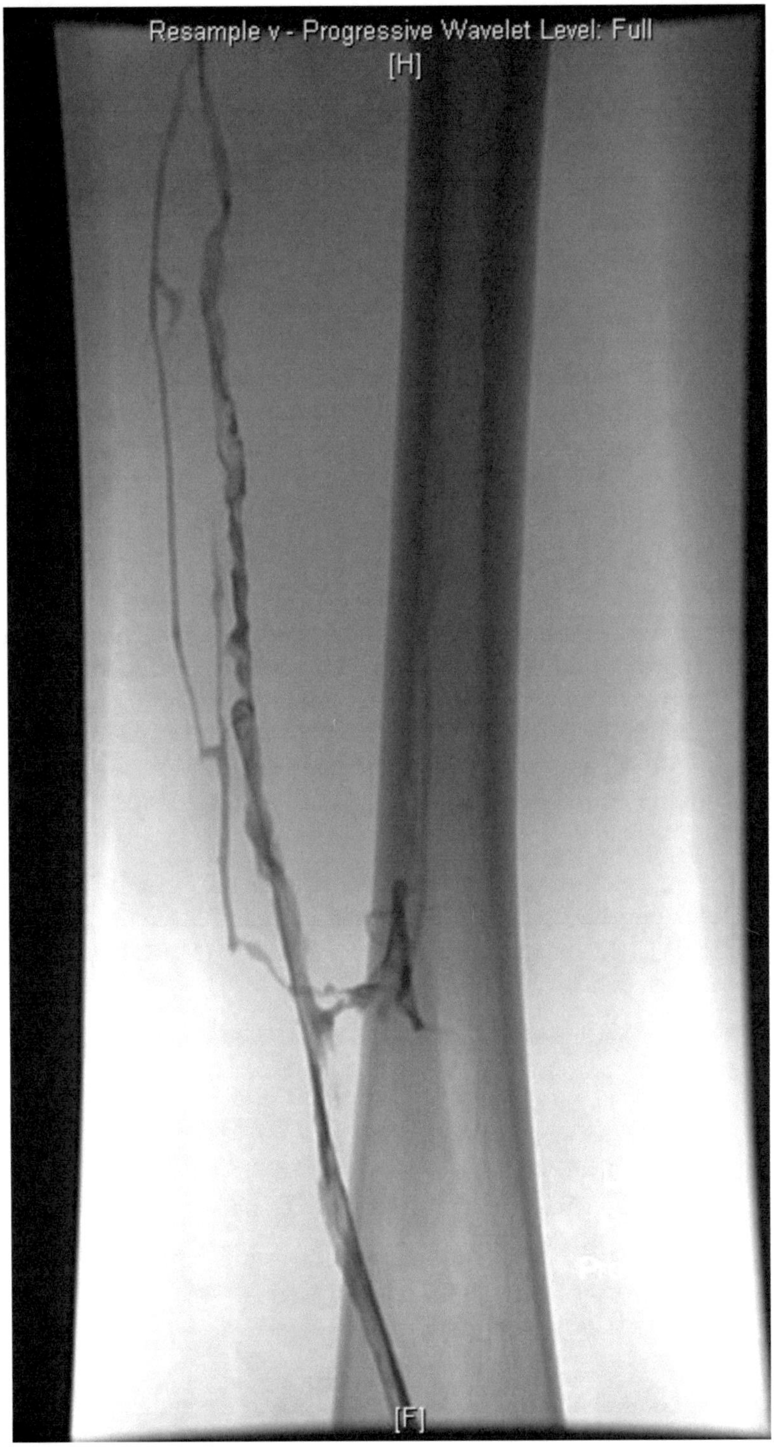

Fig. 1. 20 y.o. girl with acute DVT and swollen, dusky leg. Popliteal access has been achieved and venogram demonstrates thrombus in the femoral vein.

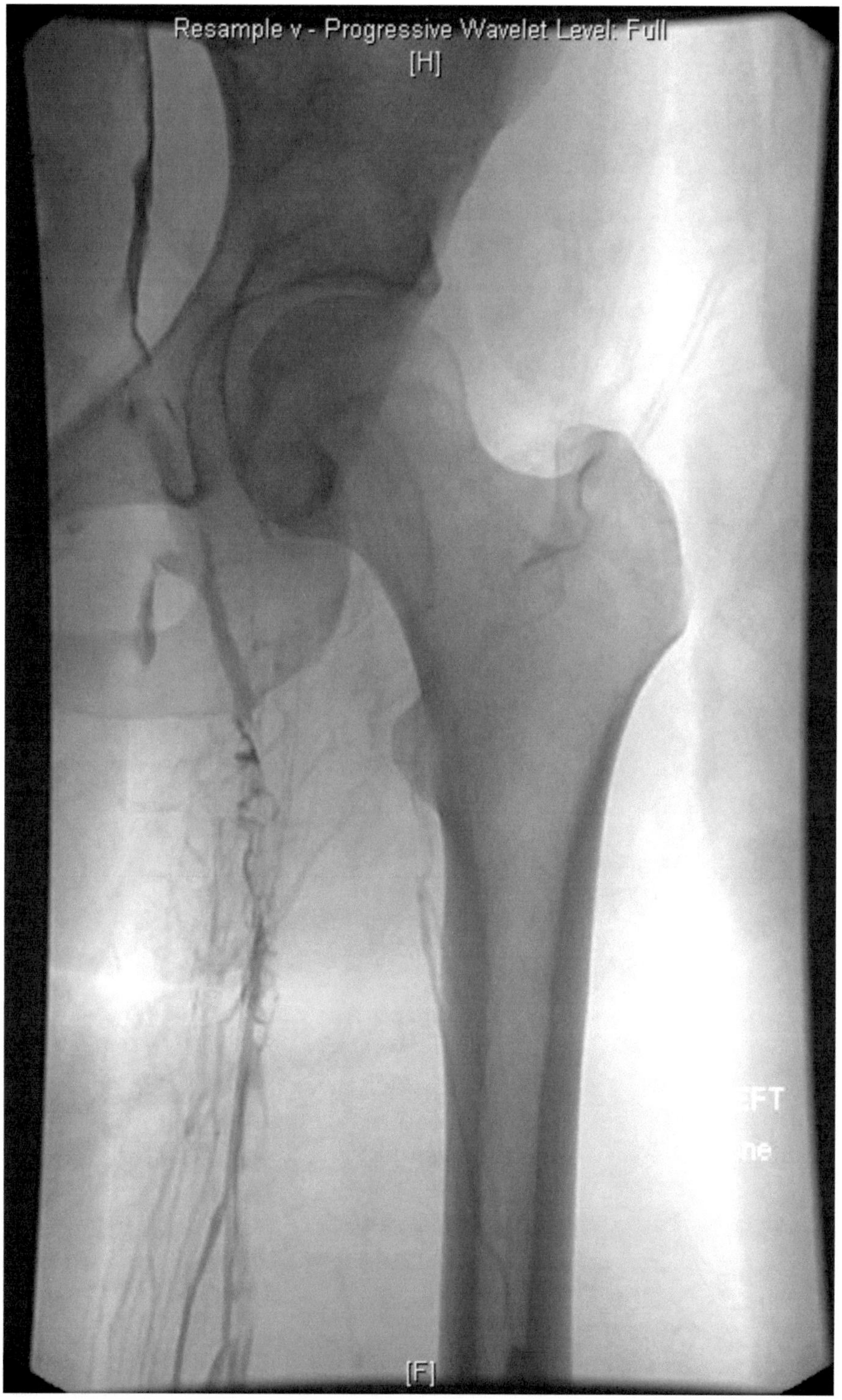

Fig. 2. Same patient. Thrombus extends into common femoral vein.

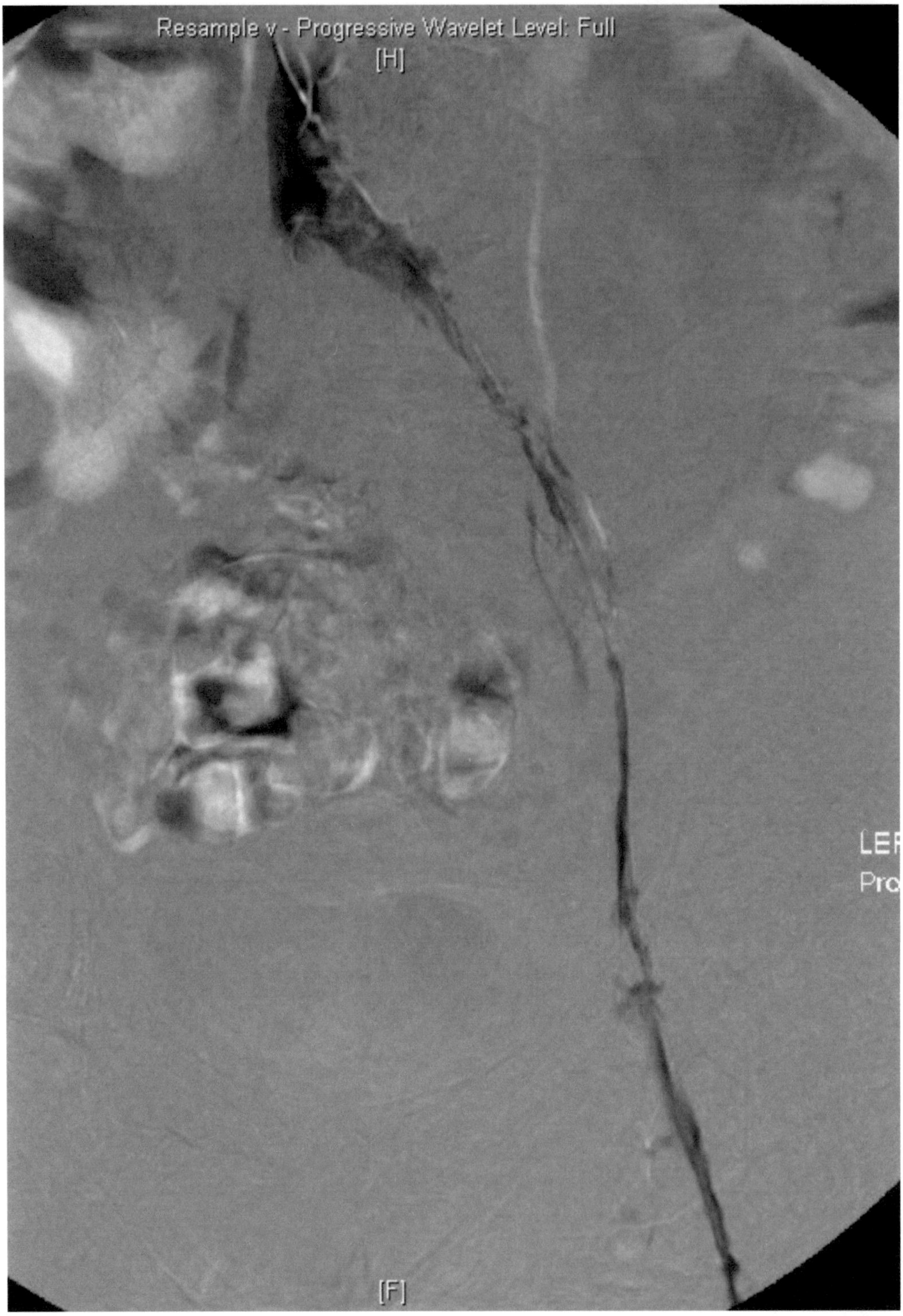

Fig. 3. Same patient. Thrombus extending into iliac veins.

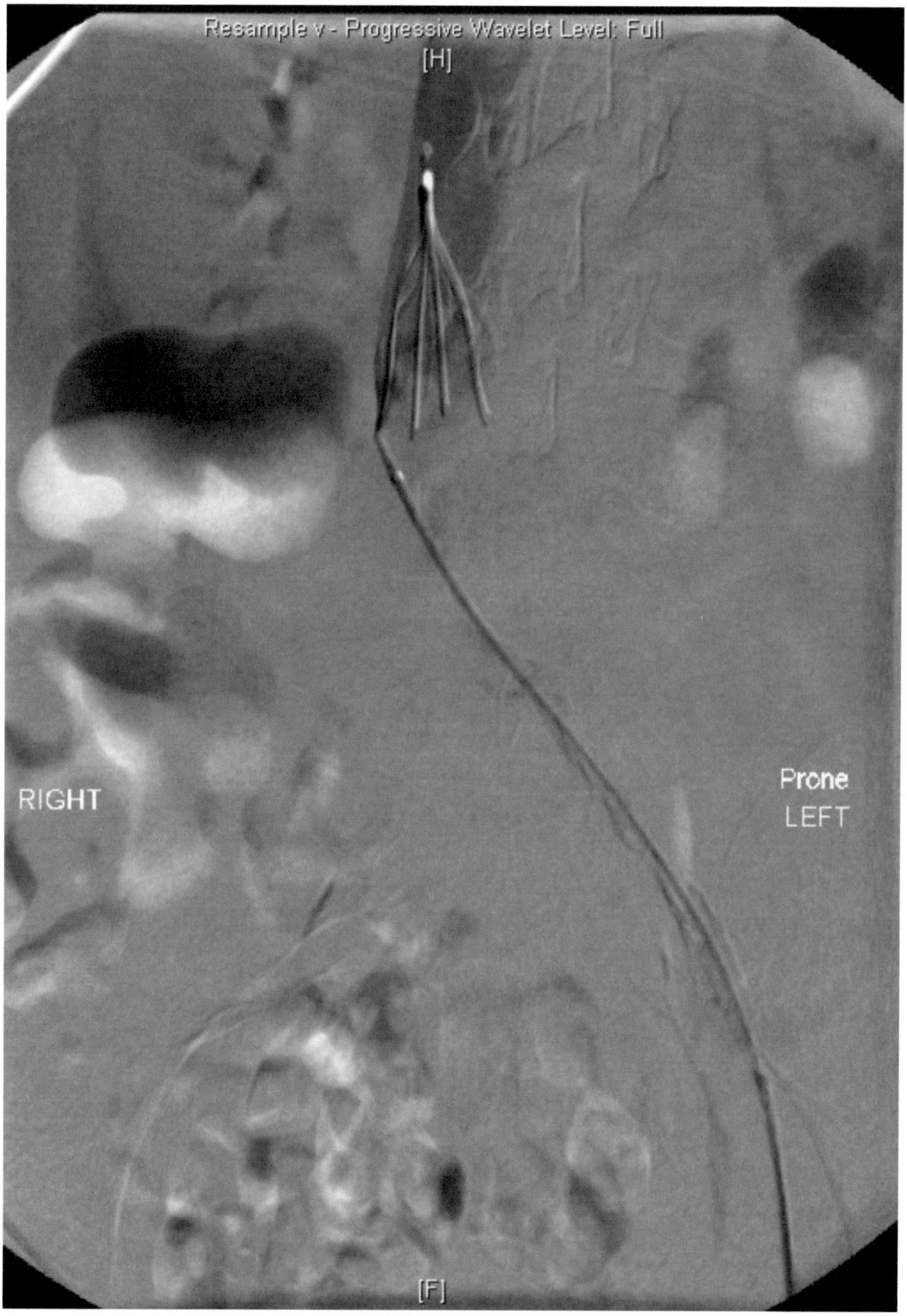

Fig. 4. Same patient. IVC filter placed prior to commencement of procedure. Infusion catheter placed through the thrombus and Urokinase infusion commenced.

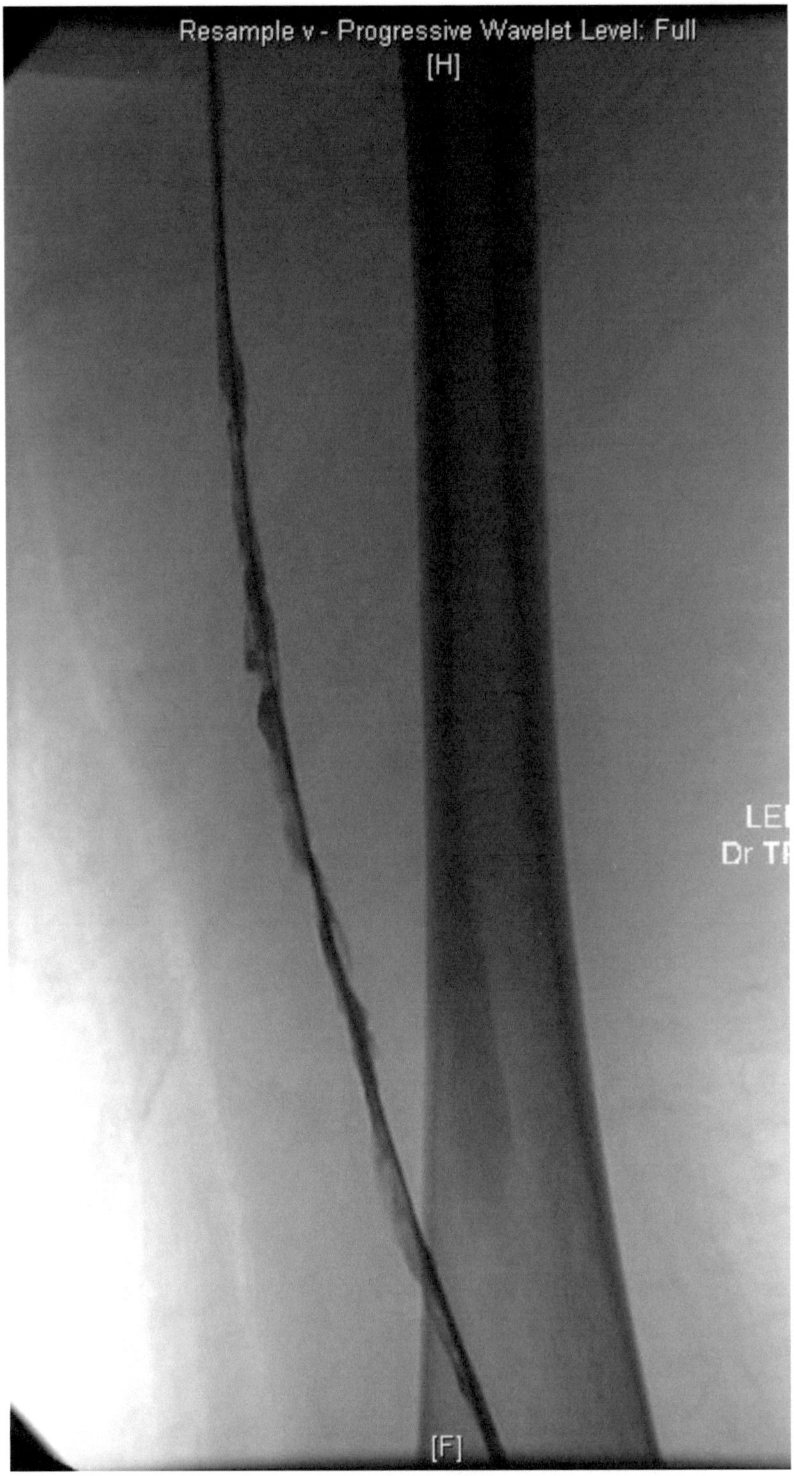

Fig. 5. Post 18 hours CDT. Thrombus still present in femoral vein.

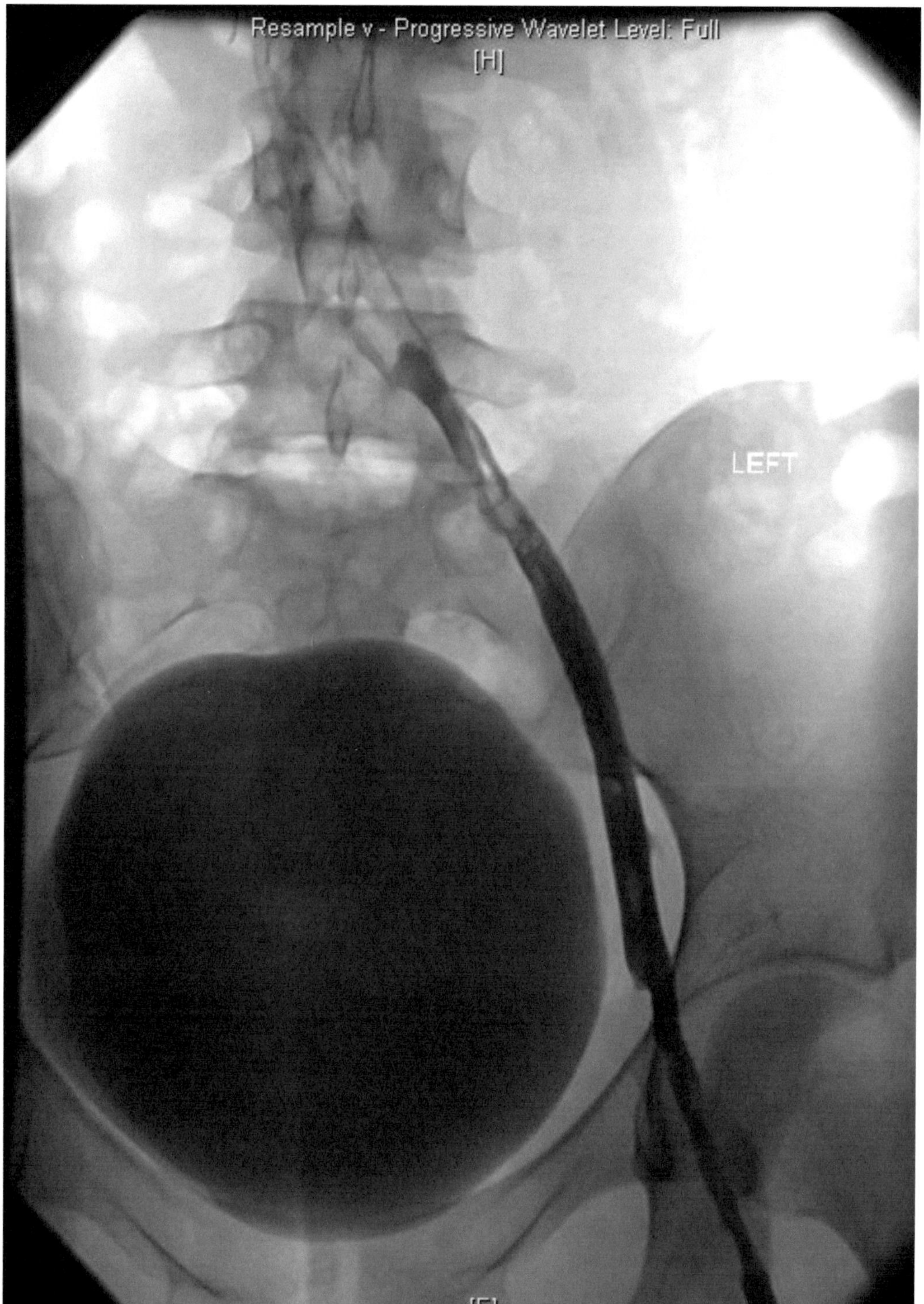

Fig. 6. Post 18 hours CDT. Persistent thrombus in iliac veins.

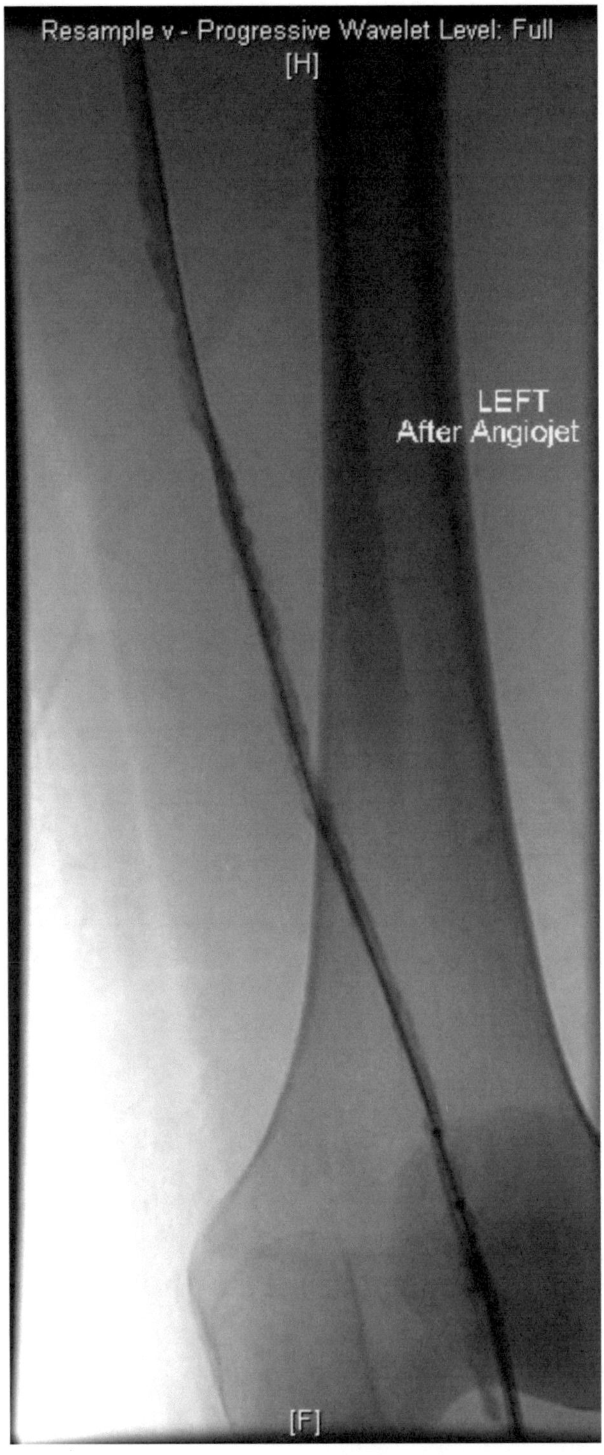

Fig. 7. Post mechanical thrombectomy with Angiojet system demonstrates clearance of thrombus.

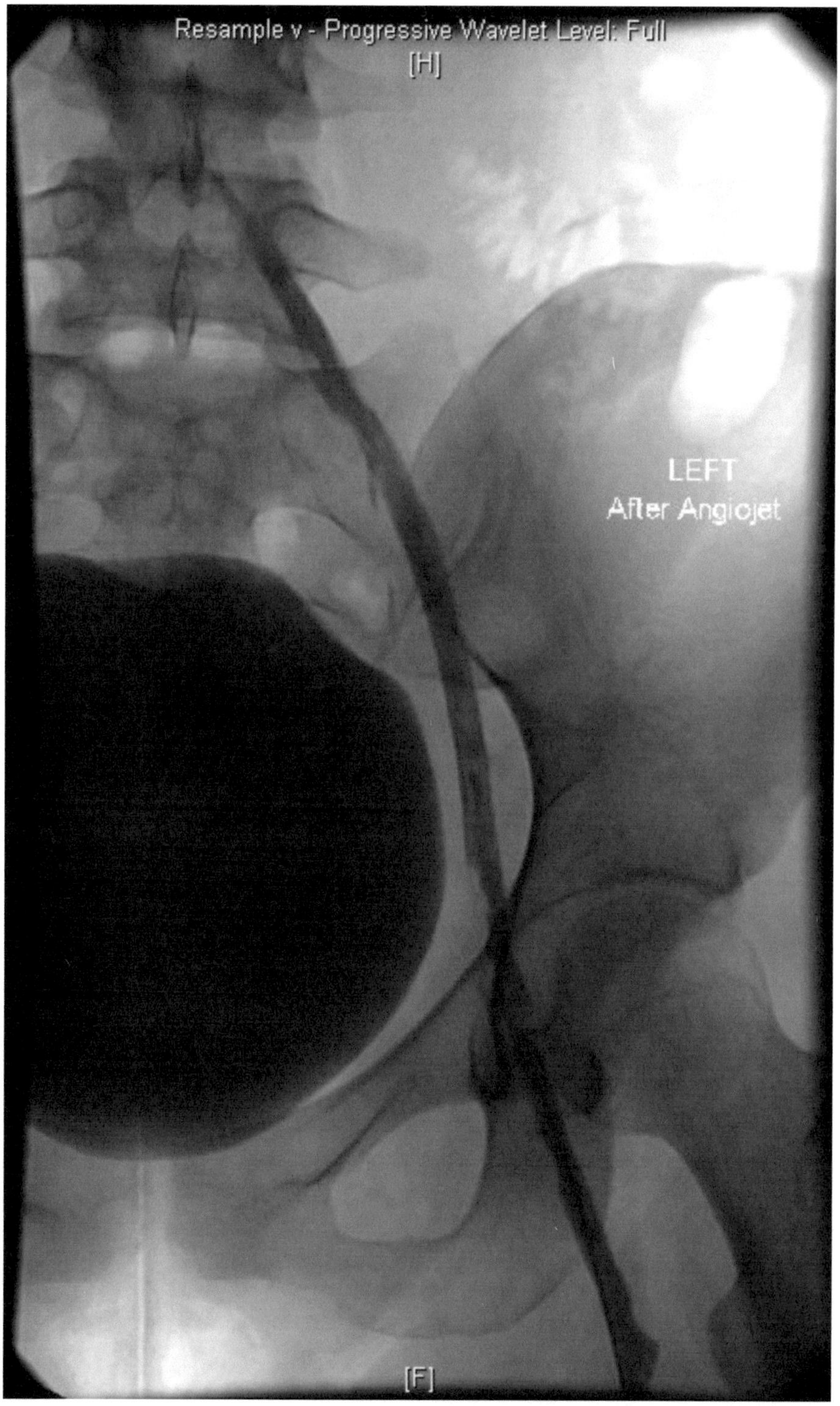

Fig. 8. Improvement of thrombus in iliac veins post Angiojet.

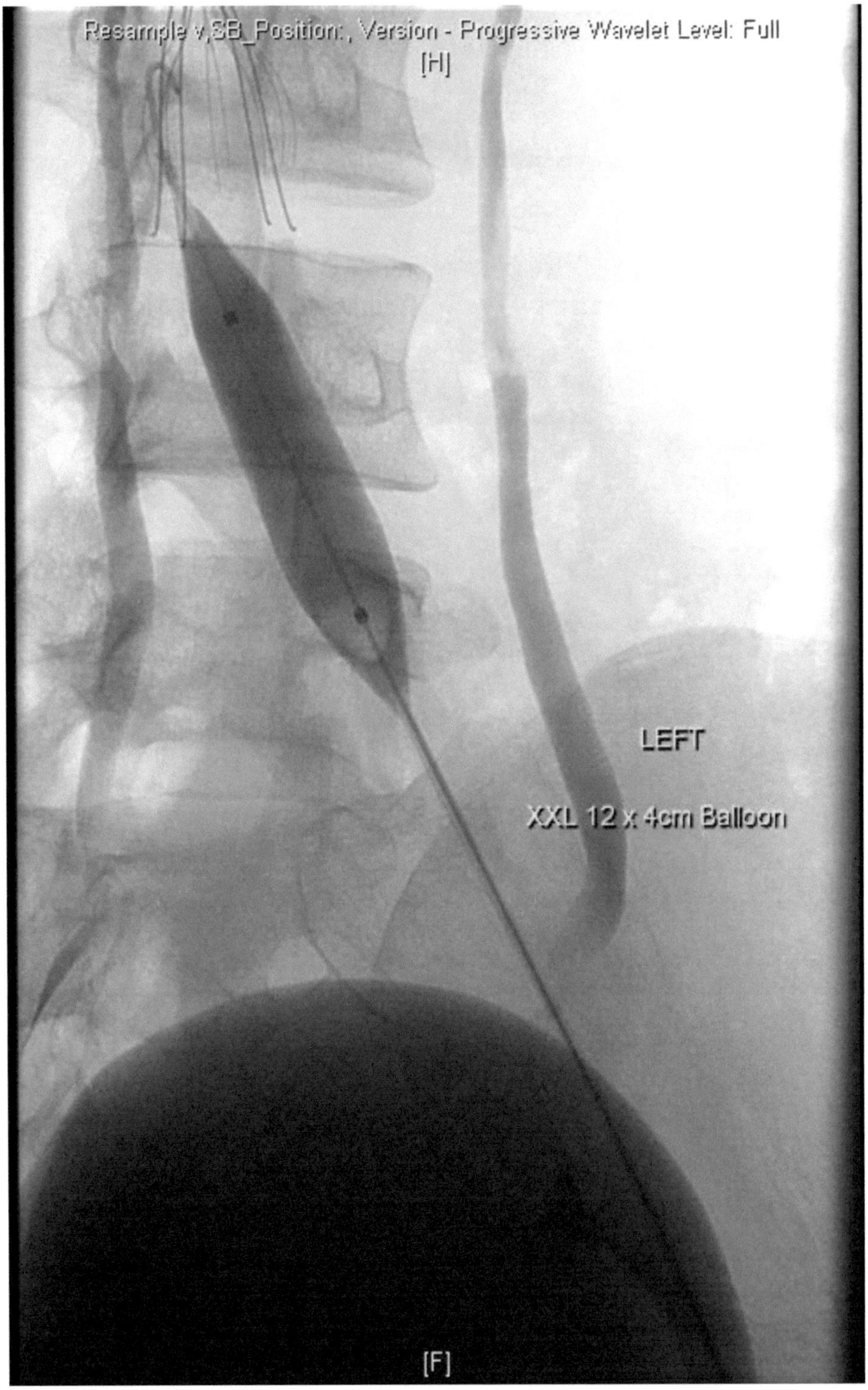

Fig. 9. Angioplasty of the common iliac vein

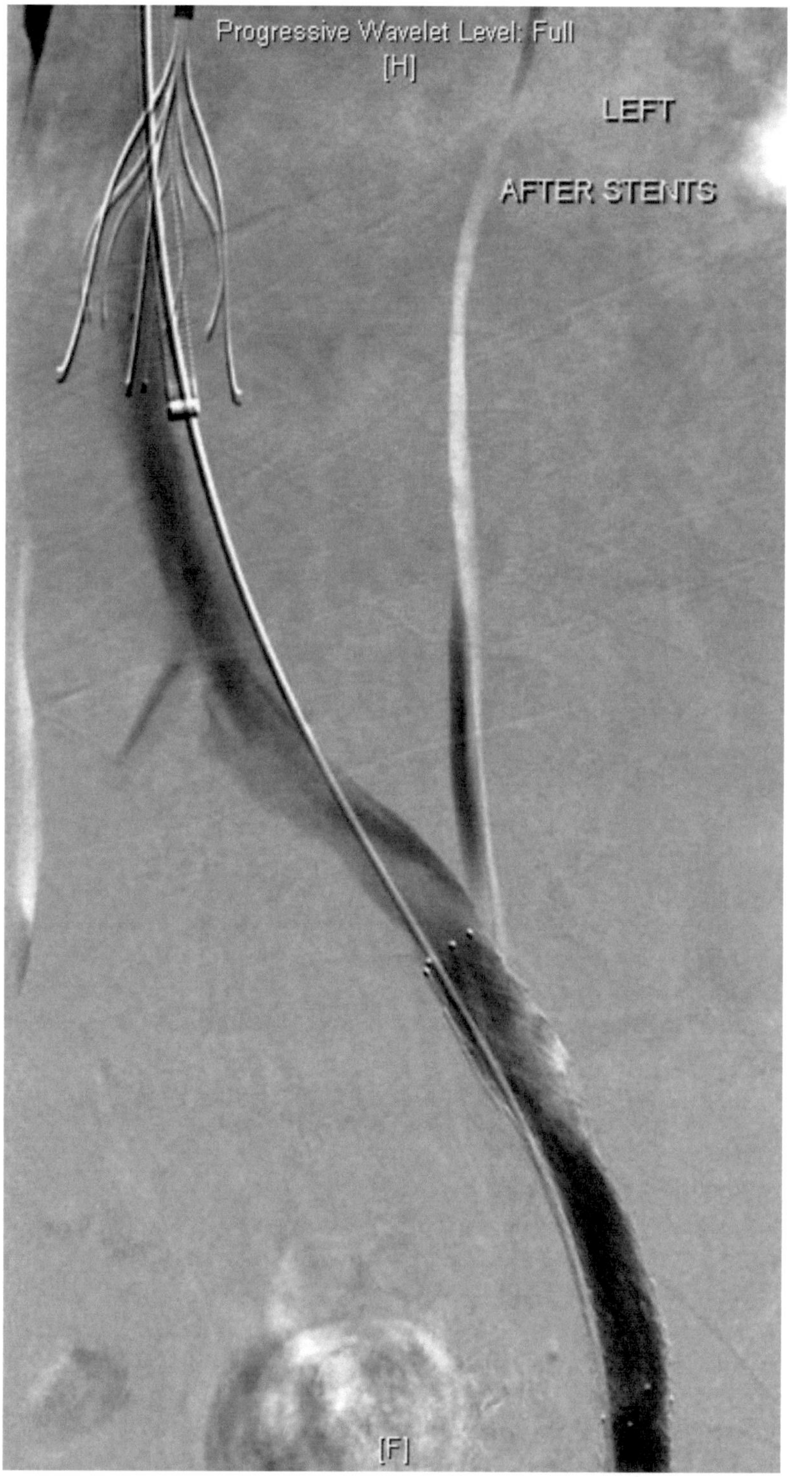

Fig. 10. Stent deployed in the left iliac vein with good flow through the vessel.

7. Conclusion

Endovascular techniques are important therapeutic options in the prevention of limb loss, recurrence and post thrombotic syndrome related to acute DVT, and have been shown to be superior to anticoagulation therapy alone. It also is advantageous in uncovering and treating underlying lesions that contribute to the DVT.

No guidelines are available currently in terms of patient selection, techniques and the use of IVC filters and at present these decisions are made on a case by case basis at the discretion of the interventionist. Large randomized controlled trials underway currently will hopefully be able to shed more insight on these issues.

8. References

Arko FR, Davis CM, Murphy EH, et al. 2007. Aggressive Percutaneous Mechanical Thrombectomy of Deep Venous Thrombosis. *Archives of Surgery.* 142 (6):513-519

Comerota AJ & Aldridge SC. 1993. Thrombolytic therapy for deep venous thrombosis: a clinical review. *Can J Surg*. 36(4): 359-64.

Francis CW, Blinc A, Lee S, Cox C. 1995. Ultrasound accelerates transport of recombinant tissue plasminogen activator into clots. *Ultrasound Med Biol*;21(3):419e24

Gallus AS, 1998. Thrombolytic therapy for venous thrombosis and pulmonary embolism. *Clin Haematol*. 11(3):663-73.

Grosman C & McPherson S. 1999. Safety and efficacy of catheter directed thrombolysis for iliofemoral venous thrombosis. *Am J Roentgenol*. 172: 667-672.

Grunwald MR and Hofmann LV. 2004. Comparison of UK, Alteplase, and reteplase for CDT of DVT. *Journal Vasc Interv Radiol*; 15:347-352

Hartung O, Otero A, Boufi M, et al. 2005. Mid term results of endovascular treatment of symptomatic chronic non-malignant iliocaval venous occlusive disease. *J Vasc Surg*. 42(6):1138-44.

Karthikesalingam, EL Young, RJ Hinchliffe, et al. 2011. A systematic review of percutaneous Mechanical thrombectomy in the treatment of DVT. *Eur J Vasc endovasc Surgery*, 41: 554-565

Lang EV, Kulis AM, Villani M, et al. 2008. Hemolysis comparison between the OmniSonics OmniWave endovascular system and the Possis AngioJet in a porcine model. *J Vasc Interv Radiol*;19(8):1215e21

Lee MS, Makkar R, Singh V et al. 2005. Pre-procedural administration of aminophylline does not prevent AngioJet rheolytic thrombectomy-induced bradyarrhythmias. *J Invasive Cardiol*;17(1):19e22

Leizorovicz A, Simonneau G, Decousus H et al. 1994. Comparison of efficacy and safety of low molecular weight heparins and unfractionated heparin in initial treatment of deep venous thrombosis: a meta analysis. *BMJ*. 309 (6950): 299-304.

Lensing AW, Prins MH, Davidson BL, et al. 1995. Treatment of deep venous thrombosis with low-molecular-weight heparins: a meta-analysis. *Arch Intern Med;* 155:601–607.

Lorch H, Welger D, Wagner V, et al. 2000. Current practice of temporary vena cava filter insertion: a multicenter registry. *J Vasc Interv Radiol.* 11(1): 83-8.

Mewissen. 1999. CDT for lower extremity Deep venous thrombosis: report of a national multicenter registry, *Radiolog;* 211:39-49

Molina JE, Hunter DW & Yedlicka JW. Thrombolytic therapy for iliofemoral venous thrombosis. 1992. *Vasc Surg.* 26:630-637.

Neglen P, Raju S. 2005. *Endovascular treatment of chronic occlusions of the iliac veins and the inferior vena cava. Rutherford RB, editor. Vascular Surgery.* 6th ed. Philadelphia: Elsevier Saunders;. pp 2321-32.

Patel K, Basson MD, Borsa JJ, et al, May 2011. Deep Venous Thrombosis. In: *Emedicine.* Available from:
http://emedicine.medscape.com/article/1911303-overview

Piccioli A, Prandoni P Goldhaber S. Epidemiologic characteristics, management and outcome of deep venous thrombosis in a tertiary-care hospital: The Brigham and Women's Hospital DVT registry. 1996. *American Heart Journal.* 132(5).

Prandoni P, Lensing A, Cogo A, et al. 1996. The Long-Term clinical course of Acute Deep Venous Thrombosis. *Annals of Internal Medicine.* 125:1-7.

Raju S, Fountain T & McPherson SH. 1998. Catheter directed thrombolysis for deep venous thrombosis. *J Miss State Med Assoc.* 39(3):81-4.

Raju S, Owen S Jr, Neglen P. 2002. The clinical impact of iliac venous stents in the management of chronic venous insufficiency. *J Vasc Surg;* 35:8-15.

Schweizer J, Kirch W, Koch R, et al. 1998. Short and long term results after thrombolytic treatment of deep venous thrombosis. *J Am Coll Cardiol.* 36:1336-1343.

Sharafuddin MJ, Sun S, Hoballah JJ, et al. 2003. Endovascular management of venous thrombotic and occlusive diseases of the lower extremities. *J Vasc Interv Radiol.* 14(4)4:405-23.

Sirgusa S, Cosmi B, Piovella F, et al. 1996. Low molecular weight heparins and unfractionated heparin in the treatment of patients with acute venous thromboembolism: results of a meta analysis. *The American Journal of Medicine.* 100(3): 269-277.

Tarry WC, Makhoul RG, Tisnado J, et al. 1994. Catheter directed thrombolysis following ven cava filtration for severe deep venous thrombosis. *Ann Vasc Surg.* 8(6):583-590.

Titus JM, Moise MA, Bena J, et al. 2011. Ilioifemoral stenting for venous occlusive disease. *J Vasc Surg.* 53(3): 706-712.

Vedantham S, Millward S, Cardella J, et al. 2006. Society of Interventional Radiology Position Statement: Treatment of Acute Iliofemoral deep Vein Thrombosis with use of Adjunctive Catheter directed Intrathrombus Thrombolysis. *J Vasc Interv Radiol.* 17:613-616.

Wells PS & Forster AJ. Thrombolysis in deep vein thrombosis: is there still an indication? 2001 *Thromb Haemost.* 86 (1):499-508.

Zhu DW. The potential mechanisms of bradyarrhythmias associated with AngioJet thrombectomy. 2008.*J Invasive Cardiol*; 20 (8 Suppl. A):2Ae4A

5

Radiological Imaging and Intervention in Venous Thrombosis

Andrew Christie, Giles Roditi,
Ananthakrishnan Ganapathy and Chris Cadman
Glasgow Royal Infirmary radiology department, Glasgow, Scotland

1. Introduction

Radiological imaging plays a central role in the diagnosis, and treatment, of deep venous thrombosis (DVT) in the upper and lower limb. The intention of this chapter is not to distract the reader with a detailed account of the physics behind generating ultrasound (US), computed tomography (CT) and MR (magnetic resonance) vascular imaging. This would demand a chapter in its own right, and this information can be readily found in textbooks. Instead, emphasis will be placed on the clinical indications for requesting imaging in the diagnosis of DVT, as well as the potential limitations of these modalities. This will be supplemented with a review of current evidence and guidelines, and examples of the common image findings. The latest advances in venous MR imaging will be discussed, as will the role of interventional radiology in the treatment of DVT. Finally, considering that it is now universally accepted that DVT and pulmonary embolus (PE) are essentially manifestations of the same disease - namely, venous thromboembolism (Moser et al., 1994) - the imaging and radiological management of PE will also be addressed.

2. Diagnostic imaging in venous thrombosis

2.1 Historical venography

Conventional venography (angiography) has traditionally been regarded as the "reference standard" for imaging the venous system (de Valois et al., 1990). This was performed by opacifying veins with iodinated contrast injected into the vessel via direct puncture, or targeted catheterisation usually from a punctured femoral vein at the groin (fig. 1). Venous imaging has always been challenging with angiography, in particular with the diagnosis of deep vein thrombosis (DVT). Completely occluded veins do not opacify and hence thrombosis has to be inferred rather than directly visualised. Unfortunately, this is compounded by the fact that even normal veins can be rendered invisible by virtue of the direction of venous flow towards the heart, which is counter to the diagnostic need. Contrast injection into an artery will reveal all the distal branches, but the same procedure in veins may not permit adequate visualisation of the tributaries. Furthermore, cannulation of peripheral veins can be hampered by the extent of limb swelling which accompanies DVT.

An additional problem is the small, but recognised, risk of actually causing thrombosis through the irritant effects of iodinated contrast medium on the vascular endothelium.

Even allowing for these limitations, the continued use of conventional angiography is not sustainable in modern clinical practice considering it is a relatively time consuming and hence expensive procedure, and there is a growing demand on hospital Radiology departments to diagnose an increasingly prevalent disorder, affecting 200 per 100,000 of those aged 70- 79 years. The argument for providing a robust and efficient means of diagnosis is augmented by evidence that the initial clinical evaluation of DVT is often ineffective (Barnes et al., 1975; Haeger, 1969, as cited in Fraser & Anderson, 1999). Other conditions including lymphoedema, cellulitis, superficial phlebitis, muscle sprain and ruptured baker's cyst can be indistinguishable from DVT. Indeed, seventy five percent of patients who present with signs and symptoms of DVT do not have the disease (Heijboer et al., 1993; Wells et al., 1995).

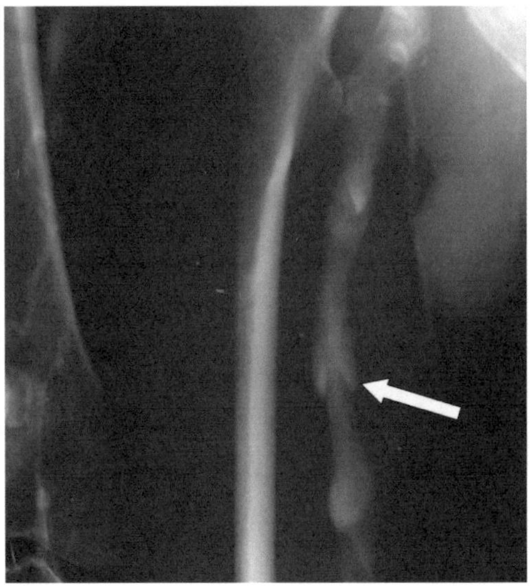

Fig. 1. Lower limb venogram showing a normal superficial femoral vein. Note the normal valves (*arrow*).

2.2 Ultrasound

Ultrasound successfully addresses many of the above requirements, and has clearly become the first line imaging modality in suspected DVT (Cronan, 1993; Dorfman & Cronan, 1992). Unlike other modalities, it can also be a portable technique, allowing assessment of critically ill patients at the bedside. Cronan et al. gathered data from multiple studies to show a sensitivity of 95% and a specificity of 98% in detecting lower limb disease. The performance of venous ultrasound in the upper limb has been less studied, mainly because of the lower incidence of upper limb thrombus. However, the frequency of upper limb venous thrombosis is increasing considering that the two major risk factors are malignancy and central venous catheter placement (Allen et al., 2000; Baron et al., 1998). The performance of upper limb venous sonography should be high as ultrasound provides the highest spatial resolution of any current imaging modality where veins are sonographically visible (Roditi & Fink, 2009). A relatively large study of upper limb venous sonography including over one hundred patients reported a sensitivity and specificity of 82% (Baarslag et al., 2002).

The most accurate ultrasound tool for diagnosing DVT is compressibility of the vein in the transverse plane; a normally patent vein simply disappears when compressed by the ultrasound transducer (fig. 2). The maximum pressure required to obliterate a vein is much less than that required to deform the adjacent artery. Fortuitously, the entire deep venous system of the lower limb consists of arteries that parallel veins. Compression should not be performed in the longitudinal plane because the transducer may slide off the vessel with compression resulting in a false - positive finding.

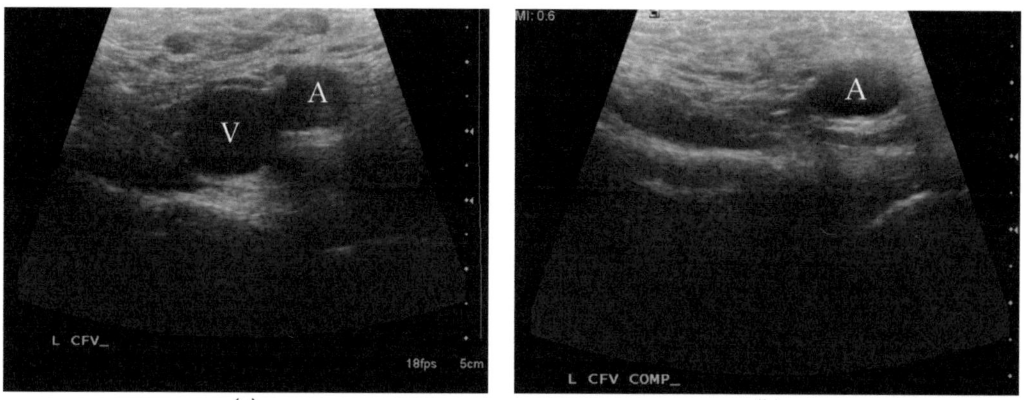

(a) (b)

Fig. 2. (a) Transverse ultrasound of a normal left common femoral vein (*V*) and common femoral artery (*A*). (b) Transducer compression obliterates the vein, leaving the accompanying artery unaffected (*A*).

Technique: In suspected lower limb DVT the veins are examined from the inguinal ligament (junction of the great saphenous vein of the superficial system with the common femoral vein of the deep system), to the popliteal vein within the popliteal fossa. There is varying opinion on the usefulness of assessing the distal calf veins, and they are not routinely scanned by the authors in whose institution's protocol employs a repeat interval scan for those with high pre-test probability (see later). There is currently no consensus on what, if any, treatment is indicated in below knee thrombus (Righini, 2007; Schellong, 2007), and the reliability of compression US in excluding calf DVT has been questioned (Dauzat et al., 1997, as cited in Johnson et al., 2010; Kearon et al., 1998). A meta - analysis reported the sensitivity for detecting isolated calf DVT to be 73% (Kearon et al., 1998). Anticoagulation of calf DVT (that might spontaneously resolve) may unnecessarily place patients at increased risk of potential side effects of such medication, with an estimated 1.1% risk of major bleeding (Krakow & Ortel, 2005, as cited in Johnson et al., 2010). This particularly applies to frailer patients vulnerable to intra - cerebral haemorrhage from even innocuous trauma.

Furthermore, the value of adding distal (calf) US to proximal US of the lower limbs for diagnosis of PE was investigated in a sub-analysis of a large, randomised trial. A total of 855 patients with suspected PE underwent investigation by pre - test probability assessment, D-dimer testing, proximal US and computed tomography pulmonary angiography (CTPA). These patients also underwent distal US, although the findings of this investigation were not used in clinical diagnosis. A total of 59 patients had isolated distal DVT and, of these 59 patients, 21 patients (36%) had no PE on CTPA. Of these 21 patients, 20 patients were not given anticoagulant therapy and had an uneventful follow-up. Thus, in patients with suspected PE, distal US has limited diagnostic value, and a high false positive rate, making it an investigation of limited value for diagnosis of PE (Righini et al., 2008). By contrast, because the vast majority of PEs arise from the pelvis or lower limb, and the treatment for proximal (above knee) DVT is identical to that for proven PE, a positive diagnosis of proximal DVT can eliminate the need to perform imaging of the pulmonary arteries. However, in clinical practice, many patients will have a CTPA, especially if they have respiratory symptoms.

Venous compression technique is known as greyscale imaging. This can be augmented by performing colour Doppler - collectively known as duplex scanning. The Doppler effect is used to analyse blood flow by detecting the change in frequency of ultrasound waves that occurs when sound interacts with moving red blood cells. In the absence of DVT, variations in the Doppler waveform can be elicited by performing simple techniques. By squeezing the calf gently, known as augmentation, the Doppler flow within the venous system proximally increases as the muscle pump drives more blood towards the heart. This helps the operator to confidently exclude clot between the calf and the vein being visualised by the transducer. Another method is to ask the patient to take a deep breath. The increased intra - abdominal pressure during deep inspiration has a compressive effect upon the normal inferior vena cava and pelvic veins, causing a noticeable reduction in Doppler flow, thereby helping to excluded DVT within these proximal veins (fig. 3).

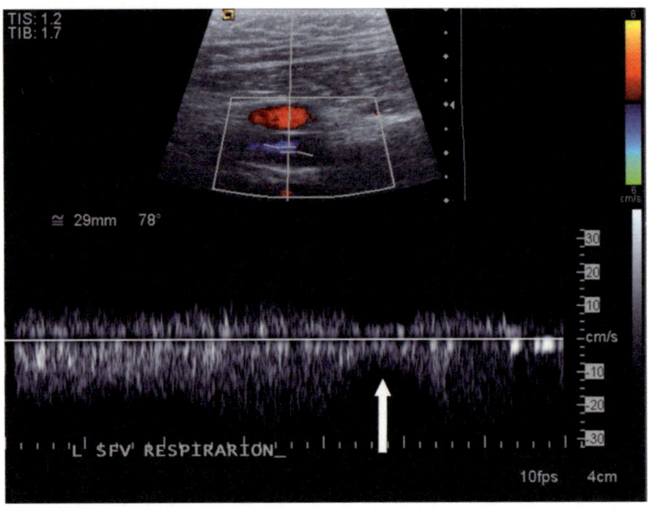

Fig. 3. Duplex US. Normal phasic variation in Doppler waveform within the superficial femoral vein during deep respiration (*arrow*).

Other indicators of thrombus include distension of the vein in acute thrombosis (typically long established clot does not expand the lumen), and visualising clot within the affected vein (fig. 4). Unfortunately, a significant number of acute clots are isoechoic i.e. of the same ultrasound density to flowing blood, rendering them invisible to the naked eye unless colour mapping is used. Differentiating acute from chronic DVT is a challenge with all imaging modalities, not just ultrasound. The maturation of thrombus from anechoic i.e. less dense than blood, through to hyperechoic i.e. more dense is very variable, and exact age determination is not possible. Six months following a DVT, 50% of patients will have persisting abnormality on US (Dougherty RS & Brant WE, 2007), making the distinction between acute-on-chronic versus chronic changes very difficult. In addition to thrombus appearance, studies have assessed change in thrombus diameter (Kearon et al., 1998), change in thrombus length (Linkins et al., 2004), and Doppler analysis of flow (Prandoni et al., 2002) in an attempt to differentiate acute from chronic changes, but there remains no consensus on which ultrasound measurement can be relied upon to solve this potentially important dilemma. A sensible approach is to obtain a baseline scan at the time of discontinuing anticoagulation to allow for comparison in the event of the patient re-presenting with recurring symptoms.

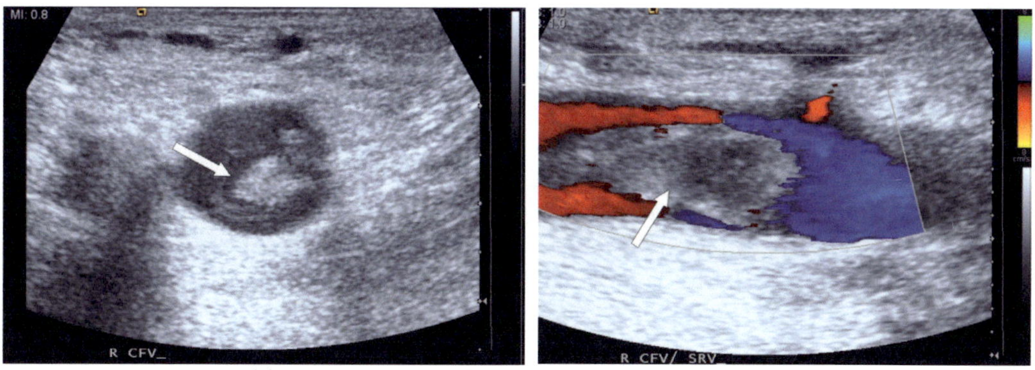

(a) (b)

Fig. 4. (a) Transverse image showing non - compressible DVT within the right common femoral vein on US. The lumen of the vein contains echogenic clot implying that it is relatively chronic (*arrow*). (b) Longitudinal Duplex image highlighting non - occlusive clot within the common femoral vein (*arrow*) with blood flowing around the thrombus.

Venous Thrombi are dynamic structures, especially within the first 1 to 2 weeks after their onset (O'shaughnessy & Fitzgerald, 2000a, 2000b). Up to 25% of calf DVTs may propagate into the proximal veins (Johnson et al., 2010). Therefore, it is routine practice to repeat a negative scan after 5 to 7 days to assess for propagation into the proximal vasculature, particularly in patients with high pre-test probability scores.

Importantly there are of course limitations to US. As discussed, the calf veins are not readily identified, especially in the swollen oedematous leg, often necessitating a repeat examination to exclude proximal clot propagation. In addition the iliac veins are not readily assessable, and the adductor canal (at the junction of the superficial femoral vein [SFV] and popliteal vein) is notoriously difficult to visualise even in thin patients. The saphenous vein or collaterals can be mistaken for the SFV. In addition, the SFV is duplicated in approximately 20% of patients, potentially leading to diagnostic error, particularly if one system is occluded and the other patent. Obesity and oedema can render examinations inconclusive. Interestingly, studies have shown that whilst US is sensitive and specific for symptomatic lower limb DVT, it has rather poor sensitivity for asymptomatic DVT compared to conventional venography, with sensitivity between 29 and 38% (Davidson et al., 1992; Turkstra et al., 1997, as cited in Roditi & Fink, 2009). US has been investigated as a potential screening test in asymptomatic patients deemed to be at high risk of DVT following surgical procedures. However, the sensitivity and specificity appear to be reduced in this setting, a randomised - controlled trial discovering no added benefit of screening patients for DVT after lower limb arthroplasty surgery (Robinson et al., 1997, as cited in Fraser & Anderson, 1999).

A final potential pit - fall is worth clarifying, especially for the referring clinician acting upon the radiological report. The superficial femoral vein is actually part of the deep venous system, and thrombus involving this vein could easily be interpreted as only a superficial phlebitis by the unaware clinician. The term should either be avoided, and replaced with the deep femoral vein (the practice of the authors), or the conclusion of the report should clearly indicate that there is DVT.

2.3 Computed tomography and pulmonary embolus

A study performed in 1994 showed that among patients with proximal DVT, approximately 40% had an associated asymptomatic PE, supporting the belief that PE and DVT are essentially manifestations of the same disease, sharing similar risk factors (Moser et al., 1994). Although PE can result from several embolic sources including air, fat, amniotic fluid and tumour, it has been estimated that PE originates from lower limb DVT in at least 90% of cases (Sevitt & Gallagher, 1961). Another common feature of these conditions is their rather non-specific presentation, with clinical signs often being of limited value in confirming a diagnosis (British Thoracic Society, 2003). Only a minority of patients presenting to the emergency department with classic pleuritic chest pain will have PE. Imaging again plays an essential role in diagnosis.

Chest radiography will be the first radiological examination obtained in almost all patients presenting with PE, but a definitive diagnosis cannot be made on chest radiography alone. The majority of patients will have non-specific abnormalities such as airspace opacification, diaphragmatic elevation, linear atelectasis, and possibly cardiac silhouette changes. Conversely, a completely normal chest radiograph can be seen in up to 40%. The principal role of the plain chest radiograph is therefore to detect conditions that can mimic PE, such as pneumonia or pneumothorax.

CTPA is now established as the first line investigation for the diagnosis of PE, surpassing ventilation/perfusion (V/Q) scans, most noticeably by reducing the number of indeterminate, non-diagnostic examinations (Johnson MS, 2002). In addition, CTPA has a superior inter - observer correlation (Blachere et al., 2000), with sensitivities of 94 - 96% and specificities of 94 - 100% being reported (Blachere et al., 2000; Remy-Jardin et al., 2000). Following targeted contrast opacification of the pulmonary arterial tree, multidetector CT allows evaluation of pulmonary vessels down to sixth order branches with the ability to reformat the original data in multiple planes to enhance the diagnostic accuracy (fig. 5). Emboli are recognised as intraluminal filling defects that partially or completely occlude the vessel. The most specific sign of acute PE is a filling defect that forms acute angles to the vessel wall. Clot forming an obtuse angle implies chronic thromboembolic disease, but this can also be seen in the acute setting. Secondary signs on CT reflect the non-specific abnormalities frequently seen on chest radiography. Pleural based wedge shaped consolidation indicates peripheral haemorrhage or infarction. Peripheral oligaemia (paucity of blood vessels distal to the occluded artery), pleural effusions and linear atelectasis (partial collapse) can also be observed.

Detailed depiction of the lung parenchyma offers additional information not provided by V/Q scans (fig. 6b). In the context of a negative test for PE, an alternative explanation for the patient's symptoms may be highlighted. A study found that as many as two - thirds of patients with an initial suspicion of PE received another diagnosis following CTPA (Hull et al., 1994, as cited in Schoepf & Costello, 2004). In another study, CTPA identified pleural or parenchymal abnormalities that explained indeterminate defects on V/Q scans in 57% of patients (van Rossum et al., 1996, as cited in Kanne et al., 2004). Although a normal V/Q scan essentially excludes PE, a high probability scan has a sensitivity of 88%, compared to 94 - 96% for CTPA (Kanne et al., 2004). Patients with intermediate or indeterminate probability scans (because of background lung or pleural abnormalities) still have a 30 - 40% incidence of PE (Klein JS, 2007). V/Q scans, however, should always be considered in young patients with low pre-test probability and normal chest radiographs in view of its lower radiation dose.

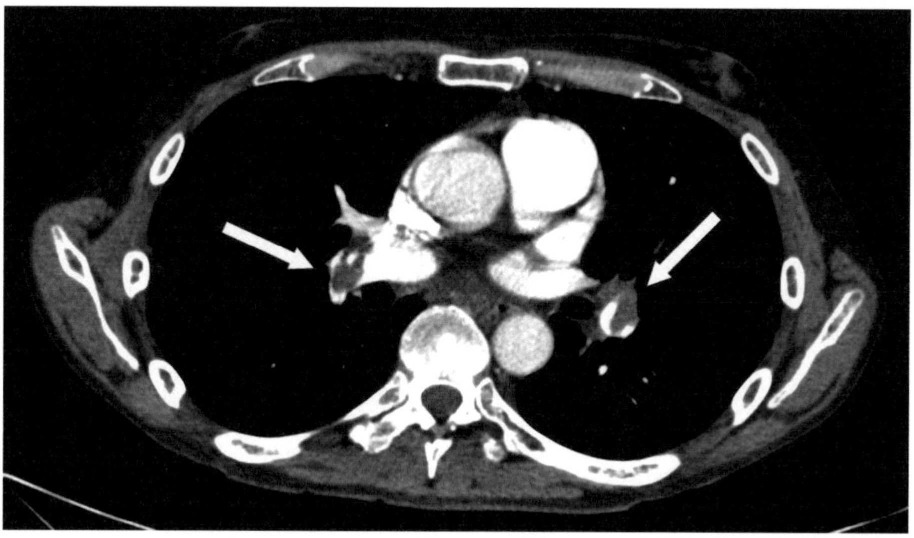

Fig. 5. CTPA in the axial (transverse) plane demonstrating bilateral filling defects within the contrast opacified pulmonary arteries diagnostic of PE (*arrows*).

The main cause of death within the first 30 days after a PE is right ventricular failure (Schoepf et al., 2004). Right ventricular enlargement on CTPA has been shown to correlate with right ventricular dysfunction on echocardiography, and to predict early death from acute PE. In patients with confirmed PE, evidence of right heart strain / dysfunction should always be sought as this can influence patient management with regards reperfusion therapy. To accurately, and reproducibly, measure ventricular size the original CT data is manipulated to allow reformatting in the 4 chamber orientation. This is simply performed at the reporting workstation. The ventricle is measured at its maximum size at a level 1 cm ahead of the corresponding atrioventricular valve. A right ventricle : left ventricle ratio of > 0.9 is indicative of right ventricular enlargement (fig 6).

CT venography (CTV) can be combined with CTPA to evaluate both PE and DVT in a single CT study (fig. 7). The lower limb veins are scanned at intervals 3 or 4 minutes following completion of the pulmonary angiogram. The sensitivity and specificity of CTV has been reported between 89 - 100% and 94 - 100% respectively (Begemann et al., 2003; Loud et al., 2001, as sited in Kanne et al., 2004). The combined study also allows evaluation of the iliac system, not afforded by US. However, a major concern is the additional radiation exposure. A study found the addition of CTV to increase the gonadal dose by a factor of 500 in women and 2000 in men (the dose is higher in men since the testes are external to the body cavity). This translates to increased likelihood of birth defects and radiation - related death, albeit at a very low added risk (Rademaker et al., 2001). Combined CTV also requires substantial contrast medium dose for adequate venous opacification, significantly greater amounts than the relatively small quantities (50 - 75 ml) required for CTPA on modern multidetector scanners. The value of this combined study is therefore debatable, and CTV is not included in the CTPA protocol in most European institutions, including our own.

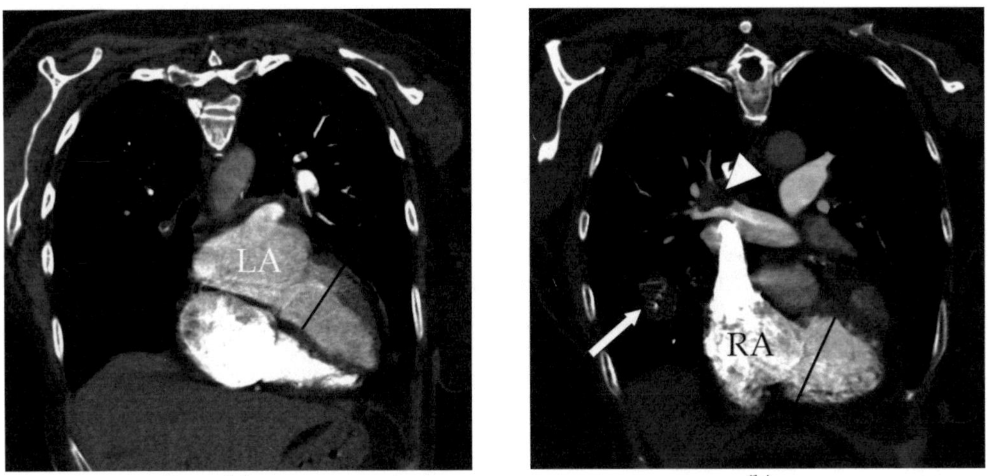

(a) (b)

Fig. 6. Coronal oblique reformatted CTPA at the level of the atrioventricular valves demonstrating right ventricular enlargement. (a) Maximum size of the left ventricle (*line*). LA = left atrium. (b) Maximum size of the right ventricle (*line*). RA = right atrium. The corresponding right ventricle : left ventricle ratio is > 0.9. Note the clot within the right pulmonary artery (*arrowhead*); and a lung tumour (*arrow*) which was not clinically suspected.

The value of adding lower limb US in the evaluation of patients undergoing CTPA has been evaluated in a large, randomised trial of 1819 patients with clinically suspected PE. Following pre - test probability assessment, 909 patients were randomised to investigation by D-dimer measurement and CTPA, and 916 patients were randomised to D-dimer measurement, CTPA and venous US of the leg. The primary outcome was 3 month thromboembolic risk in patients who were left untreated on the basis of exclusion of PE by the investigation strategy. The prevalence of PE and the 3 month risk of thromboembolism was the same in both investigation groups. Thus, venous US of the leg does not improve diagnosis of 3 month thromboembolic risk when added to investigation by D-dimer analysis and CTPA (Righini et al., 2008). Therefore, it can be argued that for patients who have undergone CTPA for the investigation of PE, US of the leg is a redundant investigation.

The diagnostic power of current CT has provoked another interesting debate with the ability to potentially identify clot down to sixth order branches with multi - detector row scanners (MDCT). Older single detector row scanners (SDCT) have limited ability in detecting isolated subsegmental PE. Whilst the treatment of embolus detected within third and even fourth order subsegmental arteries is undisputed, the clinical relevance of detecting clot within smaller, more peripheral branches is questionable (Kanne et al., 2004), and could be unnecessarily subjecting patients to the side effects of anticoagulation. A review of 20 prospective cohort studies and 2 randomised controlled trials was done to evaluate the importance of single and multiple detector row CTPA in the diagnosis of subsegmental PE. This meta-analysis showed that the diagnosis rate of sub-segmental PE was 4.7% with SDCT and 9.4% with MDCT. However, the 3 month risk of thromboembolic events in patients with suspected PE who were left untreated based upon a diagnostic algorithm that included a negative CTPA was 0.9% for SDCT and 1.1% for MDCT. Therefore, although MDCT increases the proportion of patients diagnosed with PE compared with SDCT, it does not substantially reduce the 3-month risk of thromboembolism. The authors suggest that isolated sub-segmental PE may not be clinically relevant (Carrier et al., 2006). Small peripheral emboli are believed to form even in healthy individuals (although this has never been substantiated); and it is a function of the lung to prevent these small clots from entering the arterial bed (Tetalman et al., 1973, as cited in Schoepf & Costello, 2004).

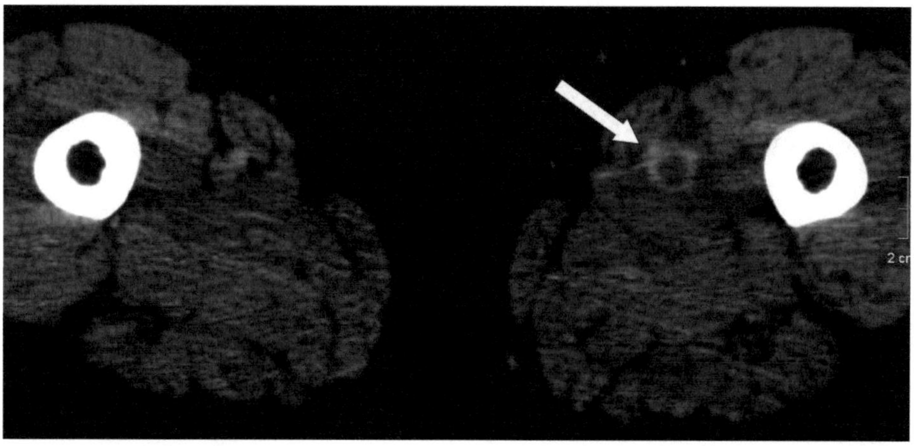

Fig. 7. CTV (combined with CTPA) demonstrating clot within the left superficial femoral vein (*arrow*).

2.4 Magnetic resonance imaging

MRI has been perhaps underutilised in DVT because it is seen as relatively expensive, less accessible and more time consuming compared to other modalities. Furthermore, this probably also relates to the variability of venous enhancement encountered using the wide variety of imaging techniques available (Roditi & Fink, 2009). Despite this, MRI is undergoing the greatest evolution in terms of venous imaging. Studies have already shown the sensitivity and specificity of MR venography (MRV) to be comparable to conventional venography in diagnosing femeropopliteal DVT (Cantwell et al., 2006; Fraser et al., 2002, as cited in Cantwell et al., 2006). Conventional venography is poor by comparison in opacifying the pelvic vessels (Cantwell et al., 2006; Spritzer, 2009). To reiterate, US also performs poorly in assessing the iliac vessels. Where MRV has perhaps until now performed less well than venography is in assessing the calf veins (Cantwell et al., 2006). With contrast enhanced MRV this was largely because of difficulties in predicting the arrival of contrast in the more distal veins to optimally time the acquisition of the images. This is confounded by the very short transit time of standard extracellular contrast agents within the vascular bed as they rapidly redistribute into the extracellular fluid space.

Recent advancements in the physical properties of contrast agents have overcome the aforementioned difficulties in imaging the calf vessels. The "blood pool" contrast agent gadofosveset trisodium (Vasovist, Bayer Schering Pharma, Berlin, Germany) binds to plasma albumin extending the blood pool residence time. Not only does this eliminate time constraints in acquiring satisfactory images, but allows very high spatial resolution imaging of both the deep and superficial venous system (fig. 8). As previously mentioned, a potential pitfall of venography and US is the not uncommon occurrence of duplicated veins. A study investigating the effects of these anatomical variants in DVT suggested that DVT was twice as likely to be missed (Liu et al., 1986, as cited in Cantwell et al., 2006). Fig. 9 shows duplication of the SFV readily identified by high resolution MRI.

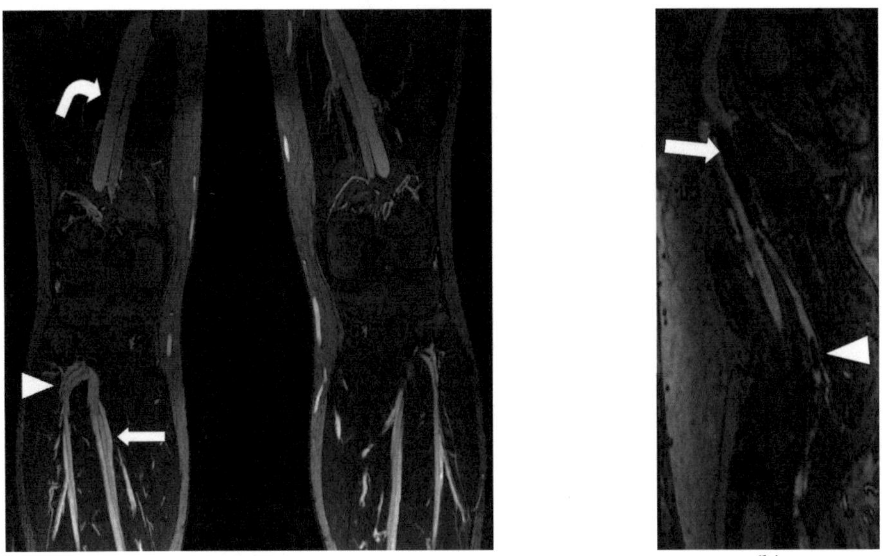

(a) (b)

Fig. 8. High resolution MRI using "blood pool" contrast allows excellent visualisation of both veins and their accompanying arteries. (a) Coronal plane. The normal anatomy of the calf arteries with their accompanying paired veins is clearly demonstrated with the anterior tibial artery and veins (*arrowhead*) and the peroneal artery and veins (*straight arrow*). The superficial (deep) femoral vein and artery are also shown (*curved arrow*). (b). Sagittal oblique view showing clot within the common femoral vein (*arrow*) and great saphenous vein (*arrowhead*).

The lack of radiation makes MRI a more attractive option than CT, particularly when there are concerns regarding pelvic DVT in younger patients as the reproductive organs are within the scanning field. For this reason, MRI should always be considered in excluding DVT in pregnancy. US is often equivocal especially in the latter stages due to technical difficulties. A further venous complication of pregnancy is ovarian vein thrombosis, or puerperal ovarian vein thrombophlebitis. Presentation is usually on the 2nd or 3rd day postpartum with lower abdominal pain and fever. The major complications are septicaemia and PE, which is reported to occur in up to 25%. MR is considered to be more sensitive than CT or US in making the diagnosis (Kubik-Huch RA et al., 1999, as cited in Spritzer, 2009).

Several studies have evaluated the performance of pulmonary contrast enhanced MRA for the diagnosis of PE. One of the larger studies (Oudkerk et al., 2002, as cited in Roditi & Fink, 2009) assessed MRA in 141 patients with an abnormal perfusion lung scintigraphy and compared the findings with those of pulmonary DSA. Sensitivity was 77%, and the demonstration of emboli in two patients with a normal angiogram resulted in a specificity of 98%. The major advantage of MR is the lack of radiation exposure. A study has shown that the radiation from a single CTPA may cause an additional attributable lifetime risk of cancer of almost 1% in young women (Einstein et al., 2007, as cited in Roditi & Fink, 2009), mainly because breast tissue is relatively radiosensitive. With the introduction of "blood pool" contrast agents a comprehensive examination can be performed for PE and DVT using a single low dose contrast injection, without the associated radiation concerns that hamper CT.

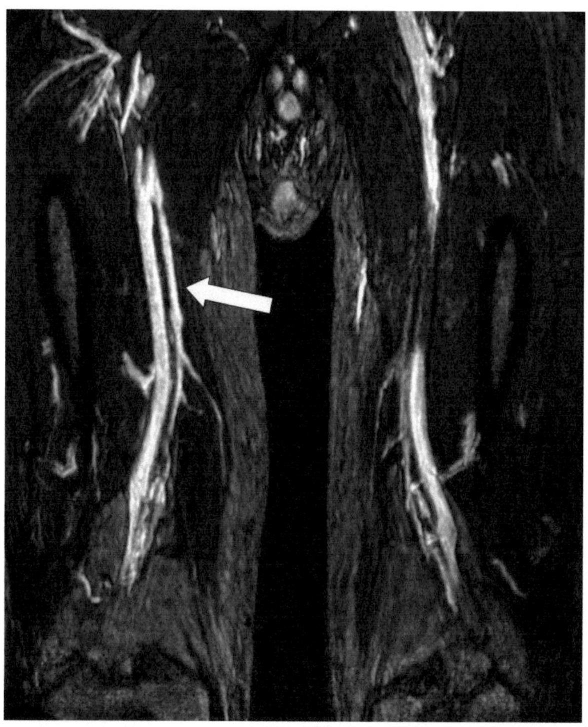

Fig. 9. High resolution MRI in the coronal plane showing duplication of the superficial femoral vein (*arrow*). Note that the superficial femoral artery is not visible because it was occluded at the groin. The patient had known claudication.

The limitations of MR are the relative expense limiting availability, and for some patients the claustrophobic environment preventing completion of the examination. At present, MRI should be considered when there is a strong clinical suspicion of pelvic DVT, and in young women requiring investigation for PE with abnormal chest X - ray precluding a V/Q scan.

3. Role of interventional radiology in venous thrombosis

3.1 Introduction

Despite advances in diagnostic techniques and therapeutic approaches, DVT remains a potentially life threatening disorder. Anticoagulation, which is the current standard of treatment for patients with acutely diagnosed above knee DVT, involves treatment with low molecular weight heparin followed by a 6 month course of warfarin (Hyers et al., 1998). This treatment is designed to stop further progression and potential embolisation, but does not treat or remove the existing thrombus and may be insufficient in treatment of extensive ilio-femoral thrombosis. A large clot burden in the proximal veins in the acute phase can lead to local complications including venous oedema, acute compartment syndrome, tissue necrosis and venous gangrene, and systemic complications such as PE.

Over time normal fibrinolytic mechanisms will result in a variable degree of recanalisation of the thrombosed segment but this may not be sufficient for resolution of clinical symptoms. Chronic DVT and venous insufficiency has been shown to diminish a person`s quality of life and socioeconomic activity (Vedantham et al., 2004).

There are a number of endovascular treatment options in DVT which aim to achieve thrombus removal, restoring patency and potentially limiting the acute complications associated with DVT. It is important to appreciate the limitations of these treatments and the relative lack of randomised controlled trials evaluating the efficacy of these interventions.

3.2 Catheter directed thrombolysis treatment

This technique involves infusion of a thrombolytic agent in and around the thrombus via an infusion catheter. This leads to high dose delivery of the thrombolytic agent locally, reducing the systemic complications, and has been shown to have almost double the venous patency rate at one year, compared to systemic thrombolysis (Comerota et al., 2007). This has been sanctioned by the American College of Chest Physicians (ACCP) as a first line treatment in "selected patients with extensive acute proximal DVT who have a low risk of bleeding" (Kearon et al., 2008). Further criteria include a young patient with a good functional status, life expectancy greater than one year and symptoms for ideally less than 14 days.

Although the administration of the thrombolytic agent is local, the lytic agent can migrate systemically and can increase the risk for major bleeding complications requiring the patient to be monitored aggressively in a high dependency/intensive care setting.

The route for catheter placement is usually decided depending on the thrombus location and burden. This may be placed via the jugular, contralateral femoral or ipsilateral popliteal vein, ideally using ultrasound guided access. Catheters with multiple side - holes and long infusion length can be used for drug delivery and although there is no single drug that has been approved for this use, streptokinase and more recently alteplase (rt-PA) have been used for this purpose. Venography at the time of the procedure can help assess the clot burden, plan adjunctive treatments (venoplasty, pharmaco-mechanical disruption) and also help define a suitable end point.

There is however a lack of prospective randomised data assessing the benefits of thrombolysis as compared to anticoagulant therapy (Pianta & Thomson, 2011). This, in combination with haemorrhagic complications and lack of awareness among physicians has limited acceptance of this procedure.

3.3 Percutaneous mechanical thrombectomy and pharmacomechanical thrombolysis

This involves use of a mechanical clot removal device such as a Trerotola (Arrow-Trerotola™ PTD®, Arrow, Reading, PA) which is a rotational device or a hydrodynamic device such as Angiojet (AngioJet® Rheolytic Thrombectomy system: Medrad Intervention, Warrendale, PA) . Other devices such as Trellis (Cividien, Santa Clara, California) or the Clot Buster Amplatzer Thrombectomy Device (ATD, Minneapolis, MN) are also available.

The aim is to achieve maceration/disruption of the clot, thus facilitating thrombus aspiration and removal. This is a much less invasive option than open surgical thrombectomy and other advantages include improved clot removal and more rapid restoration of flow. Intensive patient monitoring is also not necessary unlike catheter directed thrombolysis (fig. 10).

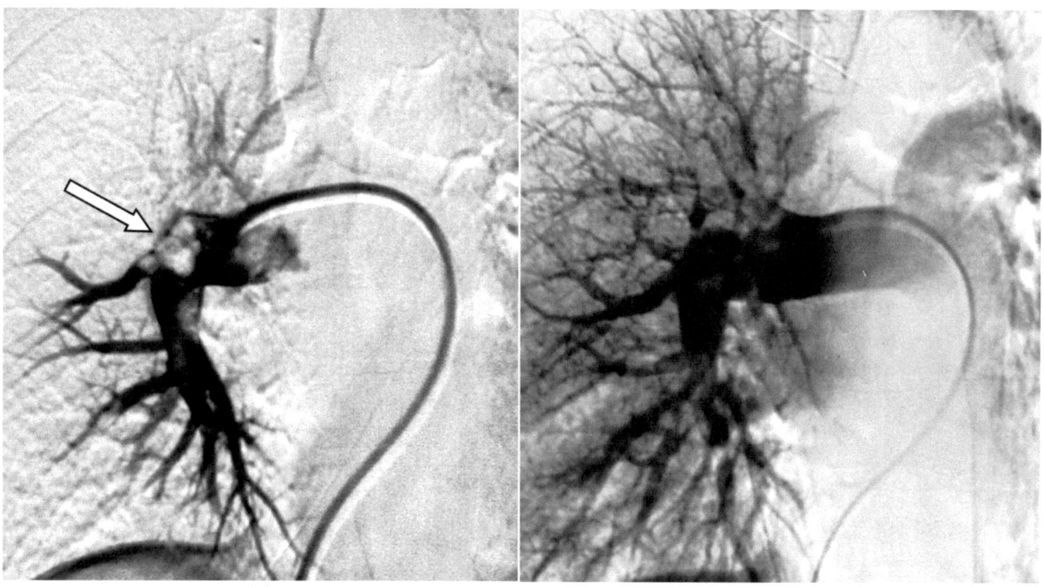

(a) (b)

Fig. 10. Catheter thrombectomy. (a) Catheter tip within the right main pulmonary artery, adjacent to embolus (*arrow*). (b) Post - treatment shows disruption of the clot. Note the striking difference in contrast opacification of the pulmonary arterial tree pre - and post - treatment.

Complications include vessel wall and valve injury and kidney failure due to haemolysis. Although patients can experience transient shortness of breath presumably due to pulmonary microemboli, experience gained from thrombectomy of clotted fistulas has shown that concomitant use of a plasminogen activator significantly reduced the risk of symptomatic pulmonary embolism from the procedure (O'Sullivan, 2010).

Pharmacomechanical thrombolysis involves the combined use of a thrombectomy device in combination with catheter directed infusion of a thrombolytic agent. The advantages of this combination include better permeation of the thrombolytic agent and a smaller duration of treatment. Although some devices can lower the systemic dose of the drug, others do not do so.

A retrospective study of 93 patients showed that pharmacomechanical thrombolysis was an effective treatment modality in patients with significant DVT and compared to catheter directed thrombolysis alone, it provided similar treatment success, reduced length of intensive care and hospital stay, and reduced hospital costs (Lin et al., 2006). However, another study has shown that that use of the Trerotola device alone constituted effective treatment of acute ilio-femoral DVT independent of adjunct pharmacological thrombolysis (Lee et al., 2006).

There is, however, a relative lack of randomised data on the use of these devices and further randomised studies are necessary.

3.4 Venoplasty and stenting

Balloon venoplasty is usually performed in patients in combination with catheter directed thrombolysis or pharmacomechanical treatment to help macerate the existing clot or to dilate a venous stenosis which may have been a contributory factor in the development of the DVT. Venous stenosis can occur due a number of aetiologies. Benign causes include May-Thurner syndrome (Ferris et al., 1983), where long standing pulsatile compression of the left common iliac vein by the left common iliac artery leads to development of a venous web. Malignant compression or invasion can be another cause. Chronic deep vein thrombosis can lead to vessel wall fibrosis and development of stenosis.

Unlike arteries, veins have a high elastic recoil and lower rates of flow which leads to less satisfactory results with long term stent patency, in the iliac veins, with a greater than 50% re-stenosis in up to 15% of patients (Hood & Alexander, 2004). These figures are much worse for patients who are hypercoagulable, have longer stent lengths and need infra-inguinal stents.

Stenting an underlying lesion has, however, shown to help prevent or prolong the interval to recurrence and can result in 50% increased patency rate than thrombolysis alone (Hood & Alexander, 2004) and lower recurrence rates of ilio-femoral DVT (up to 73% lower) in patients with May-Thurner syndrome (Oguzkurt et al., 2004). Most experience has been gained with Wallstents (Boston Scientific, Hemel Hempstead, Herts, UK) which are self expanding stents with a good radial strength. Studies have also shown the efficacy and durability of stents in the IVC (Ing et al., 2001; Razavi et al., 2000).

3.5 Inferior vena cava filters

These percutaneously implantable devices are placed in the infra-renal inferior vena cava to reduce the risk of a significant pulmonary embolism (fig. 11). Specific indications include venous thromboembolism with a contraindication to oral anticoagulation or pulmonary embolism despite adequate anticoagulation (Kaufman et al., 2006). There are further uses including patients with DVT who have cancer or burns, and also in high risk trauma and surgical patients. Case selection is paramount and the risks of device implantation and removal must be carefully assessed.

Device implantation is usually via the femoral or the internal jugular vein in a suitable infrarenal position. Cavograms are performed to delineate the renal veins, asses the extent of thrombus and exclude contraindications such as dilated IVC which may not be suitable for standard filter deployment. Suprarenal placement is undertaken if there is thrombus extension into or above the renal veins.

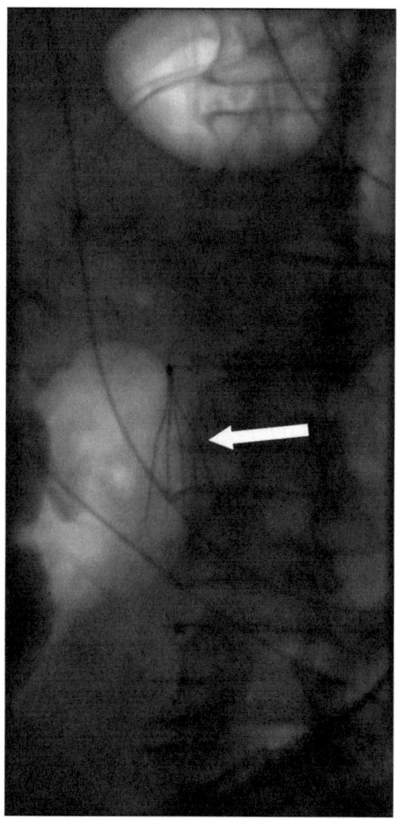

Fig. 11. Temporary IVC filter (*arrow*).

IVC filters are classified as temporary or permanent (Streiff, 2000) and there are various devices available that are approved for use. To cite a few examples, the Bird`s Nest Filter and the Trapease filter are permanent whereas the Gunther Tulip and the Cook Celect Filter are retrievable. Timely removal of retrievable filters is important to reduce the long term risk of filter deployment. In terms of safety and efficacy, there is no significant difference between the two types of devices (Nazir et al., 2009). Complications associated with the device include those encountered at the time of insertion such as access site haematoma, pneumothorax, inadvertent arterial puncture and misplacement. Delayed complications include IVC thrombosis, occlusion, venous insufficiency and pulmonary embolism.

4. Conclusion

The incidence of deep venous thrombosis is increasing, not just in the lower limb but also within the deep veins of the upper limb, where malignancy and central venous catheter placement are the major precipitating factors. Ultrasound provides a rapid and readily available assessment, and can be portably used at the bedside in critically ill patients. There is however limitations to ultrasound, particularly the poor visualisation of below knee clot. In high risk patients, a short interval repeat scan is indicated to exclude the 25% of such clots which can propagate above the knee.

The iliac veins within the pelvis are also inaccessible to ultrasound in almost every patient. If DVT is strongly suspected within the pelvis, MRI should be considered. This modality has seen the greatest advancements in recent times, with current protocols able to visualise the venous system in very high spatial resolution. CT angiography of the limbs, whilst sensitive and easily incorporated into routine CT pulmonary angiograph in suspected PE, should be avoided in view of the radiation burden. The major advantage of MRI is the lack of radiation exposure. MRI will almost certainly feature more commonly in DVT evaluation in the near future with new "blood pool" contrast agents allowing a comprehensive examination for PE and DVT in the same scan. One specific application is in relatively young patients with abnormal CXR precluding a V/Q scan. However, CT is currently the "gold standard" for diagnosing PE.

There are a number of endovascular treatment options in DVT which aim to achieve thrombus removal, restoring patency and potentially limiting the acute complications associated with DVT. It is important to appreciate there are limitations to these treatments, with a relative lack of randomised controlled trials evaluating their true efficacy. They should however be given consideration in selected patients as outlined above.

5. Acknowledgements

We would like to thank Dr Iain Robertson & Dr Richard Edwards, consultant interventional radiologists, Gartnavel hospital, Glasgow for kindly providing the images of catheter thrombectomy.

6. References

Allen AW, Megargell JL, Brown DB, Lynch FC, Singh H & Singh Y. Venous thrombosis associated with the placement of peripherally inserted central catheters. J Vasc Interv Radiol. 2000; 11: 1309-1314.

Baarslag HJ, van Beek, EJR, Koopman MMW & Reekers JA. Prospective study of color duplex ultrasonography in patients suspected of having deep venous thrombosis of the upper extremities. Annals of Int Med. 2002; 136(12): 865-872.

Baron JA, Gridley G, weiderpass E, Nyren O & Linet M. Venous thromboembolism and cancer. Lancet. 1989; 351: 1077-1088.

Blachere H, Latrabe V, Montaudon M, valli N, Couffinhal T, Raherisson C, Leccia F & Laurent F. Pulmonary embolism revealed on helical CT angiography: comparison with ventilation- perfusion radionuclide lung scanning. Am J Roentgenol. 2000; 174: 1041-1047.

British Thoracic Society guidelines for the management of suspected acute pulmonary embolism. Thorax. 2003; 58(6): 470-483.

Cantwell CP, Cradock A, Bruzzi J, Fitzpatrick P, Eustace S & Murray JG. MR venography with true fast imaging with steady- state precession for suspected lower- limb deep vein thrombosis. J Vasc Interv Rad 2006; 17: 1763-1769.

Carrier M, Righini M, Wells PS, Perrier A, Anderson DR, Rodger MA, Pleasance S & Le Gal G. Pulmonary embolism diagnoses on computer tomography: incidental and clinical implications. A systematic review and meta- analysis of the management outcome studies. J Thromb Haemost. 2010; 8(8): 1716-1722.

Comerota AJ & Paolini D. Treatment of acute ileofemoral deep venous thrombosis: a strategy of thrombus removal. Eur J Vasc Endovasc Surg. 2007; 33(3): 351-360.

Cronan JJ. Venous thromboembolic disease: the role of US. Radiology. 1993; 186: 619-630.

De Valois JC, van Schaik CC, Verzijibergen F, van Ramshorst B, Eikelboom BC & Meuwissen OJ. Contrast venography. Eur J Radiol. 1990; 11(2): 131-137.

Dorfman GS & Cronan JJ. Venous ultrasonography. Radiol Clin North Am. 1992; 30: 879-893.

Dougherty RS & Brant WE. 2007. vascular ultrasound, In: *Fundamentals of diagnostic radiology*, Brant WE & Helms CA., pp 1019-1060. Lipincott Williams & Wilkins, ISBN- 13: 978-0-7817-6518-3, Philadelphia, USA.

Ferris EJ, Lim WN, Smith PL & casali R. May-Thurner syndrome. Radiology. 1983; 147: 29-31.

Fraser JD & Anderson DR. Deep venous thrombosis: recent advances and optimal investigation with US. Radiology. 1999; 211: 9-24.

Heijboer H, Buller HR, lensing AW, Turpie AG, Colly LP & Ten Cate JW. A comparison of real-time compression ultrasonography with impedance plethysmography for the diagnosis of deep-vein thrombosis in symptomatic outpatients. N Engl J Med. 1993; 329: 1365-9.

Hood DB & Alexander JQ. Endovascular management of iliofemoral venous occlusive disease. Surg Clin N Am. 2004; 84: 1381-1396.

Hyers TM, Agnelli G & Hull RD. 1998. Antithrombotic therapy for venous thromboembolic disease. In, *Fifth American College of Chest Physicians(ACCP) consensus conference on antithrombotic therapy*, Dalen JE, Hirsh J(eds). Chest. 114(suppl):561-579.

Ing FF, Fagan TE, Grifka RG et al. Reconstruction of stenotic or occluded ilio-femoral veins and inferior vena cava using intravascular stents: re-establishing access for future cardiac catheterisation and cardiac surgery. J Am Coll Cardiol. 2001; 37: 251-257.

Johnson MS. Current strategies for the diagnosis of pulmonary embolus. J Vasc Interv Radiology. 2002;13: 13-23.

Johnson SA, Stevens SM, Woller SC, Lake, E, Donadini M, Cheng J, Labarere J & Douketis J. Risk of deep venous thrombosis following a single negative whole leg compression ultrasound. 2010; 303(5); 438-445.

Kanne JP & Lalani TA. Role of computed tomography and magnetic resonance imaging for deep vein thrombosis and pulmonary embolism. Circulation. 2004; 109: 15-21.

Kaufman JA, Kinney TB, Streiff MB, Sing R, Proctor M, Mark DB, A Cipolle, S Cornerota, Millward F, Frederick B, Rogers D, Sacks A & Venbrux C. Guidelines for the use of retrievable and convertible vena cava filters: report from the Society of Interventional Radiology multidisciplinary consensus conference. J Vasc Interv Radiol. 2006; 17: 449-459.

Kearon C, Julian JA, Newman TE & Ginsberg JS. Non- invasive diagnosis of deep venous thrombosis. Ann Int Med. 1998; 128(8): 663-677.

Kearon C, Kahn SR, Agnelli G, Goldhaber S, Raskob GE & Comerota AJ. Antithrombotic therapy for venous thromboembolic disease: American College of Chest Physicians Evidence-Based Clinical Practice Guidelines (8th Edition). Chest. 2008; 133(6 Suppl):454S-545S.

Klein JS. 2007. Pulmonary vascular disease, In: *Fundamentals of diagnostic radiology*, Brant WE & Helms CA., pp 417-432. Lipincott Williams & Wilkins, ISBN- 13: 978-0-7817-6518-3, Philadelphia, USA.

Lee KH, Han H, Lee KJ, Yoon CS, Kim SH, Won JY & Lee DY. Mechanical thrombectomy of acute iliofemoral deep vein thrombosis with the use of an Arrow Trerotola percutaneous thrombectomy device. J Vas Interv Radiol. 2006; 17(3): 487-495.

Lin PH, Zhou W, Dardik, Mussa F, Kougias P, Hedayata N, Naoum JJ, Sayed HE, Peden EK & Huynh TT. Catheter-direct thrombolysis versus pharmacomechanical thrombectomy for treatment of symptomatic lower extremity deep venous thrombosis. Am J Surg. 2006; 192(6): 782-788.

Linkins LA, Pasquale P, Paterson S & Kearon C. Change in thrombus length on venous ultrasound and recurrent dep vein thrombosis. Arch Intern Med 2004; 164: 1973-1796.

Moser KM, Fedullo PF, Littlejohn JK & Crawford R. Frequent asymptomatic pulmonary embolism in patients with deep venous thrombosis. JAMA. 1994; 271(3): 223-225.

Nazir SA, Ganeshan A, Nazir S & Uberoi R. Endovascular treatment options in the management of lower limb deep venous thrombosis. Cardiovasc Intervent Radiol. 2009; 32: 861-876.

Oguzkurt L, Ozkan U, Ulusan S, Koc Z & Tercan F. Compression of left common iliac vein in asymptomatic subjects and patients with left iliofemoral deep vein thrombosis. J Vasc Interv Radiol. 2008; 19: 366-371.

O'Shaugnessy AM & Fitzgerald DE. Determining the stage of organisation and natural history of venous thrombosis using computer analysis. Int Angiol. 2000a; 19(3): 220-227.

O'Shaugnessy AM & Fitzgerald DE. The value of computer analysis in predicting the long term outcome of deep venous thrombosis. Int Angiol. 2000b; 19(4): 308-313.

O'Sullivan GJ. The role of interventional radiology in the management of deep venous thrombosis: advanced therapy. Cardiovasc Intervent Radiol. 2011 ;34(3):445-61.

Pianta MJ & Thomson KR. Catheter-directed thrombolysis of lower limb thrombosis. Cardiovasc Intervent Radiol. 2011; 34(1):25-36.

Prandoni P, Lensing AWA & Bernardi E. The diagnostic value of compression ultrasonograpy in patients with suspected recurrent deep vein thrombosis. Thromb Haemost. 2002; 88: 402-406.

Rademaker J, griesshaber V, Hidajat N, Oestmann JW & Felix R. Combined CT pulmonary angiography and venography for diagnosis of pulmonary embolism and deep vein thrombosis: radiation dose. Journal Thoracic Imaging. 2001; 16: 297-299.

Razavi MK,Hansch EC, Kee ST, Sze DY, Semba CP & Dake MD. Chronically occluded inferior vena cavae: endovascular treatment. Radiology. 2000; 214: 133-138.

Remi- Jardin, Remy J, Baghaie F, Fribourg M, Artoud D & Duhamel A. Clinical value of thin collimation in the diagnostic work up of pulmonary embolism. Am J Roentgenol. 2000; 175: 407-411.

Righini M. Is it worth diagnosing and treating distal deep venous thrombosis? No. J Thromb Haemost. 2007; 5(suppl 1): 55-59.

Righini M, Le gal G, Aujesky D, roy PM, Sanchez O, Verschuren F, Rutschmann O, Nonent M, Cornuz J, Thys F, Le Manach CP, Revel MP, Polleti PA, Meyer G, Mottier G, Perneger T, Bounameaux H & Perrier A. Diagnosis of pulmonary embolism by multidetector CT alone or combined with venous ultrasonography of the leg: a randomised non- inferiority trial. Lancet. 2008; 371(9621): 1343-1352.

Righini M, Le Gal G, Aujesky D, Roy PM, Sanchez O & Verschuren F. Complete venous ultrasound in outpatients with suspected pulmonary embolism. J Thromb Haemost. 2009; 7(3): 406- 412.

Roditi G & Fink C. Venous MR imaging with blood pool agents. Eur Rad 2009; 18(suppl 5): 3-12.

Schellong SM. Distal DVT: worth diagnosing. Yes. J Thromb Haemost. 2007; 5(suppl 1): 51-54.

Schoepf UJ & Costello P. CT angiography for diagnosis of pulmonary embolism: state of the art. Radiology. 2004; 230(2): 329-337.

Schoepf UJ, Kucher N, Kipfmueller F, Quiroz R, Costello P & Goldhaber SZ. Circulation. 2004; 110: 3276- 3280.

Sevitt S & Gallagher N. Venous thrombosis and pulmonary embolism. A clinico-pathological study in injured and burned patients. British Journal Surgery. 1961; 48: 475-489.

Spritzer CE. Progress in MR imaging of the venous system. Perspectives in vascular surgery and endovascular therapy. 2009; 21(2): 105-116.

Streiff MB. Vena caval filters: a comprehensive review. Blood. 2000; 95: 3669-3677.

Vedantham S, Millward SF, Cardella JF, Hofmann LV, Razavi MK, Grassi CJ, Sacks D & Kinney TB. Society of Interventional Radiology position statement: treatment of acute iliofemoral deep vein thrombosis with use of adjunctive catheter directed intrathrombus thrombolysis. J vasc Interven Rad. 2004; 20 (Suppl 7):332-335.

Wells PS, Hirsh J, Anderson DR, Lensing AW, Foster G, Kearon C, Weitz J, D'Ovidio R, Cogo A, Prandoni P, Girolami A & Jinsberg A. Accuracy of clinical assessment of deep venous thrombosis. Lancet. 1995; 345: 1315-1380.

6

Emerging Issues in Deep Vein Thrombosis; (DVT) in Liver Disease and in Developing Countries

Farjah H. AlGahtani and Abdel Galil Abdel Gader
College of Medicine and King Khalid University Hospital
Kind Saud University, Riyadh
Kingdom of Saudi Arabia

1. Introduction

This chapter addresses a new and emerging aspect of health in developing countries—one that poses a serious and growing burden on individuals, health systems, and economies of poor countries but is largely preventable. Deep Vein thrombosis (DVT) is a major medical, social and economic problem in developed countries, but in developing countries scanty information is available. Blood clots such as thrombus in a deep vein in the lower limb is the most serious unexpected killer of hospitalized patients in developed countries and over the years this has led to elaboration of numerous strategies directed towards reducing the risks of formation of such thrombi and treating them when they occur. This area has been covered extensively in the literature emerging from developed countries, and little is known about the pattern and scale of problem in developing countries.

Another area that will be covered in this chapter relates to hypercoagulation in chronic liver disease which is poorly understood till recently. Because of the relatively uncommon occurrence of overt clinical thrombosis in patients with liver disease, and the complexity of the haemostatic mechanism, in addition to the fact that clinicians often perceive that these patients are at a reduced risk for venous thromboembolism, DVT in liver disease is an understudied problem. In this chapter, we aim to discuss DVT from two aspects; DVT in liver disease, and DVT in developing countries.

2. Deep vein thrombosis in liver disease

Chronic liver diseases in the United States account for 400,000 hospitalizations and 27,000 deaths (Kochanek et al., 2004, Kozak et al. 2005). This area needs to be revisited with respect to DVT in liver disease, where viral liver disease is more common in developing countries than in developed countries (Williams,2006.). Patients with advanced liver disease (a failing liver) display a complexity of haemostatic abnormalities often occurring concurrently including coagulopathic, hypercoagulable, and hyperfibrinolytic disorders and increased platelet activation. Recent literature has revealed that hypercoagulability plays an important role in many aspects of acute and chronic liver disease (Nieuwdrop et al .2005, 2004). The resulting clinical state is determined by which component of these complex haemostatic mechanisms predominates.

2.1 Pathophysiology of the coagulation mechanism

Under normal conditions, the blood circulates freely within the vascular system. However, when blood escapes to extravascular sites after blood vessel injury or it becomes pathologically challenged, haemostasis may be activated ending in the formation of blood (fibrin) clot. This process is finely regulated by positive and negative feedback loops that control fibrin clot formation .

For many decades the accepted blood coagulation mechanism has been based on the concept of the coagulation cascade model that describes the interactions of the coagulation factors along two pathways: the intrinsic pathway which is triggered by the contact of blood with a foreign surface, and the extrinsic pathway which is triggered by exposure of the blood to the transmembrane receptor tissue factor (TF) which binds to clotting factor VIIa to form TF/FVIIa complex. Both pathways meet at the level of clotting factor X after which the common pathway progresses until the generation of the thrombin and the formation of fibrin clot. However, while the cascade model delineates the interactions between the coagulation proteins and provides a framework for interpreting the common screening coagulation tests (particularly the PT and the APTT), it is gradually been realized that the cascade model suffers from many limitations, as it fails to explain convincingly how hemostatic activation occurs *in vivo*. For example, this model cannot explain why hemophiliacs bleed when they have an intact factor VIIa/TF "extrinsic" pathway.

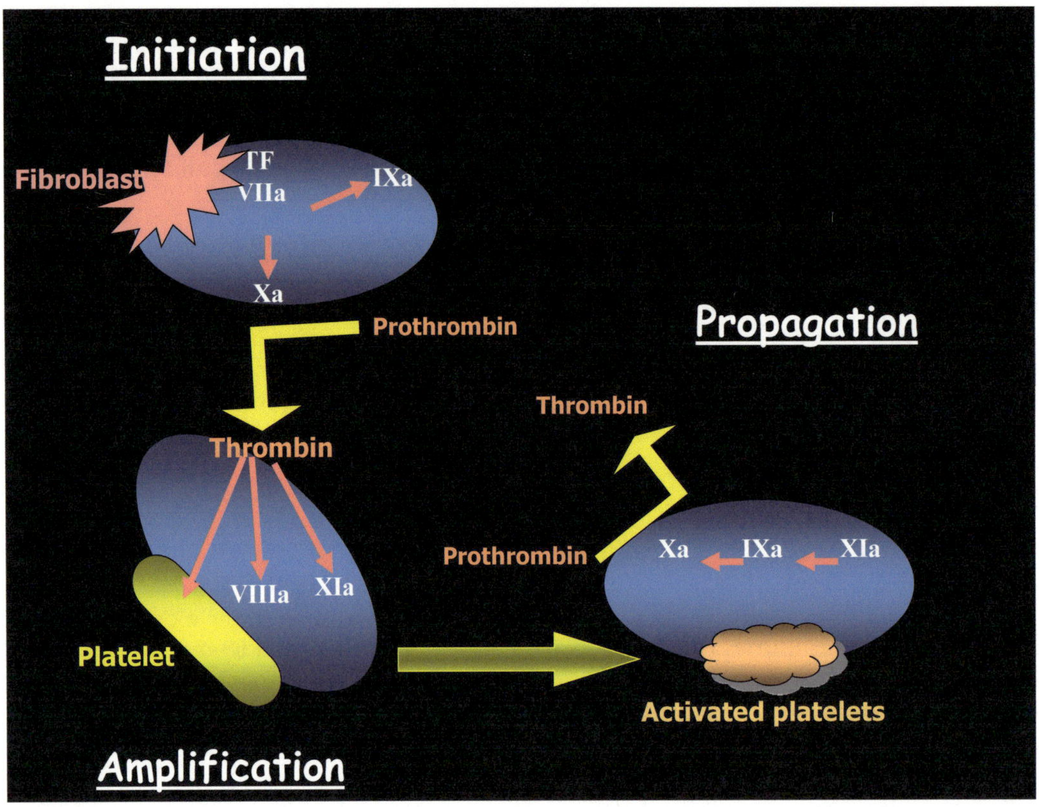

Fig. 1. Cell-based model of the mechanism of blood coagulation

The classical cascade model of the coagulation cascade is being replaced by the new, cell-based model of coagulation (Roberts et al.,2006) (Fig. 1), which emphasizes the interaction of coagulation proteins with cell surfaces of platelets, subendothelial cells and the endothelium. According to this model the coagulation is initiated (The Initiation Phase) by the formation of a complex between tissue factor (TF) exposed on the surface of fibroblasts as a result of a vessel wall injury, and activated factor VII (FVIIa), normally present in the circulating blood. The TF-FVIIa complexes convert FX to FXa on the TF bearing fibroblasts. FXa then activates prothrombin (FII) to thrombin (FIIa). The next phase is the Amplification Phase in which this limited amount of thrombin activates FVIII, FV, FXI and platelets, on the surface of blood platelets. Thrombin-activated platelets change shape, and as a result will expose negatively charged membrane phospholipids, which form the perfect template for the assembly of various clotting factors and full thrombin generation involving FVIIIa and FIXa (The Propagation Phase). According to this cell-based model the tissue factor (TF) extrinsic pathway is the principal cellular initiator of normal blood coagulation in vivo (Mackman et al. 2007), and the major regulator of haemostasis and thrombogenesis, with the intrinsic pathway, playing an amplification role.

2.2 The role extrinsic pathway in thrombosis

From the above account, it is clear for clotting to occur blood must be exposed to tissue factor. Therefore for thrombosis to set such exposure will happen when the blood vessel is injured and blood comes in contact with variety of cells that express TF, in particular monocytes and neutrophils. Endothelial cells also express TF mostly due to binding TF-expressing microparticles (MPs- see below) (Schwertz et al. 2006). More prominence has recently been given circulating TF-positive microparticles (MPs) (Morel et al. 2006). These are small membrane fragments released from activated or apoptotic vascular cells (Rauch et al., 2007).

There is strong evidence to show that TF-positive MPs contribute to thrombosis in patients with cancer (Rauch et al.,2007, Tesselaar et al.,2007), cardiovascular disease (Misumi et al., 1998), and sickle cell disease (Shet et al., 2003). Many cell types can generate circulating TF-positive MPs including leucocytes, endothelial cells, platelets and vascular smooth muscles and these MPs can be recruited to a thrombus and enhance its growth in both arterial and venous thrombosis (Schwertz et al. 2006).

2.3 Pathophysiology of coagulation mechanism in liver disease

In case of severe liver disease the protein levels that are synthesized in the liver are reduced as the synthetic capacity is lost. Thus, levels of both pro-and anticoagulant proteins decrease as liver disease progresses. A relatively balanced reduction in pro-and anticoagulant activity does not result in a net hyper-or hypocoagulable state until the loss of liver synthetic capacity is severe. However, the ability of the haemostatic system to maintain haemostasis when stressed is progressively reduced. Thus, the balance between bleeding and thrombosis becomes increasingly precarious as protein synthetic capacity is lost .

In addition, the important role of endothelial function in maintaining haemostatic balance means that local endothelial dysfunction can lead to the development of a hypercoagulable state at one anatomic site. Thrombotic complications can be seen in the portal and mesenteric systems (Mammen et al., 1992), hepatic veins (Singh et al., 2000), and peripherally in the extremities with associated pulmonary emboli (Northup et al., 2006). The prothrombotic state may be involved in other sequelae of chronic liver disease, including hepatic parenchymal extinction, fibrosis and portopulmonary hypertension. Thus, a prolonged prothrombin time does not adequately portray the levels of other clotting factors, particularly factors VIII, X and II that can be more than adequate to promote clot formation (Violi et al., 1995). As well, it is known that the coagulation disorders associated with falling liver can induce further hepatic damage, namely, parenchymal extinction. Wanless et al (Wanless et al., 1995) have clearly demonstrated the histopathologic evidence of the secondary hepatic damage caused by circulatory disturbances due to thrombotic occlusion of intrahepatic blood vessels (microvascular thrombosis).

2.4 The prevalence of deep vein thrombosis in liver disease

Deep vein thromboses in the lower extremity are common in the general medicine population without liver disease and range from 4% to 12% in inpatients (Anderson et al., 1991, Stein et al., 2002). Patients with cirrhosis share many of the same risk factors as hospitalized general medicine inpatients, including prolonged immobility, obesity, recent surgical procedures and malignancies. The presence of anticardiolipin and antiphospholipid antibodies have also been documented in patients with cirrhosis (Violi et al., 1994) and hepatitis C (Prieto et al., 1996). Hyperfibrinolysis, perhaps related to persistence of tissue plasminogen activator, is also prevalent in decompensated cirrhosis (Gunawan et al., 2006). It is not commonly symptomatic that DVT events may occur in patients with liver cirrhosis despite the coagulopathy of liver disease and clinical experience suggests this is the case. Several studies have shown lower levels of antithrombin, protein C and protein S in cirrhosis patients compared with controls (Mammen EF et al., 1992, De Caterina et al., 1993, Vukovich et al., 1995, Walker et al., 1990, Zurborn et al., 1988). Indeed, the diminution in the circulating levels of these inhibitors was noted in the early stages of liver disease and well before the setting of its chronic stages as in liver cirrhosis (Al-Ghumlas et., 2005, Abdo et al., 2010),

The literature is sparse in the area of clinical DVT in cirrhosis and is limited to case reports and a single case-controlled study (Ben Ari et al., 1997) comparing hospitalized cirrhotic patients with and without DVT. In this retrospective study, a new DVT or PE was diagnosed in appropriately 0.5% of all inpatients with documented cirrhosis despite 21% of these patients being on some form of DVT prophylaxis. While the rate of VTE is lower than expected in the general medicine population, these data show that patients with liver cirrhosis are not immune to VTE. It is plausible that this underestimates its true incidence. This could be explained as symptoms of VTE in the decompensated liver cirrhosis patients, particularly edema and dyspnea are common and not specific. Diagnosis requires a high index of suspicion and accurate radiologic testing methods.

2.5 Clinical presentation

The symptoms of DVT in the decompensated cirrhotic patient, edema, and dyspnea are common and not specific; those patients have similar risk factors as medical inpatients. Patients with liver disease can present to medical services with complaints of leg edema, leg pain dyspnea, and abdominal pain.

2.6 Diagnostic and treatment challenges

Diagnosing DVT in patients with liver disease need high level suspicion, presence of laboratory investigation such as D-dimer and radiological procedure of Duplex ultrasound; thus elevation of coagulation markers such as the prothrombin time and partial thromboplastin time does not safeguard against thrombotic events. Serum albumin level was independently associated with the occurrence of thrombosis (Ben Ari et al., 1997, Senzolo et al., 2009).

2.7 DVT prophylaxis in liver disease

Current guidelines from American College of Chest Physicians (ACCP) DVT prophylaxis do not specifically comment on the advanced liver disease patients' population (Senzolo et al., 2009). The lack of specific guidelines is because of the perceived risk of bleeding complications, sense of auto-anticoagulation, impaired laboratory tests, and most important lack of clinical trials to support the practice of routine use of DVT prophylaxis in liver disease/cirrhosis and its safety, particularly the risk of bleeding is unknown. Recently two studies (Senzolo et al., 2009, Bechman et al .,2010).) found that the prophylactic use of LMWH in patients with cirrhosis and who are at high risk of thrombosis, to be safe from the risk of bleeding. Actually Bechman et al .,2010 revealed for the first time, to our knowledge, there are apparent decreased efficacy of LMWH in cirrhotic patients, which may indeed argue for studying the appropriate dosing in cirrhotic patients (Bechman et al., 2010).

In a recent study, approximately 76% of the cirrhotic patients included in the cohort received neither pharmacological nor mechanical DVT prophylaxis. No significant differences in the incidence of VTE were observed between the group that received pharmacologic or mechanical prophylaxis and the group that did not receive prophylaxis (Abdulaziz et al., 2011). The utilization of DVT prophylaxis was suboptimal.

Until the risks and benefits of VTE prophylaxis are established in this particular population, the VTE prophylaxis cannot be withdrawn in the cirrhotic population at present time. (Senzolo et al., 2009).

3. Deep vein thrombosis in developing countries

Deep vein thrombosis is a preventable disease and the incidence of VTE is 1-3 per 100 per year (Nordstrőm et al., 1992; Anderson et al., 1991; Oger et al., 2000; Cushman et al., 2004,). DVT is a significant cause of morbidity and mortality and without prophylaxis, the risk of a DVT event is especially high in patients admitted to medical orthopedic surgery wards (Geerts et al., 2008), with an incidence of venographic DVT without prophylaxis estimated at 40% to 60% (Geerts et al., 2008). Given its silent nature; the incidence, prevalence, morbidity and mortality rates of DVT are probably under-estimated in developing countries. Although most patients survive DVT, yet serious and costly long-term complications may occur; almost one-third of patients will suffer from venous stasis syndrome (postphlebitic syndrome) (Prandoni et al., 1996). DVT is a major burden on US healthcare systems: estimates put costs at nearly $500 million per year (Hawkins, 2004).

3.1 Scale of DVT problem in the developing countries

DVT in developed counties is considered a public health problem and over the years this has led to elaboration of numerous strategies directed towards reducing the risks of DVT.

Given this to be the situation in the developed countries, the the magnitude of the problem would be much lower in the developing countries. Indeed many population studies that are carried in Western developed countries documented the lower incidence of VTE in Asians and Hispanics compared to Caucasians (Kearon 2001, White et al 2009).

Although there is strong evidence that the prevalence of venous thrombo-embolism (VTE) varies significantly among different ethnic/racial groups, the genetic, physiologic and/or clinical basis for these differences remain largely undefined (White et al ., 2009).

Identifying the scale of DVT in developing countries is difficult due to scanty and conflicting available published literature on the scale of the problem, the diagnostic tools, management and treatment challenges facing these countries. Most published information on the DVT was generated from small hospital-based studies that documented DVT as a significant complication of orthopedic surgery particularly total knee arthroplasty (Chung et al 2010, Ko et al. 2003, Leizorovicz et al 2005, Sen et al 2011, Sen et al 2011), and general hospital patients (Ogeng'o et al 2001, Angchaisuksiri et al 2007, Sakon et al. 2006, Lee et al. 2009). Essentially all these and other similar studies advocated the importance of thrombohphylaxis to avoid the risk of VTE.

As to population studies very few could be identified and almost all from Asian Far Eastern countries particularly China and Korea. In one study from Korea the incidence of VTE, DVT and PE per 100,000 individuals was found to be 8.83, 3.91 and 3.74 in 2004 and increased to 13.8, 5.31 and 7.01 in 2008 (Jang et al 2001). Another recent study from Hong Kong documented an annual incidence of of VTE at 16.6 events per 100,000 populations (Lui et al 2002). Another Chinese study reported the incidence of DVT and PE of 17.1 and 3.9 per 100,000 populations (Cheuk et al 2004). The incidence of DVT in all three studies is almost one tenth that reported from developed counties; yet the problem of DVT remains to be a health problem that clinicians should be aware of.

3.2 Challengesof DVT In developing countries

3.2.1 Health disparity in the developing world

There is remarkable disparity in standards of the health care among developing countries, especially the percentage of the Grand National Product that is expended in health care. Also, when comparing developed to developing countries, some countries like Saudi Arabia, Egypt, Jordan and the UAE could take the lead: Egypt (5.8%), Saudi Arabia (4%), Pakistan (2.4%) and India (4.8%) have limited total expenditure on health, compared to the United States (15.2%), Switzerland (11.5%), France (10.1%) and Norway (10.3%) (WHO Health Report, 2006). Such disparity shows up as unequal distribution of healthcare personnel and deficiency in training programs in the developing world. This is also reflected on the life expectancy and disease outcome and survival in these countries.

3.2.2 Registries

In reviewing the available evidence on the epidemiology of deep vein thrombosis (DVT) in the developing countries, it is quite clear that there are few on-going registries that track data on patients with DVT. Most of those registries are hospital-based rather than national. For example in Saudi Arabia there is the Saudi Thrombosis and Familial Thrombophilia (S-TAFT) Registry (Saour et al., 2009), which is considered the only registry in Gulf Region and perhaps the Middle East. In developing countries there is very scanty and non-conclusive data on the prevalence, incidence, risk factors, genetic predisposition, distribution of DVT occurrences among different age groups and gender, and the burden of DVT on different patient groups (e.g. post-surgical, pregnancy etc…). Most importantly, how physicians manage DVT is also unknown and no cost-effective analysis is available on the current treatment regimens deployed in these countries. Such registry for DVT should include demographic data and extensive medical history (past and present). Detailed information on environmental, lifestyle and occupational factors could help identifying certain groups who are at increased risk of developing DVT or its complications. There is also need to accumulate laboratory data which should include blood group, factor VIII, inherited thrombophilic defects (such as factor V Leiden and prothrombin mutations), fibrinogen level, as well as routine laboratory investigations. Screening for inherited thrombophilia and other genetic diseases that predispose to DVT is crucial and has gained popularity worldwide. The available data on the prevalence of thrombophilic risk factors for VTE, particularly factor V Leidin, prothrombin G20210A, mutations C677T methylenetetra-hydrfolate reductase and hyperhomocysteinaemia) in developing countries is scanty but agree on their rarity and much lower prevalence than in developed countries (Jun et al 2006, et al 2002, Lim et al 2004, Omar et al 2007).

3.2.3 Epidemiology

The burden of DVT in the developing world is unknown due to lack of documentation and large-scale research projects aiming at identifying the different epidemiology aspects. Some of the developing countries (Saudi Arabia, United Arab of Emirates and the rest of the Arab Gulf countries), have the financial resources to setup such registries. However, setting up registries requires substantial training to the current and future personnel who are working fulltime in maintaining them. Policymakers, represented by the governments, academic medical centers and, most importantly, local and regional funding agencies, must work together in order to consider emphasizing DVT as a public health problem so that the appropriate increasing proportion of public health resources is reallocated to address DVT and its related issues.

3.2.4 The cost and value of pharmacoeconomics research

Registries will not only allow tracking DVT in terms of its epidemiology, but also how much it burdens each country's economy. Pharmacoeconomic analysis is of great value in the evaluation of the cost of medical care. For example, cost-identification analysis seeks to identify the cost of providing the treatment of the disease. Cost-minimization analysis seeks to identify the least expensive alternative intervention to get the same outcome after treating the disease. Most importantly, cost-of-illness analysis estimates the total financial burden of DVT or its associated disability (e.g. reduced working hours, sick days, less life-expectancy etc…) to the country. This is done by estimating the total cost of diagnosing DVT, its management and the DVT-associated lost productivity. Cost-benefit analysis evaluates one or more treatment regimens in terms of pure currency expressions (e.g. dollars). This will allow the governments to identify which diseases cost higher. For example, in this form of analysis, we can compare the cost of DVT awareness, prevention and treatment to the cost of chronic kidney disease. Such analysis guides the policymakers to identify the top ranked diseases affecting the economy and allocates more dollars to combat them.

3.2.5 Awareness and education of the public

We believe that intensive awareness and educational campaigns supported by the media and endorsed by the governments will contribute in limiting the DVT problem. For example, school teachers and cashiers should be advised, and allowed, to move around during their working hours since their job entails long standing hours. Educational initiatives in the airports and airplanes in the form of brochures or brief videos are encouraged to increase travelers' awareness. With such efforts, it might be expected that there would be a reduction in the number of individuals who develop DVT which, in turn, might reduce the number of patients requiring treatment and follow up as post thrombotic syndrome long run.

3.2.6 DVT diagnosis

The use of pretest probability scoring system such as Geneva score (Kelly et al., 2003), Wells score (Wells et al., 1997) to diagnosis DVT is considered commendable efforts towards early diagnosis. This could be germane to the developing countries in reducing the economic cost that may have the impact on the scale of DVT. This will also help the researchers and clinicians, policymakers to make proper assessment of the magnitude of the problem, management, and prevention strategies.

3.2.7 Clinical and research training programs

We believe that the lack of training programs in clinical hematology in the developing countries is contributing to the problem of misdiagnosing and under-diagnosing of DVT. Unlike the Western countries, such training programs are limited to the medical schools which may not meet the need of any country to well-trained hematologists. It is important that special emphasis on undergraduate medical education, by inclusion of management and prevention strategies in the medical curriculum, will increase the early reporting of DVT by different medical specialists. On the other hand, training programs should be developed to train the allied health professionals (e.g. nurses, technicians etc…) on aiding the clinicians in diagnosing DVT. Establishing a strong research infrastructure in terms of highly trained and qualified fulltime research personnel, research facilities and budgets will help to bridge the knowledge gaps in DVT in developing countries.

3.2.8 Cultural and social issues

There are some cultural and social issues that may contribute to the underreporting of the DVT in the developing countries. Having a chronic disease may represent a stigma. Being diagnosed with DVT is considered a social disability. Women usually hide having any kind of disease especially if it is DVT-related pregnancy which may affect her ability of childbearing.

4. Conclusion

In conclusion, we believe that addressing DVT as a regional public health problem in the developing countries should take a multi-dimensional approach targeting the epidemiology of DVT and implementation of cost-effective preventive and therapeutic programs.

5. References

Abdulaziz Aldawood, Yaseen Arabi, Abdulrahman Aljumah, Alawi Alsaadi, Asgar Rishu, Hasan Aldorzi, Saad Alqahtani, Mohammad Alsultan, and Afaf Felemban. The incidence of venous thromboembolism and practice of deep venous thrombosis prophylaxis in hospitalized cirrhotic patients. Thromb J. 2011; 9: 1

Abeer K.Al-Ghumlas AK, Gader AMA, Al Faleh FZ. Haemostatic abnormalities in liver disease: could some haemostatic tests be useful as liver function tests? Blood Coag Fibrinol. 2005;16:329-335

Al Sayegh F, Almahmeed W, Al Humood S, Marashi M, Bahr A, Al Mahdi H, Bakir S, Al Farhan M. Global Risk Profile Verification in Patients with Venous Thromboembolism (GRIP VTE) in 5 Gulf countries. Clin Appl Thromb Hemost. 2009 May-Jun;15(3):289-96.

Anderson FA Jr, Wheeler HB, Goldberg RJ, Hosmer DW, Patwardhan NA, Jovanovic B, Forcier A, Dalen JE. A population-based perspective of the hospital incidence and case-fatality rates of deep vein thrombosis and pulmonary embolism. The Worcester DVT Study. Arch Intern Med 1991; 151: 933–8.

Angchaisuksiri P, Atichartakarn V, Aryurachai K, Archararit N, Rachakom B, Atamasirikul K, Tiraganjana A. Risk factors of venous thromboembolism in thai patients. Int J Hematol. 2007 Dec;86(5):397-402.

Angchaisuksiri P, Pingsuthiwong S, Sura T, Aryuchai K, Busabaratana M, Atichartakarn V. Prevalence of the C677T methylenetetra- hydrofolate reductase mutation in Thai patients with deep vein thrombosis. Acta Haematol. 2000;103(4):191-6.

Bechmann Lars P. , Matthias Sichau, Marc Wichert, Guido Gerken1, Knut Kro¨ ger, and Philip Hilgard. Low-molecular-weight heparin in patientswith advanced cirrhosis. Liver International 2010 :ISSN 1478-3223

Ben Ari Z, Panagou M, Patch D, Bates S, Osman E, Pasi J et al. (1997) Hypercoagulability in patients with primary biliary cirrhosis and primarysclerosing cholangitis evaluated by thrombelastography. J Hepato l26:554–559.

Cushman M, Tsai AW, White RH, Heckbert SR, Rosamond WD, Enright P, Folsom AR. Deep vein thrombosis and pulmonary embolism in two cohorts: the longitudinal investigation of thromboembolism etiology. Am J Med 2004; 117:19–25.

Chung LH, Chen WM, Chen CF, Chen Th, Liu CL. Deep Vein Thrombosis after total knee arthoplasty in asian patients without prophylactic antiagoagulation.Orthopedics. 2011 Jan 3;34(1):15.

Cheuk BL, Cheung GC, Cheng SW. Epidemiology of Venous Thromboembolism in a Chinese Population. Br J Surg. 2004 Apr;91(4):424-8.

De Caterina M, Tarantino G, Farina C, Arena A, Di Maro G, Esposito P, Scopacasa F. Haemostasis unbalance in Pugh-scored liver cirrhosis: characteristic changes of plasma levels of protein C versus protein S. Haemostasis, 1993; 23: 229–35.

Dhillon KS, Askander A, Doraismay S. Postoperative Deep-Vein Thrombosis in Asian patients is not a rarity: a prospective study of 88 patients with no prophylaxis. J Bone Joint Surg Br. 1996 May;78(3):427-30.

Gader AA, Haggaz AE, Adam I. Epidemiology of Deep Venous Thrombosis during pregnancy and puerperium in Sudanese Women. Vasc Health Risk Manag. 2009;5(1):85-7

Geerts WH, Bergqvist D, Pineo GF, Heit JA, Samama CM, Lassen MRet al. (2008) Prevention of venous thromboembolism: American Collegeof Chest Physicians Evidence-Based Clinical Practice Guidelines (8thedition). Chest 133 (6 Suppl.):381S–453S.

Gunawan B, Runyon B. The efficacy and safety of epsilon-aminocaproic acid treatment in patients with cirrhosis and hyperfibrinolysis. Aliment Pharmacol Ther 2006; 23: 115–20.

Hawkins D. Pharmacoeconomics of thrombosis management. Pharmacotherapy. 2004;24(7 pt 2):95S-99S.

Jang MJ, Bang SM, Oh D. Incidence of venous thromboembolism in Korea: from the Health Insurance Review and Assessment Service database. J Thromb Haemost. 2011 Jan;9(1):85-91.

Jun ZJ, Ping T, Lei Y, Li L, Ming SY, Jing W. Prevalence of factor V Leiden and prothrombin G20210A mutations in Chinese patients with deep venous thrombosis and pulmonary embolism. Clin Lab Haematol. 2006 Apr;28(2):111-6.

Kearon C. Epidemiology of venous thromboembolism. Semin Vasc Med. 2001;1(1):7-26.

Kelly J, Hunt BJ., The utility of pretest probability assessment in patients with clinically suspected venous thromboembolism. J Thromb Haemost. 2003 Sep;1(9):1888-96.

Kochanek KD, Murphy SL, Anderson RN, Scott C. Deaths: final data for 2002. Natl Vital Stat Rep. 2004; 53 (5): 1 - 115

Ko PS, Chan WF, Siu TH, Khoo J, Wu WC, Lam JJ. Deep Venous Thrombosis after total hip or knee arthroplasty in a "low-risk" Chinese population. Arthroplasty. 2003 Feb;18(2)174-9.

Kozak LJ , Owings MF , Hall MJ . National Hospital Discharge Survey: 2002 annual summary with detailed diagnosis and procedure data . Vital Health Stat 13 . 2005 ; 158 : 1 - 199 .

Lee AD, Stephen E, Agarwal S, Premkumar P. Venous Thromboembolism in India. Eur J Vasc Endovasc Surg. 2009 Apr;37(4):482-5. Epub 2009 Feb 8.

Leizorovicz A, Turpie AG, Cohen AT, Wong L, Yoo MC, Dans A; SMART Study Group. Epidemiology of venous thromboembolism in Asian patients undergoing major orthopedic surgery without thromboprophylaxis. The SMART study. J Thromb Haemost. 2005 Jan;3(1):28-34.

Lim YW, Chong KC, Chong I, Low CO, See HF, Lam KS. Deep vein thrombosis following hip fracture and prevalence of hyperhomocysteinaemia in the elderly. Ann Acad Med Singapore. 2004 Mar;33(2):235-8.

Liu HS, Kho BC, Chan JC, Cheung FM, Lau KY, Choi FP, Wu WC, Yau TK. Venous thromboembolism in the Chinese population--experience in a regional hospital in Hong Kong. Hong Kong Med J. 2002 Dec;8(6):400-5.

Mackman N, Tilly RE, Key NS. The role of the extrinisic pathway of blood coagulation in hemostasis and thrombosis. Arterioscler Thromb Vasc Biol. 2007;27:1687-1693

Mammen EF. Coagulation abnormalities in liver disease. Hematol Oncol Clin North Am 1992; 6: 1247–57.

Marco Senzolo, Maria Teresa Sartori , Ton Lisman.Should we give thromboprophylaxis to patients with liver cirrhosis and coagulopathy?.HPB 2009, 11, 459–464.

Misumi K, Ogawa H, Yasue H, Soejima H, Suefuji H, Nishiyama K, Takazoe K, Kugiyama K, Tsuji I, Kumeda K, Nakamura S. Comparison of plasma tissue factor levels in unstable and stable angina pectoris. Am J Cardiol. 1998;81:22–26

Morel O, Toti F, Hugel B, Bakouboula B et al. Procoagulant microparticles: disrupting the vascular homoestasisequation?ArteriosclerThrombVasc Biol;2006;26:2594-2604

Nieuwdorp M, Stroes ES, Meijers JC, Buller H. Hypercogulability in the metabolic syndrome. Curr Opin Pharmacol 2005; 155-9.

Nordstr¨om M, Lindblad B, Bergqvist D, Kjellstr¨om T. A prospective study of the incidence of deep-vein thrombosis within a defined urban population. J Intern Med 1992; 232:155–160.

Northup PG, McMahon MM, Ruhl AP, Altschuler SE, Volk-Bednarz A, Caldwell SH, Berg CL. Coagulopathy does not fully protect hospitalized cirrhosis patients from peripheral venous thromboembolism. Am J Gatroenterol 2006; 101: 1524-8.

Ogeng'o JA, Obimbo MM, Olabu BO, Gatonga PM, Ong'era D. Pulmonary thromboembolism in an East African tertiary referral hospital. J Thromb Thrombolysis. 2011 Jun 12. [Epub ahead of print]

Oger E. Incidence of venous thromboembolism: a community-based study in western France. ThrombHaemost 2000; 83:657–60.

Omar S, Ghorbel IB, Feki H, Souissi M, Feki M, Houman H, Kaabachi N. (Hyperhomocysteinemia is associated with deep venous thrombosis of the lower extremities in Tunisian patients. Clin Biochem. 2007 Jan;40(1-2):41-5.

Prandoni P, Lensing AW, Cogo A et al The long-term clinical course of acute deep venous thrombosis. Ann Intern Med 1996, 7-125:1

Prieto J, Yuste JR, Beloqui O, Civeira MP, Riezu JI, Aguirre B, Sangro B. Anticardiolipin antibodies in chronic hepatitis C: implication of hepatitis C virus as the cause of the antiphospholipid syndrome. Hepatology 1996; 23: 199–204.

Rauch U, Antoniak S. Tissue factor-positive micoprticles in blood associated with coagulopathy in cancer. Thromb Haemost.2007;97:9-10)

Roberts HR, Hoffman M, Monroe DM. A cell-based model of thrombin generation SeminThrombHemost. 2006 Apr;32Suppl 1:32-8.

Roger Williams. Global Challenges in Liver Disease. Heptology 2006;44:521-526.

Sakon M, Maehara Y, Yoshikawa H, Akaza H. Incidence of venous thromboembolism following major abdominal surgery: a multi-center, prospective epidemiological study in Japan. J Thromb Haemost. 2006 Mar;4(3):581-6.

Saour JN, Shoukri MM, MammoThe Saudi Thrombosis and Familial Thrombophilia Registry. Design, rational, and preliminary results. LA. Saudi Med J. 2009 Oct;30(10):1286-90.

Schwertz H, Tollley ND, Foulks JM, Denis MM, et al. Signal-dependant splicing of tissue factor pre-mRNA modulates the thrombogenicity of human platelets. J Exp Med. 2006;203:2433-2440.

Sen RK, Kumar A, Tripathy SK, Aggarwal S, Khandelwal N, Manoharan SR. Risk of postoperative venous thromboembolism in Indian patients sustaining pelvi-acetabular injury. Int Orthop. 2011 Jul;35(7):1057-63.

Sen RK, Tripathy SK, Singh AK. Is routine thromboprophylaxis justified among Indian patients sustaining major orthopedic trauma? A systematic review. Indian J Orthop. 2011 May;45(3):197-207.

Sen RK, Kumar A, Tripathy SK, Aggarwal S, Khandelwal N, Manoharan SR. Risk of Postoperative Venous Thromboembolism in Indian patients sustaining pelvi-acetabular injury. Int Orthop. 2011 Jul;35(7):1057-63. Epub 2010 Jul 24.

Shet AS, Aras O, Gupta K, Hass MJ, Rausch DJ, Saba N, Koopmeiners L, Key NS, Hebbel RP. Sickle blood contains tissue factor-positive microparticles derived from endothelial cells and monocytes. Blood. 2003;102:2678 -2683

Singh V, Sinha SK, Nain CK, Bambery P, Kaur U, Verna S, Chawla YK, Singh K, Budd-Chiari syndrome: our experience of 71 patients. J GastroenrolHepatol 2000;15: 550-4.

Stein PD, Patel KC, Kalra NK, Petrina M, Savarapu P, Furlong JW Jr, Steele RD Jr, Check FE. Estimated incidence of acute pulmonary embolism in a community/teaching general hospital. Chest 2002; 121: 802–5.

Tesselaar ME, Romijn FP, van dL, I, Prins FA, Bertina RM, Osanto S Microparticle-associated tissue factor activity: a link between cancer and thrombosis J Thromb Haemost. 2007 Mar;5(3):520-7.

Violi F, Ferro D, Basili S, Cimminiello C, Saliola M, Vezza E, Cordova C. Prognostic value of clotting and fibrinolytic systems in a follow-up of 165 liver cirrhotic patients. CALC Group. Hepatology 1995; 22: 96–100.

Violi F, Ferro D, Basili S, D'Angelo A, Mazzola G, Quintarelli C, Cordova C. Relation between lupus anticoagulant and splanchnic venous thrombosis in cirrhosis of the liver. BMJ 1994; 309: 239–40.

Vukovich T, Teufelsbauer H, Fritzer M, Kreuzer S, Knoflach P. Hemostasis activation in patients with liver cirrhosis. Thromb Res1995; 77: 271–8.

Walker FJ. Protein C deficiency in liver disease. Ann Clin Lab Sci 1990; 20: 106–12.

Wanless IR, Wong F, Blendis LM, Greig P, Heathcote EJ, Levy G. Hepatic and portal vein thrombosis in cirrhosis: possible role in development of parenchymal extinction and portal hypertension. Hepatology 1995; 21: 1238–47.

Wang CJ, Wang JW, Chen LM, Chen HS, Yang BY, Cheng SM. Deep Vein Thrombosis after total knee athroplasty. J Formos Med Assoc. 2000 Nov;99(11):848-53

Wells PS, Anderson DR, Bormanis J, Guy F, Mitchell M, Gray L, et al. Value of assessment of pretest probability of deep-vein thrombosis in clinical management. Lancet 1997;350:1796.

White RH, Keenan CR. Effects of race and ethnicity on the incidence of venous thromboembolism. Thromb Res. 2009;123 Suppl 4:S11-7).

World Health Organization The world health report 2006: Working Together For Health. ISBN 92 4 156317 6 (NLM classification: WA 530.1)

Zenzolo M, Sartori MT, Lisman T. Should we give thromboprophylaxis to patients with liver cirrhosis and coagulopathy? HPB (Oxford). 2009 Sp;11(6):459-65.

Zurborn KH, Kirch W, Bruhn HD. Immunological and functional determination of the protease inhibitors, protein C and antithrombin III, in liver cirrhosis and in neoplasia. Thromb Res 1988; 52: 325–36.

7

Venous Thromboembolism Prophylaxis in Cancer Patients

Hikmat Abdel-Razeq
King Hussein Cancer Center, Amman, Jordan

1. Introduction

Venous Thromboembolism (VTE) is a common disease, comprising the life-threatening pulmonary embolism (PE) and its precursor deep vein thrombosis (DVT). In view of the clinically silent nature of VTE; the incidence, prevalence and mortality rates are probably under estimated (Kniffin et al., 1994). Although VTE is a common disease, fortunately it is preventable; identifying high risk patients and the application of suitable prophylactic measures is the best way to decrease the incidence of VTE and its associated complications. Using unfractionated heparin (UFH), the rate of radiologically detected DVT was reduced by 67% without significant bleeding complications (Belch et al., 1981).

Although most patients survive DVT, they often suffer serious and costly long-term complications. Venous stasis syndrome (postphlebitic syndrome) with painful swelling and recurrent ulcers is well known complication following DVT (Prandoni et al., 1996). Additionally, PE is associated with substantial morbidity and mortality both tend to be higher among cancer patients and those who survive such event may develop chronic complications like pulmonary hypertension (Carson et al., 1992; Pengo et al., 2004). In a large study, Sørensen et al. examined the survival of patients with cancer and VTE compared to those without VTE matched for many factors including the type and duration of cancer diagnosis; the one year survival rate for cancer patients with VTE was 12% compared to 36% in the control group ($P<0.001$). Furthermore, the risk of VTE recurrence was higher in cancer patients compared to those without (Sørensen et al., 2000).

2. Cancer as a risk factor for VTE

The association between cancer and thrombosis is well-established since the first observation made by Armand Trousseau more than hundred years ago (Prandoni et al., 1992). Cancer and its treatment are recognized risk factors for VTE; in a population-based case-control study of 625 Olmsted County patients, the risk of VTE was six- fold higher in cancer patients compared to those without (Heit et al., 2000). Thrombosis is the most frequent complication and the second cause of death in patients with overt malignant diseases. Increasing evidence suggests that thrombotic episodes may also precede the diagnosis of cancer by months or years (Donati, 1995). The risk of VTE varies by cancer type; higher in patients with malignant brain tumors and adenocarcinoma of the pancreas, colon, stomach, ovary, lung, prostate, and kidney (Chew et al., 2006; Gerber DE, et al., 2006; Marras et al., 2000; Sallah et al., 2002; Thodiyil& Kakkar, 2002), but lower in sites like skin and breast (Andtbacka et al., 2006; Chew HK et al., 2007). In addition to primary tumor type, other cancer-related factors play important role in VTE rates; the risk of VTE is highest during the first 3–6 months after the initial diagnosis of cancer (Blom et al., 2005). Such risk also varies with the stage of the disease; much higher with advanced stage compared to early stage disease (Blom JW et al., 2005) and among cancer patients on active treatment with chemotherapy or radiotherapy (Haddad & Greeno, 2006).

Certain anti-cancer therapies are known to increase the risk of VTE in cancer patients. The rate of VTE increases by two to five folds in women with breast cancer treated with tamoxifen, a selective estrogen receptor modulator (SERM), and this risk was even higher when tamoxifen was combined with chemotherapy, a practice that was abandoned many years ago (Fisher et al., 2005; Pritchard et al., 1996). Aromatase inhibitors (AI), however, like anastrozole, letrozole and exemestane are less thrombogenic (Breast International Group (BIG) 1-98 Collaborative Group, 2005; ATAC (Arimidex Tamoxifen Alone or in Combination Trialists' Group), 2002).

Cancer type:
High: Brain, Ovary, Pancreas, Colon, Stomach, Lung, Prostate, Kidney
Low: Skin, Thyroid, Breast
Duration since cancer diagnosis:
High: First 6 months
Low: After 12 months
Stage of disease:
High: Locally-advanced and metastatic disease
Low: Early-stage
Anticancer therapy:
High: Chemotherapy, radiotherapy, surgery
Low: No active treatment
Hormonal therapy:
High: Tamoxifen
Low: Aromatase inhibitors like letrozole, anastrozole and exemestene
Antiangiogenesis and immune modulators:
Thalidomide
Lenalidomide
Bevacizumab
Sorafenib
Sunitinib

Table 1. Cancer-related risk factors for thrombosis

The recent introduction of immune modulators and antiangiogenesis drugs in clinical practice resulted in higher rates of VTE among cancer patients receiving such therapy. Thalidomide, lenalidomide, bevacizumab, sorafenib and sunitinib are approved by the US Food and Drug Administration (FDA) for many types of cancers; all are associated with increased risk of VTE (Zangari et al., 2009). Up to 23% of patients using bevacizumab in combination with chemotherapy to treat colorectal and gastric cancers experienced thrombotic events (Kabbinavar et al., 2007; Shah et al, 2005). Lower rates, however, wereobserved when different combination chemotherapy were used in the treatment of non-small cell lung cancer (Johnson et al., 2004). In addition to thrombosis, bevacizumab was associated with significant increase risk of bleeding; a fact that complicates decision making (Kabbinavar et al., 2003) . However, the highest incidence of VTE was observed in multiple myeloma patients treated with thalidomide, dexamethasone and doxorubicin-containing chemotherapy [Zangari et al., 2002). Higher VTE rates were also observed with thalidomide derivatives; lenalidomide and pomalidomide when used in combination with dexamethasone (Zonder et al., 2006 & Dimopoulos et al., 2007). Cancer-related risk factors are summarized in table-1.

Different antithrombotics including low molecular weight heparin (LMWH), low-dose warfarin, full-dose warfarin with target international normalized ratio (INR) of 2 to 3, and aspirin (ASA) were all tried to reduce the risk of VTE in cancer patients undergoing such therapy (Baz et al., 2005; Cavo M et al., 2004; Minnema et al., 2004). Specific recommendations in these clinical settings are beyond the scope of this review. However, in a recent trial that included a total of 667 patients with previously untreated multiple myeloma who received thalidomide-containing regimens and had no clinical indication or contraindication for a specific antiplatelet or anticoagulant therapy were randomly assigned to receive ASA (100 mg/d), fixed-dose warfarin (1.25 mg/d), or LMWH (enoxaparin 40 mg/d). A composite primary end point included serious thromboembolic events, acute cardiovascular events, or sudden deaths during the first 6 months of treatment; of 659 analyzed patients, 43 (6.5%) had serious thromboembolic events, acute cardiovascular events, or sudden death during the first 6 months (6.4% in the ASA group, 8.2% in the warfarin group, and 5.0% in the LMWH group). Compared with LMWH, the absolute differences were +1.3% (95% CI, - 3.0% to 5.7%; P =.544) in the ASA group and +3.2% (95% CI, - 1.5% to 7.8%; P = .183) in the warfarin group (Palumbo et al., 2011).

In addition to chemotherapy agents, drugs that are commonly used to support cancer patient while on active treatment may increase the risk of VTE. Erythropoiesis-stimulating agents (ESA); erythropoietin and darbepoietin are both associated with higher VTE rates. A meta-analysis of 35 trials in 6,769 cancer patients concluded that such treatment increased the risk of thromboembolic events by 67% compared with patients not receiving this therapy (Bohlius et al., 2006).

3. Making the decision

Despite its proven success, many registry studies have shown low compliance rates with published VTE prophylaxis guidelines. In a national Canadian multi-center survey study (the CURVE study), the medical records of patients in 20 teaching and 8 community hospitals were reviewed to assess the adherence to the established sixth American College of Chest Physicians (ACCP) consensus guidelines for VTE prophylaxis. In this study, 1894 eligible patients were included; thromboprophylaxis was administered only to 23% of all patients and to 37% of patients who were bedridden for more than 24 hours. However, only 16% of the patients had appropriate prophylaxis; in particular, patients with cancer had a significantly reduced likelihood of receiving prophylaxis (OR = 0.40, 95% CI (0.24–0.68)

(Kahn et al., 2007). Similar findings were also reported in the IMPROVE study in which only 45% of cancer patients who either met the ACCP criteria for requiring prophylaxis or were eligible for enrollment in randomized clinical trials that have shown the benefits of pharmacologic prophylaxis actually received prophylaxis [Tapson et al., 2007]. In another study conducted by our group, two hundred cancer patients with established diagnosis of VTE were identified; majority (91.8%) had advanced-stage cancer at time of VTE diagnosis. In addition to cancer, many patients had multiple coexisting risk factors for VTE with 137 (68.5%) patients had at least three, while 71 (35.5%) had four or more. Overall, 111(55.5%) patients developed lower-extremity DVT while 52 (26%) patients developed PE, other sites accounted for 18%. Almost three quarters of the patients (73.5%) had not received any antecedent prophylaxis. Prophylaxis rate was 23% among patients with >3 risk factors and 50% among the highest risk group with >5 risk factors (Abdel-Razeq et al., 2011).

Compared to surgical patients, decisions on when to offer prophylaxis in cancer patients admitted to medical units is difficult to make (Monreal et al., 2004); medical patients typically have many risk factors, the interaction of which is difficult to quantify. In a recent survey, The Fundamental Research in Oncology and Thrombosis (FRONTLINE), marked differences were seen in the use of thromboprophylaxis for surgical and medical cancer patients, with over 50% of surgeons reporting that they initiated thromboprophylaxis routinely, while most medical oncologists reported using thromboprophylaxis in less than 5% of medical cancer patients (Kakkar et al., 2003). These studies and many others (Chopard et al., 2005; Ageno et al., 2002), demonstrate that VTE prophylaxis in cancer patients is still underutilized.

Many factors may contribute to the low VTE prophylaxis rate in cancer patients. Obviously, concerns about bleeding especially in patients undergoing active treatment with chemotherapy that can lead to low blood counts is one of these reasons; this issue was evident in our study patients where 113 (18.6%) had prolonged PT and or PTT and another 92 (15.2%) had platelet counts < 100 K (Abdel-Razeq et al., 2001). While these may not represent absolute or even relative contraindications for using anticoagulants for VTE prophylaxis, nevertheless, such factors may prevent physicians from prescribing anticoagulant prophylaxis for cancer patients. Other reasons may include concerns about higher bleeding risks from tumor metastasis in vital structures like the brain. Such patients can be offered mechanical methods if anticoagulants deemed contraindicated. However, the absence of a suitable risk assessment model may also contribute to such low prophylaxis rate; such risk assessment model should take into account the additive or even the synergistic effect of the many other additional risk factors that cancer patients are typically admitted with.

Caprini et al. had established a risk assessment model to help health professionals in making the decision on when and how to prescribe VTE prophylaxis (Caprini et al., 2001 ; Motykie et al., 2000). Though we found it useful, we faced several limitations when we tried to apply such model in cancer patients. All cancer patients were given the same risk score; while in fact type of cancer, stage, nature of anti-cancer therapy and time since cancer diagnosis are, as discussed above, important factors that affect VTE rate in cancer patients (Abdel-Razeq et al., 2010).

4. Published guidelines

Several clinical and scientific groups including the ACCP (Geerts et al., 2008), the American Society of Clinical Oncology (ASCO) (Lyman et al., 2007) and the National Comprehensive Cancer Network (NCCN) (Wagman et al., 2008) have established guidelines for VTE prophylaxis in cancer patients. All have different and somewhat conflicting recommendations but all lack a risk assessment model. While the ACCP guidelines were very conservative and advised prophylaxis for cancer patients who are bedridden with an acute medical illness, the NCCN, on the other hand, lowered their threshold for VTE prophylaxis; their most recent updated guidelines stated: "The panel recommends prophylactic anticoagulation therapy for all inpatients with a diagnosis of active cancer (or for whom clinical suspicion of cancer exists) who do not have a contraindication to such therapy (category 1)." Their recommendation was based on an assumption that ambulation in hospitalized cancer patients is inadequate to reduce VTE risk (Wagman et al., 2008). The ASCO guidelines published in 2007 have taken a more neutral position by stating in their summary conclusions: "Hospitalized patients with cancer should be considered candidates for VTE prophylaxis with anticoagulants in the absence of bleeding or other contraindications to anticoagulation" (Lyman et al., 2007).

5. Ambulatory cancer patients

Cancer patients treated in the outpatient setting can also be at high risk for VTE. Current guidelines do not recommend anticoagulant prophylaxis for ambulatory cancer patients. Khorana et al tried to establish a risk assessment model for VTE prophylaxis in ambulatory cancer patients after the initiation of chemotherapy. Five predictive variables were identified in a multivariate model: site of cancer (2 points for very high-risk site, 1 point for high-risk site), platelet count of 350 x 10^9/L or more, hemoglobin less than 100 g/L (10 g/dL) and/or use of erythropoiesis-stimulating agents, leukocyte count more than 11 x 10^9/L, and body mass index of 35 kg/m^2 or more (1 point each). Rates of VTE in the validation part of their study were 0.3% in low-risk (score = 0), 2.0% in intermediate-risk (score = 1-2), and 6.7% in high-risk (score $\geq$3) category over a median of 2.5 months. The application of this model can identify patients with a nearly 7% short-term risk of symptomatic VTE and may be used to select cancer outpatients for studies of thromboprophylaxis (Khorana et al., 2008).

More recently, researchers focused on biomarkers that can predict the occurrence of VTE. P-selectin, found in the α granules of platelets and endothelial cells and expressed on the cell surface on activation, mediates the adhesion of leukocytes, platelets, and cancer cells in inflammation, thrombosis, and cancer growth and metastasis (Chen et al., 2006). Recent studies have demonstrated that high plasma levels of soluble P-selectin are strongly associated with VTE (Rectenwald et al., 2005). In a prospective cohort study, P-selectin was also shown to be a risk factor for recurrent VTE (Kyrle et al., 2007).

In a recent study, the Vienna Cancer and Thrombosis Study (VCATS) group reported that elevated serum P-selectin levels predicts VTE in 687 newly diagnosed cancer patients. The cumulative probability of VTE after 6 months of follow up was 11.9% in patients with serum P-selectin above and 3.7% in those below the 75th percentile (P = 0.002). Authors postulated that such biomarker could identify cancer patient who may benefit from prophylaxis (Ay et al., 2008).

The concept of VTE prophylaxis for ambulatory cancer patients was tested in a recent double-blind study; patients with metastatic or locally advanced cancer of lung, colo-rectal, stomach, ovary, pancreas, or bladder who are initiating a new chemotherapy course, were randomized to receive subcutaneous semuloparin (a new ultra low molecular weight heparin) or placebo. The drug was given at a dose of 20 mg subcutaneously and continued until change of chemotherapy. Twenty of the 1,608 patients treated with semuloparin (1.2%) and 55 of the 1,604 patients treated with placebo (3.4%) had a thromboembolic event, representing a 64% risk reduction in such event rate (hazard ratio [HR] = 0.36, 95% confidence interval [CI] 0.21–0.60, p<0.0001, intent-to-treat analysis). Nineteen of 1,589 patients (1.2%) in the semuloparin and 18 of the 1,583 patients (1.1%) in the placebo group had a major bleeding (HR=1.05, 95%CI 0.55 to 1.99) (Agnelli et al., 2011).

More work is needed before taking findings of these studies to clinical practice; as such ambulatory cancer patients on active chemotherapy may be considered for VTE prophylaxis based on risk level and clinical judgment.

6. VTE Prophylaxis in cancer patients undergoing surgery

Surgical interventions, both elective and emergency, increase VTE risk in cancer patients compared to similar interventions in non-cancer patients (Gallus, 1997; Kakkar et al., 2005; White et al., 2003;). Despite the utilization of VTE prophylaxis, one multicenter prospective study showed that VTE was the most frequent cause of 30-day mortality in cancer patients undergoing surgical procedures (Agnelli et al., 2006). Though low dose unfractionated heparin (LDUH) is effective in VTE prophylaxis, the drug should be given at the 5000 IU three times a day (not twice) in high risk surgical procedures like pelvic gynecological cancer procedures. LMWH, given once daily, is at least as effective as UFH for this indication (Clark-Pearson et al., 1990).

The issue of extended out-of-hospital prophylaxis in high risk surgical patients was addressed in major clinical trials (Gallus, 1997; Kakkar et al., 2005). In one double-blind, multicenter trial (ENOXACAN II), 322 patients undergoing planned curative open surgery for abdominal or pelvic cancer received enoxaparin (40 mg subcutaneously) daily for 6 to 10 days and were then randomly assigned to receive either enoxaparin (at the same dose) or placebo for another 21 days. Bilateral venography was performed between days 25 and 31, or sooner if symptoms of VTE occurred. In an intention-to-treat analysis and following the double-blind phase, VTE occurred in 4.8% in the extended enoxaparin group compared to 12.0% in the placebo group (P=0.02). This difference persisted at three months (13.8 % vs. 5.5%, P=0.01). There were no significant differences in the rates of bleeding or other complications during the double-blind or follow-up periods (Bergqvist et al., 2002).

In another open-label randomized trial designed to evaluate the efficacy and safety of thromboprophylaxis with dalteparin, another LMWH, administered for 28 days after major abdominal surgery compared to 7 days treatment. A total of 590 patients undergoing major abdominal surgery (60% for cancer) were recruited. The cumulative incidence of VTE was reduced from 16.3% with short-term (7days) thromboprophylaxis to 7.3% after prolonged thromboprophylaxis; a relative risk reduction (RR) of 55%; 95% confidence interval 15-76; P=0.012. The number that needed to be treated to prevent one case of VTE was 12 (95%

confidence interval 7-44). Bleeding events were not increased with prolonged compared with short-term thromboprophylaxis (Rasmussen et al., 2006).

A recent meta-analysis of eligible clinical studies compared safety and efficacy of extended use of LMWH (for three to four weeks after surgery) versus conventional in-hospital prophylaxis among patients undergoing major abdominal surgeries. The indication for surgery was neoplastic disease in 70.6% (780/1104) of patients. The administration of extended LMWH prophylaxis significantly reduced the incidence of VTE, 5.93% versus 13.6%, RR 0.44 (CI 95% 0.28 - 0.7); DVT 5.93% versus 12.9%, RR 0.46 (CI 95% 0.29 - 0.74); proximal DVT 1% versus 4.72%, RR 0.24 (CI 95% 0.09 - 0.67). These superior efficacy results were obtained with no significant difference in major or minor bleeding between the two groups: 3.85% in the extended thrombo-prophylaxis group versus 3.48% in the conventional prophylaxis group; RR 1.12 (CI 95% 0.61 - 2.06) (Bottaro et al., 2008). Given the results of these studies, one can conclude that extended thromboprophylaxis with LMWH should be considered as a safe and useful strategy to prevent VTE in high-risk major abdominal and pelvic surgeries especially in cancer patients. Similar conclusions were reached in a more recent Cochrane database analysis (Rasmussen et al., 2009). Results of these studies are summarized in Figure-1.

7. Central venous catheters

Central venous catheters (CVC) are commonly inserted in cancer patient and are utilized to deliver chemotherapy, blood and blood component transfusion and occasionally for blood sampling. Central catheter per se is a risk factor for VTE, this risk is even higher when such catheters are placed in cancer patients especially so when used for active chemotherapy (Bona, 1999; Rooden et al., 2005; Rosovsky & Kuter, 2005).

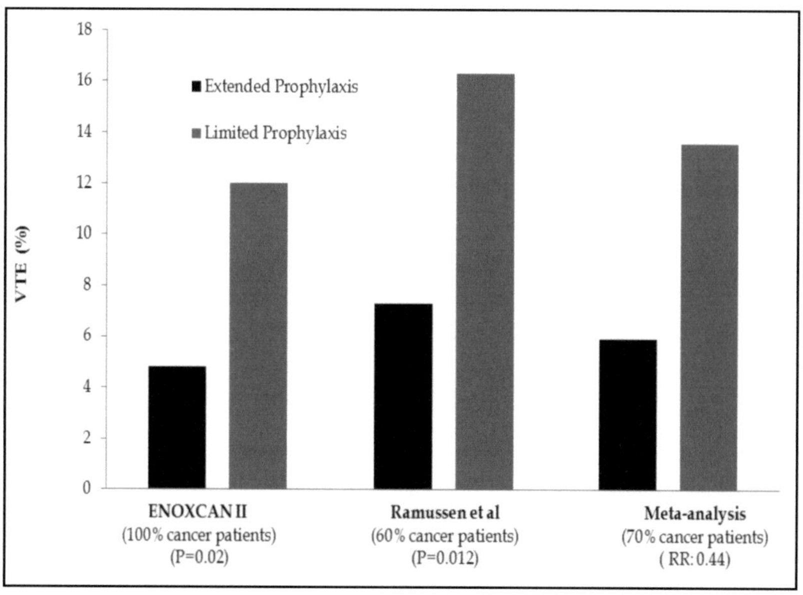

Fig. 1. Extended out-of-hospital VTE prophylaxis for cancer patients undergoing major surgery

Several clinical trials have addressed the issue of VTE prophylaxis in such patients. One study showed a benefit in reducing VTE events when low fixed-dose warfarin (1mg/day) was used for prophylaxis (Bern et al., 1990). However, two subsequent clinical trials failed to show any benefit [Heaton et al., 2002: Couban et al., 2005).

Low molecular weight heparin was also tried in two large, double-blind clinical trials (Verso et al., 2005; Karthaus et al., 2006). The first trial failed to show beneficial effect of enoxaparin when used at a dose of 40 mg once daily versus placebo in a group of 385 cancer patients with CVC (Verso et al., 2005). In the second trial, dalteparin at 5,000 units once daily was tested against placebo in 439 cancer patients who were receiving chemotherapy through such catheters; clinically relevant VTE occurred in 3.7% and 3.4% in the dalteparin and placebo recipients, respectively (Karthaus et al., 2006). Nadroparin, another LMWH, showed no advantage when tested against low fixed dose of warfarin (1 mg/day) in a small randomized trial that involved 45 evaluable patients (Mismetti et al., 2003).

Given the results of these studies, thromboprophylaxis with anticoagulants for patients with central venous catheters is not recommended.

8. Inferior Vena Cava (IVC) filters in cancer patients

Treatment of VTE typically includes initial anticoagulation with unfractionated heparin, LMWH or a pentasaccharide like fondaparinux, (Buller et al., 2004) along with vitamin K antagonists like warfarin. Occasionally, specific clinical situations present in which the risk of PE is very high or systemic anticoagulation might be associated with high risk of bleeding; in these instances, IVC filters are utilized to provide mechanical thromboprophylaxis to prevent PE, the life-threatening complication of VTE. Such filters are inserted using a relatively noninvasive technique to maintain central flow. Thanks to newer technology, the IVC filters are becoming a very attractive option and can function with anticoagulation to optimize the prophylaxis strategy. Inferior Vena Cava filters are usually utilized in many clinical situations detailed in table-2 (Schwarz et al., 1996; Saour et al., 2009).

However, many of such indications are subjective and consensus might occasionally be difficult to reach. In a community-based study, researchers at McMaster University reviewed 1547 local county residents with confirmed diagnosis of acute VTE and without a prior IVC filter. Following the VTE, 203 (13.1%) patients had an IVC filter placed. In reviewing the indications for IVC filter placement, panel members unanimously agreed that the use of IVC filter was appropriate in 51% of the cases and inappropriate in 26%; no consensus was reached in the remaining 23% of the cases (Spencer et al., 2010).

The clinical benefit of IVC filter placement was addressed in one prospective trial (the PREPIC study) in which 400 patients with proximal DVT who were at risk for PE, were randomized to receive IVC filter (200 patients) or no filter (200 patients). Both groups were anticoagulated with LMWH or unfractionated heparin. At day 12, two (1.1%) patients assigned to receive filters, as compared with nine (4.8%) patients assigned to receive no filters, had symptomatic or asymptomatic PE (odds ratio, 0.22; 95 percent confidence interval, 0.05 to 0.90). However, at two years, 37 (20.8%) patients assigned to the filter group, as compared with 21 (11.6%) patients assigned to the no-filter group, had recurrent DVT (odds ratio, 1.87; 95% CI, 1.10 to 3.20) (Decousus et al., 1998). This study was updated 8 years later; patients with IVC filters experienced a greater cumulative incidence of symptomatic DVT (35.7%versus 27.5%; HR 1.52, CI 1.02 to 2.27; P = 0.042), but significantly fewer symptomatic pulmonary emboli (6.2%versus 15.1%; HR 0.37, CI 0.17 to 0.79; P = 0.008) (The PREPIC Study Group, 2005). The conclusion from this long-term follow-up was similar to the original report; that is, with an IVC filter there is an equivalent trade-off of fewer PE at the cost of more DVTs. There was no difference in long-term morbidity or mortality in both groups.

Main Indications:
Failure of anticoagulation: Recurrent VTE despite anticoagulation
Contraindications and/or severe complications of anticoagulation:
High risk for bleeding
Real bleeding (GI,GU,GYN, CNS)
Thrombocytopenia (Depends on count and etiology)
Immediate post-operative VTE
Large CNS Tumor: Primary or metastatic
Other indications:
Large, free-floating iliocaval thrombus
Limited cardiopulmonary reserve (Cor Pulmonale)
Poor compliance with medications
Patients at risk for falls while on anticoagulation therapy

IVC: Inferior Vena Cava, GI: Gastrointestinal, GU: Genitourinary, GYN: Gynecological, CNS: Central Nervous System, VTE: Venous Thromboembolism

Table 2. Indications for IVC filter placement

Given the lack of long term benefits of IVC filters; temporary, retrievable filters had gained increasing interest. Many different retrievable filters had recently received approval for temporary insertion. Recent data suggest that the use of these filters may be associated with low rates of PE and insertion complications (Imberti & Prisco, 2008). Nevertheless; no randomized clinical trials have been performed. In one large retrospective study that included 252 evaluable patients who had retrievable filter placed for different indications; only 47 filters were successfully retrieved yielding a retrieval rate of 18.7% (Dabbagh et al., 2010). Similar or higher retrieval rates were reported by others (Mismetti et al., 2007).

Regardless of the type of the filter placed, the most recent American Colleague of Chest Physicians (ACCP) guidelines recommend systemic anticoagulation, when possible, even with the filter in place (Kearon et al., 2008).

Cancer itself, or its treatment, might result in certain clinical complications that make systemic anticoagulation very risky (Abdel-Razeq et al., 2011). Venous thromboembolic disease is a frequent complication in patients with intracranial malignancies. Many of the primary brain tumors like gliomas or secondary metastatic tumors to the brain are either bulky or very vascular thus increasing the risk of bleeding with or without systemic anticoagulation (Ruff & Posner, 1983). Brain metastases from melanoma, choriocarcinoma, thyroid carcinoma, and renal cell carcinoma have particularly high propensities for spontaneous hemorrhage while metastatic tumors from sites like lung and breast are less likely to bleed spontaneously (Mandybur, 1993). However, not all patients with intracranial malignancies are at higher risk of bleeding with anticoagulation. Complication rate of IVC filters in patients with brain tumors is higher than commonly perceived and may outweigh the risk of anticoagulation. Researchers at Brigham and Women's Hospital in Boston reviewed the records of 49 patients with intracranial malignancies and venous thromboembolic disease to determine the effectiveness and complications resulting from systemic anticoagulation or IVC filter placement. Of the 42 patients received IVC filters, a strikingly high percentage (62%) developed one or more complications; 12% developed recurrent PE, while 57% developed filter thrombosis, recurrent DVT, or post-phlebitic syndrome. These complications severely reduced the quality of life of affected patients. Only 15 (31%) patients were treated with anticoagulation, and seven of these received it because of continued thromboembolic disease. None of these 15 patients had proven hemorrhagic complications (Levin et al., 1993).

Many recent studies questioned the need to insert IVC filters in cancer patients particularly those with advanced-stage disease whose survival is short and prevention of PE may be of little clinical benefit and could be a poor utilization of resources. In one retrospective study performed to determine the clinical benefit of IVC filter placement in patients with malignancy, 116 patients who had such filters inserted were included. Ninety one (78%) patients had stage IV disease, 42 (46%) of them died of cancer within 6 weeks and only16 (14%) were alive at one year (Jarrett et al., 2002).

The benefits of IVC filter placement on overall survival, as measured from the time of VTE was addressed in a recent retrospective study that examined 206 consecutive cancer patients with VTE. Patients were classified into 3 treatment groups: anticoagulation-only (n= 62), IVC filter-only (n=77), or combination of both IVC filter and anticoagulation (n=67). Median overall survival was significantly greater in patients treated with anticoagulation (13 months) compared with those treated with IVC filters (2 months) or combination of both (3.25 months; $P < 0.0002$). IVC patients were at 1.9 times more risk of death than anticoagulation only (hazard ratio=0.528; 95% confidence interval=0.374 to .745). Multivariate analysis revealed that performance status and type of thrombus were not confounders and had no effect on overall survival (Barginear et al., 2009).

In another study, the survival benefit of IVC filters in patients with late-stage malignancy was evaluated in a group of 5,970 patients who were treated with a primary diagnosis of malignancy at a tertiary care facility. Retrospective analysis identified 55 consecutive patients with stage III or IV malignant disease and VTE who received IVC filters. In a case control study, 16 patients with VTE but without IVC filter were matched for age, sex, type of malignancy, and stage of disease. Filter placement prevented PE in 52 (94.5%) patients, however, four (7.3%) of patients had complications related to the procedure; 13 (23.6%) patients with late-stage cancer survived less than 30 days following placement of the filter; another 13 (23.6%) patients of this group, however, survived more than one year. Ambulatory status differed significantly ($P = 0.01$) between these two subgroups. Authors concluded that IVC filter placement conferred no survival benefit compared to the control group and that the survival of such patients with advanced-stage cancer was limited primarily by the malignant process (Schunn et al., 2006). Researchers at M.D. Anderson Cancer center concluded, in a study that included 308 cancer patients with VTE and IVC filters, that such filters are safe and effective in preventing PE-related deaths in selected patients with cancer. However, patients with a history of DVT and bleeding or advanced disease had the lowest survival after IVC filter placement (Wallace et al., 2004).

9. Conclusions and future directions

Despite its proven efficacy, VTE prophylaxis in cancer patients is clearly underutilized. Strategies to improve prophylaxis rate in such high risk patients are highly needed (Abdel-Razeq, 2010). Establishment of "VTE prophylaxis multidisciplinary team" addressing this issue supported by hospital administration might help. Recently, many health advocacy groups and policy makers are paying more attention to VTE prophylaxis. The National Quality Forum (NQF) recently endorsed strict VTE risk assessment evaluation for each patient upon admission and regularly thereafter (National Quality Forum (NQF), 2011). Additionally, the Joint Commission has recently approved new measure sets that included VTE prophylaxis; this standard mandates that a VTE prophylaxis method is in place within 24 hours of hospital admission, otherwise, a risk assessment and contraindications for prophylaxis should be documented for each and every hospitalized medical or surgical patient (The Joint Commission Manual for Performance Improvement Measures, 2011). Recently, Maynard and Stein (2011) have published their experience and recommendations following their extensive efforts to better utilize VTE prophylaxis in high-risk patients. Such recommendations are worth careful attention and are summarized in table-3.

Support by hospital administration for better VTE prophylaxis initiative.

Establishment of VTE Prophylaxis "Multidisciplinary Team"; this team should:

- Standardize the process of providing VTE prophylaxis
- Facilitates implementation of guidelines.
- Audit and monitor outcomes.
- Report regularly to hospital administration or a "Quality Council".

Better guidelines:

- Simple, yet efficient in daily use; two to three VTE risk levels are enough!
- Provide clear link between risk level and prophylaxis choice.
- Provide guidance to manage patients with contraindications.

Continuous education and training of all health care providers.

Table 3. Strategies to improve VTE prophylaxis in high risk cancer patients.

In conclusion, though published guidelines are somewhat different; hospitalized cancer patients, in the absence of bleeding or absolute contraindications, should be considered for thromboprophylaxis. Certain cancers, like Multiple Myeloma when treated with drugs like thalidomide or other immune modulators may benefit from prophylaxis. However, current guidelines do not recommend prophylaxis for ambulatory cancer patients or patients with central venous catheter.

Extended thromboprophylaxis with LMWH (21-28days) should be considered in cancer patients undergoing major pelvic/abdominal surgeries.

10. Acknowledgments

The authors would like to thank Ms. Haifa Al-Ahmad and Mrs. Alice Haddadin for their help in preparing this manuscript.

11. References

Abdel-Razeq H. (2010). Venous thromboembolism prophylaxis for hospitalized medical patients, current status and strategies to improve. *Ann Thorac Med.* 5:195-200.

Abdel-Razeq, HN.; Hijjawi, SB.; Jallad, SG.; Ababneh, BA. (2010). Venous thromboembolism risk stratification in medically-ill hospitalized cancer patients. A comprehensive cancer center experience. *J Thromb Thrombolysis.* 30: 286-93.

Abdel-Razeq, H.; Mansour, A.; Ismael, Y.; Abdulelah, H. (2011) Inferior vena cava filters in cancer patients: to filter or not to filter. *Ther Clin Risk Manag.* 7:99-102.

Abdel-Razeq, H.; Albadainah, F.; Hijjawi, S.; Mansour, A.; Treish, I. (2011). Venous Thromboembolism (VTE) in Hospitalized Cancer Patients: Prophylaxis Failure or Failure to Prophylax. *J Thromb Thrombolysis.* 3: 107-12.

Ageno, W.; Squizzato, A.; Ambrosini, F. *et al.* (2002). Thrombosis prophylaxis in medical patients: a retrospective review of clinical practice patterns. *Haematologica* 87:746–50.

Agnelli, G.; Bolis, G.; Capussotti, L. *et al.* (2006). A clinical outcome based prospective study on venous thromboembolism after cancer surgery: the ARISTOS project. *Ann Surg* 243:89–95.

Agnelli, G.; George, D.; Fisher, K.; Kakkar, AK. *et al.* (2011). The ultra-low molecular weight heparin (ULMWH) semuloparin for prevention of venous thromboembolism (VTE) in patients with cancer receiving chemotherapy: SAVE ONCO study. *J Clin Oncol 29*: (suppl; abstr LBA9014)

Andtbacka, RH.; Babiera, G.; Singletary, SE. *et al.* (2006). Incidence and prevention of venous thromboembolism in patients undergoing breast cancer surgery and treated according to clinical pathways. *Ann Surg* 243:96–101.

ATAC (Arimidex Tamoxifen Alone or in Combination) Trialists' Group. (2002). Anastrozole alone or in combination with tamoxifen versus tamoxifen alone for adjuvant treatment of postmenopausal women with early breast cancer: first results of the ATAC randomised trial. *Lancet* 359: 2131-2139

Ay, C.; Simanek, R.; Vormittag, R. *et al.* (2008). High plasma levels of soluble P-selectin are predictive of venous thromboembolism in cancer patients: results from the Vienna Cancer and Thrombosis Study (CATS). *Blood* 112:2703–8.

Barginear, MF.; Lesser, M.; Akerman, ML. *et al.* (2009). Need for inferior vena cava filters in cancer patients: a surrogate marker for poor outcome. *Clin Appl Thromb Hemost.* 15:263-269.

Baz, R.; Li, L.; Kottke-Marchant, K. *et al.* (2005). The role of aspirin in the prevention of thrombotic complications of thalidomide and anthracycline-based chemotherapy for multiple myeloma. *Mayo Clin Proc* 80:1568-74.

Belch, JJ.; Lowe, GDO.; Ward, AG.; Forbes, CD.; Prentice, CRM. (1981). Prevention of deep vein thrombosis in medical patients by low-dose heparin. *Scott Med J* 26:115–7.

Bergqvist, D.; Agnelli, G.; Cohen, AT. *et al.* (2002). Duration of prophylaxis against venous thromboembolism with enoxaparin after surgery for cancer. *N Engl J Med* 346:975- 80.

Bern, MM.; Lokich, JJ.; Wallach, SR. *et al.* (1990). Very low doses of warfarin can prevent thrombosis in central venous catheters: a randomized prospective trial. *Ann Intern Med* 112,423-8.

Blom, JW.; Doggen, CJ.; Osanto, S.; Rosendaal, FR. (2005). Malignancies, prothrombotic mutations, and risk of venous thrombosis. *JAMA* 293:715–22.

Bohlius, J.; Wilson, J.; Seidenfeld, J. *et al.* (2006). Recombinant human erythropoietins and cancer patients: updated meta-analysis of 57 studies including 9353 patients. *J Natl Cancer Inst* 98:708–14.

Bona, RD. (1999). Thrombotic complications of central venous catheters in cancer patients. *Semin Thromb Haemost* 25,147-55.

Bottaro, FJ.; Elizondo, MC.; Doti, C. *et al.* (2008). Efficacy of extended thrombo-prophylaxis in major abdominal surgery: what does the evidence show? A meta-analysis. *Thromb Haemost.* 99:1104-11.

Breast International Group (BIG) 1–98 Collaborative Group. (2005). A comparison of letrozole and tamoxifen in postmenopausal women with early breast cancer. *N Engl J Med* 353, 2747-57.

Buller, HR.; Davidson, BL.; Decousus, H. *et al.* (2004). Fondaparinux or enoxaparin for the initial treatment of symptomatic deep venous thrombosis: a randomized trial. *Ann Intern Med.* 140: 867-873.

Caprini, J.; Arcelus, J.; Reyna, J. (2001). Effective risk stratification of surgical and nonsurgical patients for venous thromboembolic disease. *Semin Hematol* 38:12–19.

Carson, JL.; Kelley, MA.; Duff, A. *et al.* (1992). The clinical course of pulmonary embolism. *N Engl J Med* 326:1240–5.

Cavo, M., Zamagni, E., Tosi, P., *et al.* (2004). First-line therapy with thalidomide and dexamethasone in preparation for autologous stem cell transplantation for multiple myeloma. *Haematologica* 89:826-31.

Chen, M., Geng, JG., P-selectin. (2006). mediates adhesion of leukocytes, platelets, and cancer cells in inflammation, thrombosis, and cancer growth and metastasis. *Arch Immunol Ther Exp* 54:75-84.

Chew, HK.; Wun, T.; Harvey, D.; Zhou, H.; White, RH. (2006). Incidence of venous thromboembolism and its effect on survival among patients with common cancers. *Arch Intern Med* 166:458–64.

Chew, HK.; Wun, T.; Harvey, DJ.; Zhou, H.; White, RH. (2007). Incidence of venous thromboembolism and the impact on survival in breast cancer patients. *J Clin Oncol* 25:70–6.

Chopard, P.; Dörffler-Melly, J.; Hess, U. *et al.* (2005). Venous thromboembolism prophylaxis in acutely ill medical patients: definite need for improvement. *J Intern Med* 257:352–7.

Clark-Pearson, DL.; DeLong, E.; Synan, IS.; Soper, JT.; Creasman, WT.; Coleman, RE. (1990). A controlled trial of two low-dose heparin regimens for the prevention of postoperative deep vein thrombosis. *Obstet Gynecol* 75:684–9.

Couban, S.; Goodyear, M.; Burnell, M. *et al.* (2005). Randomized placebo-controlled study of low-dose warfarin for the prevention of central venous catheter-associated thrombosis in patients with cancer. *J Clin Oncol* 23, 4063-9.

Dabbagh, O.; Nagam, N.; Chitima-Matsiga, R.; Bearelly, S.; Bearelly, D. (2010). Retrievable inferior vena cava filters are not getting retrieved: where is the gap? *Thromb Res.* 126:493-497.

Decousus, H.; Leizorovicz, A.; Parent, F. *et al.* (1998). A clinical trial of vena caval filters in the prevention of pulmonary embolism in patients with proximal deep-vein thrombosis: Prevention duRisque d'Embolie Pulmonaire par Interruption Cave Study Group. *N Engl J Med.* 338:409–415.

Dimopoulos, M.; Spencer, A.; Attal, M. *et al.* (2007). Lenalidomide plus dexamethasone for relapsed or refractory multiple myeloma. *N Engl J Med* 357:2123-32.

Donati, MB. (1995). Cancer and thrombosis: from Phlegmasia alba dolens to transgenic mice. *Thromb Haemost* 74:278.

Fisher, B.; Costantino, JP.; Wickerham, DL. *et al.* (2005). Tamoxifen for the prevention of breast cancer: current status of the National Surgical Adjuvant Breast and Bowel Project P-1 study. *J Natl Cancer Inst* 97: 1652-62.

Gallus, AS. (1997). Prevention of post-operative deep leg vein thrombosis in patients with cancer. *Thromb Haemost* 78:126–32.

Geerts, WH.; Bergqvist, D.; Pineo, GF. *et al.* (2008). Prevention of venous thromboembolism: American College of Chest Physicians evidence- based clinical practice guidelines (8th edition). *Chest* 133:381–453.

Gerber, DE.; Grossman, SA.; Streiff, MB. (2006). Management of venous thromboembolism in patients with primary and metastatic brain tumors. *J Clin Oncol* 24:1310–8.

Haddad, TF.; Greeno, EW. (2006). Chemotherapy-induced thrombosis. *Thromb Res* 118:547–666

Heaton, DC.; Han, DY.; Inder, A. (2002). Minidose (1 mg) warfarin as prophylaxis for central vein catheter thrombosis. *Intern Med J* 32: 84-8.

Heit, JA.; Silverstein, MD.; Mohr, DN.; Petterson, TM.; O'Fallon, WM.; Melton, LJ .; 3rd. (2000). Risk factors for deep vein thrombosis and pulmonary embolism: a population based case-control study. *Arch Intern Med* 160:809–15.

Imberti, D.; Prisco, D. (2008). Retrievable vena cava filters: key considerations. *Thromb Res.* 122:442-449.

Jarrett, BP.; Dougherty, MJ.; Calligaro, KD. (2002). Inferior vena cava filters in malignant disease. *J Vasc Surg.* 36:704-707.

Johnson, DH.; Fehrenbacher, L.; Novotny, WF. *et al.* (2004). Randomized phase II trial comparing bevacizumab plus carboplatin and paclitaxel with carboplatin and paclitaxel alone in previously untreated locally advanced or metastatic non-small-cell lung cancer. *J Clin Oncol* 22:2184-91.

Kabbinavar, F.; Hurwitz, HI.; Fehrenbacher, L. *et al.* (2003). Phase II, randomized trial comparing bevacizumab plus fluorouracil (FU)/leucovorin (LV) with FU/LV alone in patients with metastatic colorectal cancer. *J Clin Oncol* 21:60-5.

Kahn, SR.; Panju, A.; Geerts, With. *et al.* (2007). Multicenter evaluation of the use of venous thromboembolism prophylaxis in acutely ill medical patients in Canada. *Thromb Res* 119:145–55.

Kakkar, AK.; Levine, M.; Pinedo, HM.; Wolff, R.; Wong, J. (2003). Venous thrombosis in cancer patients: insights from the FRONTLINE survey. *Oncologist* 8:381-8.

Kakkar, AK.; Haas, S.; Wolf, H.; Encke, A. (2005). Evaluation of perioperative fatal pulmonary embolism and death in cancer surgical patients: the MC-4 cancer substudy. *Thromb Haemost* 94:867–71.

Karthaus, M.; Kretzschmar, A.; Kröning, H. *et al.* (2006). Dalteparin for prevention of catheter-related complications in cancer patients with central venous catheters: final results of a double-blind, placebo-controlled phase III trial. *Ann Oncol* 17: 289-96.

Kearon, C.; Kahn, SR.; Agnelli, G.; Goldhaber, S.; Raskob, GE.; Comerota, AJ. (2008).American College of Chest Physicians. Antithrombotic therapy for venous thromboembolic disease: American College of Chest Physicians Evidence-Based Clinical Practice Guidelines (8th Edition). *Chest.* 133(6 Suppl):454S-545S.

Khorana, AA.; Kuderer, NM.; Culakova, E.; Lyman, GH.; Francis, CW. (2008). Development and validation of a predictive model for chemotherapy-associated thrombosis. *Blood* 111:4902–7.

Kniffin, WD.; Baron, JA.; Barret, J.; Bikmeyer, JD.; Anderson, FA. (1994). The epidemiology of pulmonary embolism and deep venous thrombosis in the elderly. *Arch Intern Med* 154:861–6.

Kyrle, PA.; Hron, G.; Eichinger, S.; Wagner, O. (2007). Circulating P-selectin and the risk of recurrent venous thromboembolism. *Thromb Haemost* 97:880-883

Levin, JM.; Schiff, D.; Loeffler, JS.; Fine, HA.; Black, PM.; Wen, PY. (1993). Complications of therapy for venous thromboembolic disease in patients with brain tumors. *Neurology.* 43:1111-1114.

Lyman, GH.; Khorana, AA.; Falanga, A. *et al.* (2007). American Society of Clinical Oncology Guideline: Recommendations for venous thromboembolism prophylaxis and treatment in patients with cancer. *J Clin Oncol* 25:5490–5505.

Mandybur, TI. (1977). Intracranial hemorrhage caused by metastatic tumors. *Neurology.* 27:650-655.

Marras, LC.; Geerts, WH.; Perry, JR. (2000). The risk of venous thromboembolism is increased throughout the course of malignant glioma: an evidence-based review. *Cancer* 89:640–6.

Maynard,G.; Stein, J. (2010). Designing and implementing effective venous thromboembolism prevention protocols: Lessons from collaborative efforts. *J Thromb Thrombolysis* 29:159-66

Minnema, MC.; Breitkreutz, I.; Auwerda, JJ. *et al.* (2004). Prevention of venous thromboembolism with low molecular-weight heparin in patients with multiple myeloma treated with thalidomide and chemotherapy. *Leukemia* 18:2044-6.

Mismetti, P.; Mille, D.; Laporte, S. *et al.* (2003). Low-molecular-weight heparin (nadroparin) and very low doses of warfarin in the prevention of upper extremity thrombosis in cancer patients with indwelling long-term central venous catheters: a pilot randomized trial. *Haematologica* 88,67-73.

Mismetti, P.; Rivron-Guillot, K.; Quenet, S. *et al.* (2007). A prospective long-term study of 220 patients with a retrievable vena cava filter for secondary prevention of venous thromboembolism. *Chest.* 131:223-229.

Monreal, M.; Kakkar, AK.; Caprini, JA. *et al.* (2004). The outcome after treatment of venous thromboembolism is different in surgical and acutely ill medical patients. Findings from the RIETE registry. *J Thromb Haemost* 2:1889–91.

Motykie, G.; Zebala, L.; Caprini, J. *et al.* (2000). A guide to venous thromboembolism risk factor assessment. *J Thromb Thrombolysis* 9:253–62.

National Quality Forum (NQF) . (2011). at (NQF). Available from: http://www.qualityforum.org/Measures_List.aspx#k=THROMBOSIS [last cited on Apr 06, 2011].

Palumbo, A.; Cavo, M.; Bringhen, S. *et al.* (2011). Aspirin, Warfarin, or Enoxaparin Thromboprophylaxis in Patients with Multiple Myeloma Treated With Thalidomide: A Phase III, Open-Label, Randomized Trial. *J Clin Oncol* 29:986-993.

Pengo, V.; Lensing, AW.; Prins, MH. *et al.* (2004). Incidence of chronic thromboembolic pulmonary hypertension after pulmonary embolism. *N Engl J Med* 350:2257–64.

Prandoni, P.; Lensing, AWA.; Buller, HR. *et al.* (1992). Deep-vein thrombosis and the incidence of subsequent symptomatic cancer. *N Engl J Med* 327:1128-33

Prandoni, P.; Lensing, AW.; Cogo, A. *et al.* (1996). The long-term clinical course of acute deep venous thrombosis. *Ann Intern Med* 125:1–7.

Pritchard, KI.; Paterson, AH.; Paul, NA.; Zee, B.; Fine, S.; Pater, J. (1996). Increased thromboembolic complications with concurrent tamoxifen and chemotherapy in a randomized trial of adjuvant therapy for women with metastatic breast cancer. *J Clin Oncol* 14: 2731-7.

Rasmussen, MS.; Jorgensen, LN.; Wille-Jørgensen, P. *et al.* (2006). Prolonged prophylaxis with dalteparin to prevent late thromboembolic complications in patients undergoing major abdominal surgery: a multicenter randomized open-label study. *J Thromb Haemost* 4:2384–90.

Rasmussen, MS.; Jørgensen, LN.; Wille-Jørgensen, P. (2009). Prolonged thromboprophylaxis with low molecular weight heparin for abdominal or pelvic surgery. *Cochrane Database Syst Rev.* 1):CD004318.

Rectenwald, JE.; Myers, DD Jr.; Hawley, AE. *et al. (2005).* D-dimer, P-selectin, and microparticles: novel markers to predict deep venous thrombosis. A pilot study. *Thromb Haemost* 94:1312-1317

Rooden, CJ.; Tesselaar, ME.; Osanto, S.; Rosendaal, FR.; Huisman, MV. (2005). Deep vein thrombosis associated with central venous catheters: a review. *J Thromb Haemost* 3: 2409-19.

Rosovsky, RP.; Kuter, DJ. (2005). Catheter-related thrombosis in cancer patients: pathophysiology, diagnosis, and management. *Hematol Oncol Clin N Am* 19: 183-202.

Ruff, RL.; Posner, JB. (1983). The incidence and treatment of peripheral venous thrombosis in patients with glioma. *Ann Neurol.* 13:334-336.

Sallah. S.; Wan, JY.; Nguyen, NP. (2002). Venous thrombosis in patients with solid tumors: determination of frequency and characteristics. *Thromb Haemost* 87:575–9.

Saour, J.; Al Harthi, A.; El Sherif, M.; Bakhsh, E.; Mammo, L. (2009). Inferior vena caval filters: 5 years of experience in a tertiary care center. *Ann Saudi Med.* 29:446-449.

Schunn, C.; Schunn, GB.; Hobbs, G.; Vona-Davis, LC.; Waheed ,U. (2006). Inferior vena cava filter placement in late-stage cancer. *Vasc Endovascular Surg.* 40:287-294.

Schwarz, RE.; Marrero, AM.; Conlon, KC.; Burt, M. (1996). Inferior vena cava filters in cancer patients: indications and outcome. *J Clin Oncol.* 14:652-657.

Shah, MA.; Ilson, D.; Kelsen, DP. (2005). Thromboembolic events in gastric cancer: High incidence in patients receiving irinotecan- and bevacizumabbased therapy. *J Clin Oncol* 23:2574-6.

Sørensen, HT.; Mellemkjaer, L.; Olsen, JH.; Baron, JA. (2000). Prognosis of cancers associated with venous thromboembolism. *N Engl J Med* 343:1846–50.

Spencer, FA.; Bates, SM.; Goldberg, RJ. *et al.* (2010). A population-based study of inferior vena cava filters in patients with acute venous thromboembolism. *Arch Intern Med.* 170:1456-1462.

Tapson, VF.; Decousus, H.; Pini, M. *et al.* (2007). Venous thromboembolism prophylaxis in acutely ill hospitalized medical patients: findings from the international medical prevention registry on venous thromboembolism. *Chest* 132:936–45.

The Joint Commission Manual for Performance Improvement Measures. (2011). Available from: http://www.jointcommission.org/venous_thromboembolism/ [last cited on, Apr 06, 2011].

The PREPIC Study Group. (2005). Eight-year follow-up of patients with permanent vena cava filters in the prevention of pulmonary embolism: the PREPIC (Pre´vention du Risque d'Embolie Pulmonaire par Interruption Cave) randomized study. *Circulation.* 112:416–422.

Thodiyil, PA.; Kakkar, AK. (2002). Variation in relative risk of venous thromboembolism in different cancers. *Thromb Haemost* 87:1076–7.

Verso, M.; Agnelli, G.; Bertoglio, S. et al. (2005). Enoxaparin for the prevention of venous thromboembolism associated with central vein catheter: a double-blind, placebo-controlled, randomized study in cancer patients. *J Clin Oncol* 23, 4057-62.

Wagman, LD.; Baird, MF.; Bennett, CL. *et al.* (2008). Venous thromboembolic disease. NCCN. Clinical practice guidelines in oncology. *J Natl Compr Canc Netw* 6:716–53.

Wallace, MJ.; Jean, JL.; Gupta, S. *et al.* (2004). Use of inferior vena caval filters and survival in patients with malignancy. *Cancer.* 101:1902-1907.

White, RH.; Zhou, H.; Romano, PS. (2003). Incidence of symptomatic venous thromboembolism after different elective or urgent surgical procedures. *Thromb Haemost* 90:446–55.

Zangari, M.; Siegel, E.; Barlogie, B. *et al.* (2002). Thrombogenic activity of doxorubicin in myeloma patients receiving thalidomide: implications for therapy. *Blood* 100:1168-71.

Zangari, M.; Fink, LM.; Elice, F.; Zhan, F.; Adcock, DM.; Tricot, GJ. (2009). Thrombotic events in patients with cancer receiving antiangiogenesis agents. *J Clin Oncol* 27: 4865-73

Zonder, JA.; Barlogie, B.; Durie, BG.; McCoy, J.; Crowley, J.; Hussein, MA. (2006). Thrombotic complications in patients with newly diagnosed multiple myeloma treated with lenalidomide and dexamethasone: Benefit of aspirin prophylaxis. *Blood* 108:403.

8

Deep Vein Thrombosis of the Arms

Peter Marschang
Innsbruck Medical University
Austria

1. Introduction

Deep vein thrombosis is often regarded as a disease limited of the veins of the lower extremities, which may sometimes - in more severe cases - extend to the pelvic veins. Although this holds true for over 90% of all thromboses, clinically relevant thromboses may be found in virtually every vein system of the body. Of these uncommon localisations of thromboses, deep vein thrombosis of the arms is one of the most frequent entities, accounting for about 5% of all thromboses (Munoz et al., 2008; Isma et al., 2010). Most cases of deep arm vein thrombosis develop secondary in patients with indwelling central venous catheters, pacemakers, malignant disease, or after surgery. Conversely, primary upper extremity deep venous thrombosis is observed in patients after strenuous arm exercise ("thrombosis par effort"), in thoracic outlet syndrome and inherited or acquired thrombophilia (Bernardi et al., 2006). Acute and long-time complications of upper extremity thrombosis may be significant and include pulmonary embolism, post-thrombotic syndrome and recurrent thromboembolism. In this chapter, the clinical presentation, diagnostic procedures, treatment and prevention of thromboses of the upper extremity will be reviewed. It is not unusual to find thromboses of proximal arm veins and deep veins of the neck region at the same time. Therefore, thromboses of the internal jugular vein, which are also most often observed in the presence of indwelling central venous catheters, will also be discussed. In this review, special emphasis will be given to the practical aspects of the disease, like risk factors, clinical presentation, diagnosis, and treatment of arm vein thrombosis. For a detailed, comprehensive overview of pathophysiological mechanisms, the reader will be referred to other, excellent reviews within this field.

2. Epidemiology

The frequency of deep arm vein thrombosis relative to all deep thromboses has been reported to be between 1 and 14% (Hill & Berry, 1990; Joffe et al., 2004; Spencer et al., 2007). Recently, the prospective RIETE registry and the population based Malmö thrombophilia study reported both very similar rates of upper extremity deep vein thrombosis (4.4% and 5% of all thrombosis, respectively (Munoz et al., 2008; Isma et al., 2010). Therefore, it can be assumed that about 5% of all thrombosis will involve the deep arm veins, which corresponds to an annual incidence of approximately 3 per 100.000 patients per year (Bernardi et al., 2006). Less than 50% of these arm vein thromboses can be expected to extend into the internal jugular vein (Gbaguidi et al., 2011). About one third of patients with deep arm vein thrombosis will have primary thrombosis, i.e. idiopathic and effort-related thrombosis (Paget-von Schroetter syndrome). The remaining two thirds of patients will have secondary upper extremity thrombosis with exogenous (e.g. central venous catheters) or endogenous (e.g. cancer) risk factors. In intensive care patients as well as in patients suffering from malignant disease with central venous catheters, rates of asymptomatic thrombosis as high as 30% to over 60% have been reported (Timsit et al., 1998; Van Rooden et al., 2005). There appears to be an increase in upper extremity deep vein thrombosis in the last decades, which may reflect the increasing use of central venous catheters (S. Mustafa et al., 2003; Czihal & Hoffmann, 2011), improved diagnostic methods, or both.

3. Anatomy of the deep arm veins

The anatomy of the deep veins of the upper extremity is shown schematically in Figure 1. The two brachiocephalic veins (also known as innominate veins) join to form the superior vena cava. Each brachiocephalic vein is formed by the confluence of the subclavian with the internal jugular vein. The subclavian vein arises from (usually more than one) axillary veins, which originate from the usually paired brachial veins. The main superficial arm veins, the cephalic and basilic veins, usually drain into the sublcavian and axillary vein, respectively. The other, smaller arm veins (radial and ulnar veins) are only rarely involved in clinically significant deep vein thrombosis. Superficial thrombophlebitis may involve the cephalic and basilic veins as well as the smaller superficial veins in the cubital region or forearm. Of note, the subclavian vein passes between the clavicle and the first rib ventral of the anterior scalenus muscle, where it may be compressed in some patients especially during strenuous arm exercise. In some patients, this space is further limited by muscular hypertophy (anterior scalenus or suclavius muscle) or bone abnormalities (clavicle, first rib, cervical rib), resulting in venous thoracic outlet syndrome (Illig & Doyle, 2010).

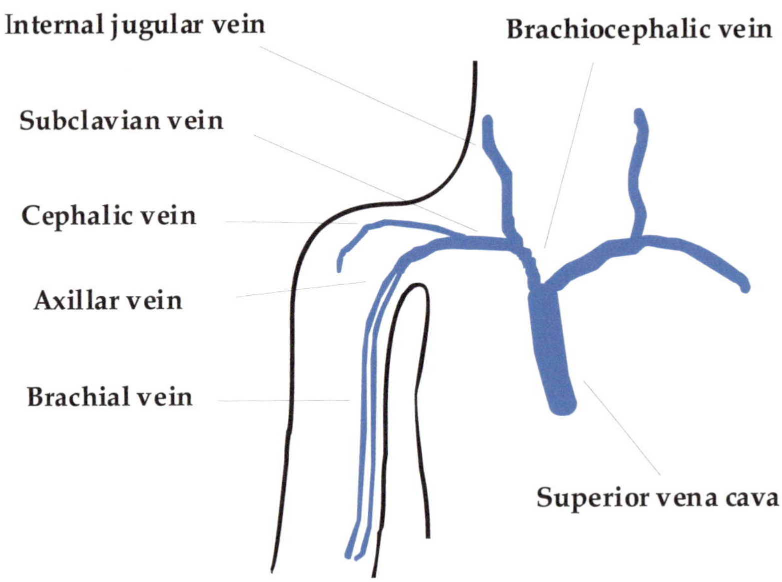

Fig. 1. Schematic view of the principal neck and arm veins.

4. Risk factors for arm vein thrombosis

Compared to deep vein thrombosis of the legs, local factors play a dominant role in deep arm vein thrombosis. By far the highest risk for thrombosis in this region is caused by foreign material in the lumen of the arm veins, most importantly indwelling central venous catheters and pacemaker leads. The odds ratio for arm vein thrombosis of patients carrying these intravascular devices compared to patients that do not has been reported to be as high as 10 to more than 1000 (Joffe et al., 2004; Blom et al., 2005), Table 1. This large variation in risk may in part be explained by specific features of the central venous catheter, as e.g. catheter type and material, site, technique and level of insertion as reviewed by Van Rooden et al., 2005. Additional factors that have an impact on the risk of thrombosis in patients with central venous catheters include the number of punctures during catheter insertion, the duration of catheterization, the fluid administered, and catheter related infections (Koksoy et al., 1995; Hernandez et al., 1998; Martin et al., 1999). In addition, wrong placement of the catheter tip in the upper half of the superior vena cava, subclavian or innominate veins results in a higher risk of thrombosis (Luciani et al., 2001; Verso et al., 2008). Implanted port a cath systems and pacemaker leads significantly increase the risk of arm vein thrombosis as well (Van Rooden et al., 2004; Goltz et al., 2010). The major pathogenetic mechanism appears to be the thrombogenicity of the foreign material itself. Other possible factors include injury of the vascular wall and disturbances of venous blood flow (Beathard, 2001). Different types of thrombi associated with central venous catheters have been described, ranging from fibrin sleeves that may be embolized following catheter removal, nonocclusive mural thrombi and complete venous obstruction (Brismar et al., 1981; Martin et al. 1999; Beathard, 2001). The second major risk factor for arm vein thrombosis is the presence of active malignant disease. Since chemotherapeutic agents are frequently delivered via central venous catheters, both major risk factors are often present in cancer patients. However, malignant disease carries a significant risk also in the absence of foreign material in the arm veins. The mechanisms by which malignant tumors promote thrombosis in various venous segments include local arrosion or invasion of blood vessels, hypercoagubility of the blood by the expression of tumor antigens, and stasis by tumor compression of venous segments proximal to the site of thrombosis (Sood, 2009; Martinelli et al., 2010). It is the experience of clinicians treating patients with thrombosis that this disease is most aggressive and difficult to treat in tumor patients. Hospitalisation has also been cited as a strong risk factor, which may be explained by the increasing frequency of complex therapeutic regimens requiring central venous lines for various indications (Joffe et al., 2004; Mai & Hunt, 2011). Other major risk factors are listed in Table 1 and include local factors (arm surgery, arm injury and immobilisation of the upper extremities by plaster casts), unusual strenuous arm exercise ("thrombosis par effort"), a family history of venous thromboembolism and inherited forms of thrombophilia, and the use of estrogen containing contraceptive drugs (Martinelli et al., 2004; Joffe et al., 2004; Blom et al., 2005). Although cited frequently, a thoracic outlet syndrome is diagnosed in comparably few cases (Blom et al., 2005). Several unusual risk factors for arm vein thrombosis have been reported in case reports, including backpacking (Schoen et al., 2007), portable computer games (Phipps & Joo, 2008), ambulatory blood pressure monitoring (Marschang et al., 2008), intravenous calcium guconate injection (Chen et al., 2009), and infraclaviculary lipoma (Palamari et al., 2010). Interestingly, two known risk factors for lower extremity deep vein thrombosis, namely age and obesity, do not appear to confer additional risk for upper deep vein thrombosis (Joffe et al., 2004; Mai & Hunt, 2011). Isolated thrombosis of the internal jugular vein may be observed in the context of two distinct clinical entities, namely after recent oropharyngeal infections with anaerobic bacteria (fusobacterium necrophorum) and in the ovarian hyperstimulation syndrome (Gbaguidi et al., 2011). For the latter syndrome, the increased risk of thrombosis has been explained by the drainage of excessive estrogen concentrations in the peritoneal fluid via the thoracic and right lymphatic duct into the confluence region of the large neck veins (Bauersachs et al., 2007).

Risk factor	Odds ratio	95 % Confidence interval	Reference
Central venous catheter	1136	153 - 8448	Blom et al. 2005
	9.7	7.8 – 12.2	Joffe et al. 2004
Active cancer	18.1	9.4 – 35.1	Blom et al. 2005
Arm surgery	13.1	2.1 – 80.6	Blom et al. 2005
Plaster cast	7.0	1.7 – 29.5	Blom et al. 2005
Factor V Leiden*	6.2	2.5 – 15.7	Martinelli et al. 2004
Prothrombin G20210A*	5.0	2.0 – 12.2	Martinelli et al. 2004
Protein C, Protein S	4.9	1.1 – 22.0	Martinelli et al. 2004
Family history of VTE	2.8	1.6 – 4.9	Blom et al. 2005
Arm injury	2.1	0.7 – 6.2	Blom et al. 2005
Oral contraceptives	2.0	1.1 -3.8	Blom et al. 2005
Unusual arm exercise	1.5	1.0 – 2.1	Blom et al. 2005

*heterozygous mutation. VTE venous thromboembolism

Table 1. Major risk factors for arm vein thrombosis with odds ratios adjusted for age and sex.

5. Clinical presentation

The presence of typical symptoms (swelling of the upper extremity, localized pain, and superficial collaterals) will raise the suspicion of the clinician to consider deep vein thrombosis of the arms. The most frequent symptom is edema of the upper extremity, which has been reported in 80% of cases by Joffe and coworkers . In addition, about 40% of patients report localized pain or aching discomfort in the involved extremity (Joffe et al., 2004). Other symptoms include reddish-blue discoloration, a sensation of heat or heaviness in the respective arm, or dilated superficial collateral veins on the upper arm, shoulder girdle, neck, and anterior chest wall (Prandoni et al., 1997a; Kommareddy et al., 2002; Bernardi et al., 2006). In at least 5% of cases, deep vein thrombosis of the arms will be completely asymptomatic (Mai & Hunt, 2011). In some cases, patients will become symptomatic only after the occurrence of complications, like dyspnea in the case of pulmonary embolism, or rarely venous gangrene (Kaufman et al., 1998). In dialysis patients, arm vein thrombosis may become symptomatic only by catheter dysfunction, like the inability to draw blood, increased dialysis pressure or arm swelling after dialysis (Hernandez et al., 1998).

In addition, classical syndromes have been described which share some but not all of their symptoms with the clinical picture described above. Superior vena cava syndrome has been described as a complication especially of catheter related arm vein thrombosis, but may also be caused by other mechanisms, e.g. venous compression by chest tumors (Lepper et al., 2011). It comprises usually bilateral edema of the face, neck, and upper extremities, together with cyanosis, plethora, and dilated subcutaneous vessels. Paget von Schroetter´s syndrome, which was first described at the end of the 19th century, is defined as a primary thrombosis of the subclavian vein at the costoclavicular junction. This syndrome is usually precipitated by musculoskeletal compression and / or repetitive microtrauma by strenuous arm exercise (thrombosis par effort) (Constans et al., 2008; Illig & Doyle, 2010). In some cases, a compression of the subclavian vein by muscular hypertophy (anterior scalenus muscle, subclavian muscle) or by the clavicle and the first rib with extreme arm movements (hyperabduction and elevation) may be responsible (thoracic outlet syndrome). Likewise, the syndrome has been linked to certain sport activities, as e.g. weight lifters, baseball pitchers or tennis players (Sheeran et al., 1997; van Stralen et al., 2005). It is observed more frequently in young patients, men (2:1), and in the dominant extremity (Illig & Doyle, 2010). The typical clinical presentation of this syndrome is a sudden onset of the typical symptoms of deep vein thrombosis described above (Illig & Doyle, 2010). Isolated thrombosis of the internal jugular vein is a rare disease which may be due to local (central venous catheters, recent oropharyngeal infections with anaerobic bacteria like fusobacterium necrophorum) or systemic factors (cancer, thrombophilia, ovarian hyperstimulation syndrome) (Sheikh et al., 2002; Gbaguidi et al., 2011). Lemierre´s syndrome, first described in 1910, is a severe condition of septic thrombosis following oropharyngeal infections, mostly due to fuosbacterium necrophorum. This syndrome is also known as human necrobacillosis or post-anginal septicaemia. Besides local symptoms (cervical edema, localized pain, dilated superficial collateral veins, erythrocyanosis, indurated vein), severe systemic complications like septicaemia and septic pulmonary embolism may occur (Vargiami & Zafeiriou, 2010; Gbaguidi et al., 2011).

When evaluating patients for clinical signs of deep arm vein thrombosis, it is important to bear in mind possible alternative diagnoses. These include e.g. superficial thrombophebitis, paravasates after peripheral infusions, lymphedema, cellulitis, haematoma, venous compression and traumatic injuries (Kommareddy et al., 2002; Bernardi et al., 2006).

6. Diagnostic procedures

As in thrombosis of the lower extremities, there are no reliable clinical symptoms to diagnose deep arm vein thrombosis. Therefore, diagnostic test are necessary to diagnose or rule out upper extremity thrombosis. Contrast venography is the gold standard diagnostic method, allowing an unparalleled overview of all arm veins with high resolution (Fig 2). However, venography is invasive, inconvenient for the patient and suffers from moderate inter-observer agreement rates (between 71 and 83%) in upper extremity deep vein thrombosis (Baarslag et al., 2003). Furthermore, possible complications as contrast agent mediated kidney damage, allergic reactions and even venography-induced thrombosis can occur (Bernardi et al., 2006).

Ultrasound has several advantages compared to invasive methods and has become the diagnostic method of choice in lower extremity deep vein thrombosis (Kearon et al., 1998; Goodacre et al., 2006). The main strengths of ultrasound are its non-invasive nature, general availability, as well as the lack of radiation and contrast material. However, ultrasound suffers generally from some disadvantages, including observer variability and usually lack of standardized documentation. In arm vein thrombosis, an additional obstacle is the portion of the subclavian vein behind the clavicle, impeding compression manoeuvres in this clinically important region. In addition, the brachiocephalic veins and the superior vena cava cannot be examined directly. In a substantial number of cases it will therefore be necessary to rely on indirect signs, as e.g. lack of Doppler signals (Fig. 3B) or characteristic changes in the Doppler flow distal of the occluded segment (Fig. 4). Nevertheless, several studies have shown high sensitivity and specificity of different ultrasound modalities (continuous wave ultrasound, compression ultrasound, colour Doppler ultrasound) in patients with suspected arm vein thrombosis (Prandoni et al., 1997a; B. O. Mustafa et al., 2002; Di Nisio et al., 2010); see Table 2. Despite these impressive numbers, the clinician should bear in mind that all these studies of arm vein thrombosis have been performed in relatively few patients. Therefore, the reported confidence intervals are wide and the safety of withholding therapy in a patient with negative ultrasound has not been proven prospectively in an adequately powered study (B.O. Mustafa et al. 2002). Even with these limitations, ultrasound is a valuable tool for the diagnosis of deep arm vein thrombosis in the hand of an experienced operator, and should be performed in most cases as the first imaging test. For magnetic resonance imaging, a study with 44 patients comparing time of flight and Gadolinium-enhanced imaging reported a moderate sensitivity and specificity (Baarslag et al., 2004). Computed tomography scanning for the diagnosis of deep arm vein thrombosis has only been described in a small case series (Kim et al., 2003), although this modality is often used to detect thrombi in clinical practice (Fig. 3A).

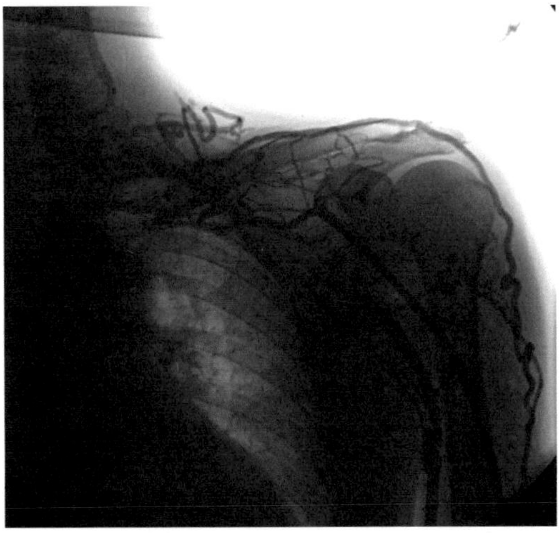

Fig. 2. Venogram of a chronic occlusion of the left subclavian vein with extensive collateralization (Department of Radiology, Innsbruck Medical University).

Since there is no imaging method combining optimal accuracy and minimal burden for the patient, alternative methods have been searched for. An interesting clinical prediction score for arm vein thrombosis, reminiscent of the Wells score for lower extremity thrombosis (Wells et al., 1997), has been published by Constans and coworkers (Constans et al., 2008). This simple score assigns one point each for a central venous catheter or pacemaker lead, localized pain and unilateral edema. One point is subtracted in the case that an alternative diagnosis would seem at least as likely as deep arm vein thrombosis. D-dimer testing has also been evaluated in a cohort of patients with suspected deep arm vein thrombosis (Merminod et al., 2006). Although nearly 100% sensitive, D-dimer suffers from a low specificity.

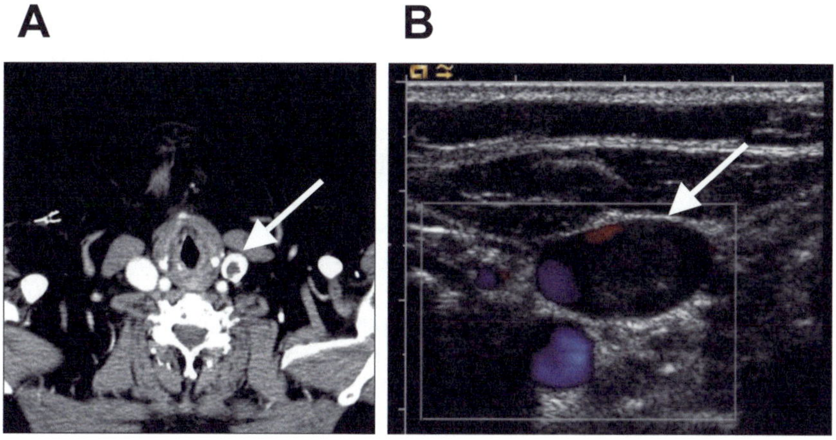

Fig. 3. Computed tomography scan (A, Department of Radiology, Innsbruck Medical University) and colour duplex ultrasound (B) of the same patient showing a floating thrombus in the left internal jugular vein.

Test	Sensitivity	Specificity	Advantage	Disadvantage	Reference
Clinical score	78%	64%	simplicity	performance	Constans et al. 2008
D-Dimer	100%	14%	sensitivity	specficity	Merminod et al. 2006
CUS	96%	94%	noninvasive	operator-dependent	Di Nisio et al. 2010
CUS + CD	100%	93%	noninvasive	operator-dependent	Di Nisio et al. 2010
MRI	71%	89%	overview	cost	Baarslag et al. 2004
Venography	100%	100%	overview	invasive	Baarslag et al. 2003

Table 2. Strengths and weaknesses of diagnostic tests for suspected deep arm vein thrombosis. CUS compression ultrasound. CD colour Doppler ultrasound. MRI magnetic resonance imaging.

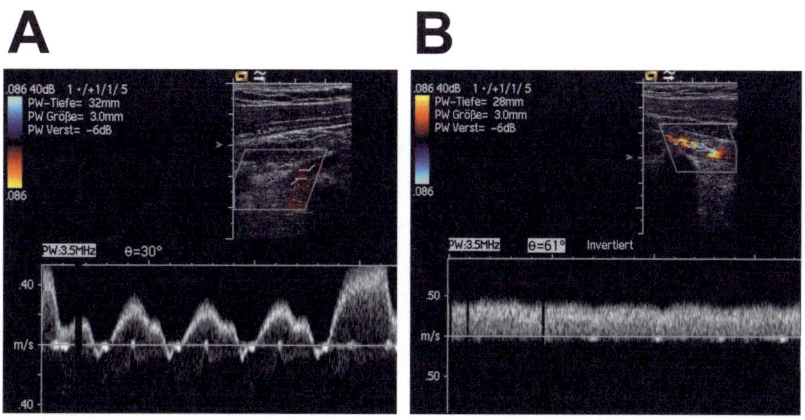

Fig. 4. Indirect sonographic diagnosis of a non-recent thrombosis of the left sublcavian vein with partial recanalisation. Normal venous flow with cardiac and respiratory modulation in the right subclavian vein (A) compared to linear flow in the left subclavian vein (B).

7. Natural history and complications

Compared to lower extremity deep vein thrombosis, relatively little is known about the natural history of deep arm vein thrombosis. The follow-up of patients not receiving anticoagulant treatment was reviewed by Thomas & Zierler, who found high rates of post-thrombotic syndrome (74%) and pulmonary embolism (12%) in patients treated only with physical methods (rest, heat, elevation) (Thomas & Zierler, 2005). These findings underscore the importance of a correct and fast diagnosis of upper extremity deep vein thrombosis and challenge the common view of arm vein thrombosis as a relatively harmless disease. However, even patients that are treated according to current guidelines have a significant risk of severe complications (Table 3). Compared to lower extremity deep vein thrombosis, patients with deep arm vein thrombosis present less frequently with concomitant pulmonary embolism (9% versus 30%) (Munoz et al., 2008; Lechner et al., 2008). However, pulmonary embolism caused by deep vein thrombosis can even be fatal in rare cases (Monreal et al., 1994). With the exception of patients with malignancies, the recurrence rate tends to be lower than in deep vein thrombosis (Spencer et al., 2007; Munoz et al., 2008). However, the total mortality of patients with upper extremity and lower extremity thrombosis appears to be similar and is mainly related to the underlying disease (Spencer et al., 2007; Munoz et al., 2008). Contrary to common believe, post-thrombotic syndrome is not a rare complication in deep arm vein thrombosis and may lead to functional disability and significant impaired quality of life in these patients (Prandoni et al., 2004; Kahn et al., 2005; Vik et al., 2009). Two modified versions of a validated score system for post-thrombotic syndrome in lower extremity thrombosis (Prandoni et al., 1997b) have been adapted to arm vein thrombosis (Table 4).

Complication	Frequency	References
Recurrence	78 / 1060 (7.4%)	Martinelli et al. 2004, Bernardi et al. 2006, Spencer et al. 2007, Munoz et al. 2008, Isma et al. 2010
Pulmonary embolism	186 / 2094 (8.9 %)	Kommareddy et al 2002, Bernardi et al. 2006, Spencer et al. 2007, Munoz et al. 2008, Lechner et al. 2008
Fatal pulmonary embolism	10 / 1156 (0.87%)	Bernardi et al. 2006, Munoz et al. 2008
Post-thrombotic syndrome	141 / 610 (23%)	Bernardi et al. 2006

Table 3. Common complications of deep arm vein thrombosis.

8. Treatment

Due to the lack of adequately powered, randomized clinical trials the current guidelines for the treatment of arm vein thrombosis are mainly based on small cohort studies, expert opinion or extrapolation of data derived from larger studies performed in patients with lower extremity deep vein thrombosis. Nevertheless, the eight edition of the American college of chest physicians' (ACCP) guidelines cover several important aspects of the treatment of patients with upper extremity deep vein thrombosis (Kearon et al., 2008). For the initial treatment, therapeutic doses of low molecular weight heparin, unfractionated heparin or fondaparinux are recommended. Overlapping with this initial treatment, long-term anticoagulation with a vitamin K antagonist should be started and continued for a minimum of 3 months. No studies are available that have addressed the ideal duration of anticoagulant therapy in patients with arm vein thrombosis. There is no specific recommendation in the ACCP guidelines on the treatment of cancer patients with upper extremity deep vein thrombosis. In cancer patients with deep arm vein thrombosis, the use of low molecular weight heparins instead of vitamin K antagonist as long-term treatment has been suggested in analogy to lower extremity thrombosis, but there are currently no studies supporting this approach (Shivakumar et al., 2009). Although various degrees of post-thrombotic syndrome have to be expected in the long term follow up of about 1 in 4 patients with upper extremity deep vein thrombosis, the ACCP guidelines do not advocate the routine use of elastic bandages or compression sleeves for the arm, unless patients report severe symptoms like persistent edema and pain.

A number of studies have described case series of deep arm vein thrombosis treated with a variety of invasive therapeutic options, including catheter-guided thrombolysis, percutaneous angioplasty with or without venous stent insertion, surgical thrombectomy and surgical decompression of costoclavicular narrowing to correct thoracic inlet syndrome, e.g. by first rib resection (Zimmermann et al., 1981; Becker et al., 1983; Machleder, 1993; Urschel & Razzuk, 1998). Some investigators recommend such an invasive approach routinely e.g in patients with effort related thrombosis (Paget von Schroetter´s syndrome) (Kommareddy et al., 2002). Here, the ACCP guidelines clearly do not recommend invasive procedures routinely, but only in selected patients and in specially equipped centers. It remains to be determined in adequately designed, randomized clinical trials whether these invasive procedures, which carry a substantial risk of major bleeding and other serious complications, provide a benefit compared to standard anticoagulation with optimal mechanical compression using elastic bandages.

Subjective symptoms	**Objective Signs**	**Subjective symptoms**	**Objective Signs**
Heaviness	Edema	Heaviness	Edema
Pain	Skin induration	Pain	Prominent veins on arm
Pruritus	Discoloration	Pruritus	Prominent veins over shoulder or anterior chest wall
Physical limitation	Venous ectasia	Cramps	Dependent cyanosis
Paraesthesia	Redness	Paraesthesia	Redness
	Pain during compression		Tenderness
Prandoni et al. 2004, Vik et al. 2009		Kahn et al. 2005	

Table 4. Two suggested modifications of the Villalta scale for the assessment of post-thrombotic syndrome in deep arm vein thrombosis. Each sign or symptom is graded as 0 (absent), 1 (mild), 2 (moderate) or 3 (severe). A score of 5 or higher is classified as post-thrombotic syndrome and score of 15 or higher as severe post-thrombotic syndrome.

Another point of debate is the question whether central venous catheters should be removed when a diagnosis of deep vein thrombosis has been confirmed in the respective vessel. Most experts opt against catheter removal, if the catheter is still needed and still functional. In a cohort study of 74 cancer patients with acute upper extremity thrombosis, the catheters were not removed and patients were treated for 3 months with standard anticoagulation without recurrent episodes of venous thromboembolism (Kovacs et al., 2007). If the catheter is removed, the ACCP guidelines recommend not to shorten the anticoagulation period below 3 months (Kearon et al., 2008).

9. Prevention

Patients with central venous catheters carry a high risk of deep arm vein thrombosis, which may exceed 60 % in certain patient groups (ICU patients, oncological and hematological patients) Van Rooden et al., 2005. Therefore, approaches to prevent catheter-related thrombosis by means of pharmacological prophylaxis e.g. in cancer patients, appear attractive. However, despite an early study showing benefit of low dose warfarin in this context (Bern et al., 1990), subsequent studies with warfarin and heparins could not confirm this protective effect. A recent meta-analysis did show a trend, but no significant reduction of symptomatic deep vein thrombosis with any form of thromboprophylaxis (Akl et al., 2008). In accordance with these data, the current guidelines for the prevention of venous thromboembolism do not recommend routine use of thromboprophyaxis in cancer patients with indwelling central venous catheters (Geerts et al., 2008).

The placement of superior vena cava filters has been reported in case reports and small case series. Although effective in preventing pulmonary embolism from thrombi in the upper extremities, these filters may cause severe complications, like cardiac tamponade and aortic perforation (Owens et al., 2010) and do not protect from thrombi in the lower extremities. Therefore, the placement of these filters should be limited to special situations (Kucher, 2011).

10. Conclusions / open questions

About 5% of all thromboses are expected to occur in the deep veins of the upper extremities. Besides effort-related thromboses, most patients with arm vein thrombosis have typical risk factors, like central venous catheters or malignancies. Typical clinical syndromes include edema and localized pain, whereas other patients are asymptomatic or present with complex syndromes. Today, diagnosis will most often be performed by ultrasound; in some cases additional testing (e.g. computed tomography scanning, magnetic resonance imaging) will be necessary. The most important complications are recurrent thrombosis, pulmonary embolism and post-thrombotic syndrome. Treatment should be initiated without delay and consist in most cases of standard anticoagulation treatment with heparins followed by a vitamin K antagonist for at least 3 months. In selected cases, invasive therapeutic regimes including catheter-guided thrombolysis and surgical procedures may be applied. Routine prevention of catheter-related thrombosis or embolic complications by anticoagulants in prophylactic doses or implantation of superior vena cava filters is not recommended. Compared to deep vein thrombosis of the lower extremities, deep vein thrombosis of the arm veins has been studied much less intensely. For example, the optimal duration of anticoagulant therapy and the value of compression therapy are not precisely known for arm vein thromboses. Therefore, many of the current recommendation are in fact extrapolations from data on deep leg vein thrombosis. Specific studies are needed to better understand the pathogenesis of deep vein thrombosis of the arms and to improve diagnostic and therapeutic strategies.

11. References

Akl, E.A.; Kamath, G.; Yosuico, V.; Kim, S.Y.; Barba, M.; Sperati, F.; Cook, D.J. & Schunemann, H.J. (2008) Thromboprophylaxis for patients with cancer and central venous catheters. *Cancer* 112, 2483-2492.

Baarslag, H.J.; Van Beek, E.J.R.; Tijssen, J.G.P.; van Delden, O.M.; Bakker, A.J. & Reekers, J.A. (2003) Deep vein thrombosis of the upper extremity: intra- and interobserver study of digital subtraction venography. *European Radiology* 13, 251-255.

Baarslag, H.J.; Van Beek, E.J.R. & Reekers, J.A. (2004) Magnetic resonance venography in consecutive patients with suspected deep vein thrombosis of the upper extremity: Initial experience. *Acta Radiologica* 45, 38-43.

Bauersachs, R.M.; Manolopoulos, K.; Hoppe, I.; Arin, M.J. & Schleussner, E. (2007) More on: the 'ART' behind the clot: solving the mystery. *Journal of Thrombosis and Haemostasis* 5, 438-439.

Beathard, G.A. (2001) Catheter thrombosis. *Seminars in Dialysis* 14, 441-445.

Becker, G.J.; Holden, R.W.; Rabe, F.E.; Castanedazuniga, W.R.; Sears, N.; Dilley, R.S. & Glover, J.L. (1983) Local thrombolytic therapy for subclavian and axillary vein-thrombosis - treatment of the thoracic inlet syndrome. *Radiology* 149, 419-423.

Bern, M.M.; Lokich, J.J.; Wallach, S.R.; Bothe, A.; Benotti, P.N.; Arkin, C.F.; Greco, F.A.; Huberman, M. & Moore, C. (1990) Very low-doses of warfarin can prevent thrombosis in central venous catheters - a randomized prospective trial. *Annals of Internal Medicine* 112, 423-428.

Bernardi, E.; Pesavento, R. & Prandoni, P. (2006) Upper extremity deep venous thrombosis. *Semin.Thromb.Hemost.* 32, 729-736.

Blom, J.W.; Doggen, C.J.; Osanto, S. & Rosendaal, F.R. (2005) Old and new risk factors for upper extremity deep venous thrombosis. *J.Thromb.Haemost.* 3, 2471-2478.

Brismar, B; Hardstedt, C & Jacobson, S. (1981). Diagnosis of thrombosis by catheter phlebography after prolonged central venous catheterization. *Annals of Surgery* 194,779-783.

Chen, S.C.; Chang, J.M.; Wang, C.S.; Wu, H.C. & Chen, H.C. (2009) Upper limb deep vein thrombosis following calcium gluconate injection. *Nephrology* 14, 621.

Constans, J.; Salmi, L.R.; Sevestre-Pietri, M.A.; Perusat, S.; Nguon, M.; Degeilh, M.; Labarere, J.; Gattolliat, O.; Boulon, C.; Laroche, J.P.; Le Roux, P.; Pichot, O.; Quere, I.; Conri, C. & Bosson, J.L. (2008) A clinical prediction score for upper extremity deep venous thrombosis. *Thromb.Haemost.* 99, 202-207.

Czihal, M. & Hoffmann, U. (2011) Upper extremity deep venous thrombosis. *Vascular Medicine* 16, 191-202.

Di Nisio, M.; van Sluis, G.L.; Bossuyt, P.M.M.; Buller, H.R.; Porreca, E. & Rutjes, A.W.S. (2010) Accuracy of diagnostic tests for clinically suspected upper extremity deep vein thrombosis: a systematic review. *Journal of Thrombosis and Haemostasis* 8, 684-692.

Gbaguidi, X.; Janvresse, A.; Benichou, J.; Cailleux, N.; Levesque, H. & Marie, I. (2011) Internal jugular vein thrombosis: outcome and risk factors. *Qjm-An International Journal of Medicine* 104, 209-219.

Geerts, W.H.; Bergqvist, D.; Pineo, G.F.; Heit, J.A.; Samama, C.M.; Lassen, M.R. & Colwell, C.W. (2008) Prevention of venous thromboembolism. *Chest* 133, 381S-453S.

Goltz, J.P.; Scholl, A.; Ritter, C.O.; Wittenberg, G.; Hahn, D. & Kickuth, R. (2010) Peripherally placed totally implantable venous-access port systems of the forearm: clinical experience in 763 consecutive patients. *Cardiovascular and Interventional Radiology* 33, 1159-1167.

Goodacre, S.; Sampson, F.; Stevenson, M.; Wailoo, A.; Sutton, A.; Thomas, S.; Locker, T. & Ryan, A. (2006) Measurement of the clinical and cost-effectiveness of non-invasive diagnostic testing strategies for deep vein thrombosis. *Health Technology Assessment* 10, 1-168.

Hernandez, D.; Diaz, F.; Rufino, M.; Lorenzo, V.; Perez, T.; Rodriguez, A.; De Bonis, E.; Losada, M.; Gonzalez-Posada, J.M. & Torres, A. (1998) Subclavian vascular access stenosis in dialysis patients: Natural history and risk factors. *Journal of the American Society of Nephrology* 9, 1507-1510.

Hill, S.L. & Berry, R.E. (1990) Subclavian vein thrombosis: a continuing challenge. *Surgery* 108, 1-9.

Illig, K.A. & Doyle, A.J. (2010) A comprehensive review of Paget-Schroetter syndrome. *Journal of Vascular Surgery* 51, 1538-1547.

Isma, N.; Svensson, P.J.; Gottsater, A. & Lindblad, B. (2010) Upper extremity deep venous thrombosis in the population-based Malmo thrombophilia study (MATS). Epidemiology, risk factors, recurrence risk, and mortality. *Thrombosis Research* 125, E335-E338.

Joffe, H.V.; Kucher, N.; Tapson, V.F. & Goldhaber, S.Z. (2004) Upper-extremity deep vein thrombosis: a prospective registry of 592 patients. *Circulation* 110, 1605-1611.

Kahn, S.R.; Elman, E.; Bornais, C.; Blostein, M. & Wells, P.S. (2005) Post-thrombotic syndrome, functional disability and quality of life after upper extremity deep venous thrombosis in adults. *Thrombosis and Haemostasis* 93, 499-502.

Kaufman, B.R.; Zoldos, J.; Bentz, M. & Nystrom, N.A. (1998) Venous gangrene of the upper extremity. *Annals of Plastic Surgery* 40, 370-377.

Kearon, C.; Ginsberg, J.S. & Hirsh, J. (1998) The role of venous ultrasonography in the diagnosis of suspected deep venous thrombosis and pulmonary embolism. *Annals of Internal Medicine* 129, 1044-1049.

Kearon, C.; Kahn, S.R.; Agnelli, G.; Goldhaber, S.; Raskob, G.E. & Comerota, A.J. (2008) Antithrombotic therapy for venous thromboembolic disease: American College of Chest Physicians Evidence-Based Clinical Practice Guidelines (8th Edition). *Chest* 133, 454S-545S.

Kim, H.C.; Chung, J.W.; Park, J.H.; Yin, Y.H.; Park, S.H.; Yoon, C.J. & Choi, Y.H. (2003) Role of CT venography in the diagnosis and treatment of benign thoracic central venous obstruction. *Korean Journal of Radiology* 4, 146-152.

Koksoy, C.; Kuzu, A.; Erden, I. & Akkaya, A. (1995) The risk-factors in central venous catheter-related thrombosis. *Australian and New Zealand Journal of Surgery* 65, 796-798.

Kommareddy, A.; Zaroukian, M.H. & Hassouna, H.I. (2002) Upper extremity deep venous thrombosis. *Semin.Thromb.Hemost.* 28, 89-99.

Kovacs, M.J.; Kahn, S.R.; Rodger, M.; Anderson, D.R.; Andreou, R.; Mangel, J.E.; Morrow, B.; Clement, A.M. & Wells, P.S. (2007). A pilot study of central venous catheter survival in cancer patients using low-molecular-weight heparin (dalteparin) and warfarin without catheter removal for the treatment of upper extremity deep vein thrombosis (the catheter study). *Journal of Thrombosis and Haemostasis* 5:1650-1653

Kucher, N. (2011) Deep-vein thrombosis of the upper extremities. *New England Journal of Medicine* 364, 861-869.

Lechner, D.; Wiener, C.; Weltermann, A.; Eischer, L.; Eichinger, S. & Kyrle, P.A. (2008) Comparison between idiopathic deep vein thrombosis of the upper and lower extremity regarding risk factors and recurrence. *Journal of Thrombosis and Haemostasis* 6, 1269-1274.

Lepper, P.M.; Ott, S.R.; Hoppe, H.; Schumann, C.; Stammberger, U.; Bugalho, A.; Frese, S.; Schmucking, M.; Blumstein, N.M.; Diehm, N.; Bals, R. & Hamacher, J. (2011) Superior vena cava syndrome in thoracic malignancies. *Respiratory Care* 56, 653-666.

Luciani, A.; Clement, O.; Halimi, P.; Goudot, D.; Portier, F.; Bassot, N.; Luciani, J.A.; Avan, P.; Frija, G. & Bonfils, P. (2001) Catheter-related upper extremity deep venous thrombosis in cancer patients: A prospective study based on Doppler US. *Radiology* 220, 655-660.

Machleder, H.I. (1993) Evaluation of a new treatment strategy for Paget-Schroetter syndrome - spontaneous thrombosis of the axillary-subclavian vein. *Journal of Vascular Surgery* 17, 305-317.
Mai, C. & Hunt, D. (2011) Upper extremity deep venous thrombosis: a review. *American Journal of Medicine* 124, 402-407.
Marschang, P.; Niederwanger, A.; Gasser, R.W.; Daniaux, M. & Sturm, W. (2008) Symptomatic upper extremity deep vein thrombosis as a complication of ambulatory blood pressure monitoring. *Thromb.Haemost.* 100, 711-712.
Martin, C.; Viviand, X.; Saux, P. & Gouin, F. (1999) Upper-extremity deep vein thrombosis after central venous catheterization via the axillary vein. *Critical Care Medicine* 27, 2626-2629.
Martinelli, I.; Battaglioli, T.; Bucciarelli, P.; Passamonti, S.M. & Mannucci, P.M. (2004) Risk factors and recurrence rate of primary deep vein thrombosis of the upper extremities. *Circulation* 110, 566-570.
Martinelli, I.; Bucciarelli, P. & Mannucci, P.M. (2010) Thrombotic risk factors: Basic pathophysiology. *Critical Care Medicine* 38, S3-S9.
Merminod, T.; Pellicciotta, S. & Bounameaux, H. (2006) Limited usefulness of D-dimer in suspected deep vein thrombosis of the upper extremities. *Blood Coagulation & Fibrinolysis* 17, 225-226.
Monreal, M.; Raventos, A.; Lerma, R.; Ruiz, J.; Lafoz, E.; Alastrue, A. & Llamazares, J.F. (1994) Pulmonary embolism in patients with upper extremity DVT associated to venous central lines - a prospective-study. *Thrombosis and Haemostasis* 72, 548-550.
Munoz, F.J.; Mismetti, P.; Poggio, R.; Valle, R.; Barron, M.; Guil, M. & Monreal, M. (2008) Clinical outcome of patients with upper-extremity deep vein thrombosis - Results from the RIETE registry. *Chest* 133, 143-148.
Mustafa, B.O.; Rathbun, S.W.; Whitsett, T.L. & Raskob, G.E. (2002) Sensitivity and specificity of ultrasonography in the diagnosis of upper extremity deep vein thrombosis - A systematic review. *Archives of Internal Medicine* 162, 401-404.
Mustafa, S.; Stein, P.D.; Patel, K.C.; Otten, T.R.; Holmes, R. & Silbergleit, A. (2003) Upper extremity deep venous thrombosis. *Chest* 123, 1953-1956.
Owens, C.A.; Bui, J.T.; Knuttinen, M.G.; Gaba, R.C. & Carrillo, T.C. (2010) Pulmonary embolism from upper extremity deep vein thrombosis and the role of superior vena cava filters: A review of the literature. *Journal of Vascular and Interventional Radiology* 21, 779-787.
Palamari, B.; Breen, J.F. & Wysokinski, W.E. (2010) Lipoma causing upper extremity deep vein thrombosis: A case report. *Journal of Thrombosis and Thrombolysis* 30, 109-111.
Phipps, C. & Joo, H. (2008) Upper limb deep vein thrombosis and portable computer games. *American Journal of Medicine* 121, E3.
Prandoni, P.; Polistena, P.; Bernardi, E.; Cogo, A.; Casara, D.; Verlato, F.; Angelini, F.; Simioni, P.; Signorini, G.P.; Benedetti, L. & Girolami, A. (1997a.) Upper-extremity deep vein thrombosis - Risk factors, diagnosis, and complication. *Archives of Internal Medicine* 157, 57-62.
Prandoni, P.; Villalta, S.; Bagatella, P.; Rossi, L.; Marchiori, A.; Piccioli, A.; Bernardi, E.; Girolami, B.; Simioni, P. & Girolami, A. (1997b.) The clinical course of deep-vein thrombosis. Prospective long-term follow-up of 528 symptomatic patients. *Haematologica* 82, 423-428.
Prandoni, P.; Bernardi, E.; Marchiori, A.; Lensing, A.W.; Prins, M.H.; Villalta, S.; Bagatella, P.; Sartor, D.; Piccioli, A.; Simioni, P.; Pagnan, A. & Girolami, A. (2004) The long term

clinical course of acute deep vein thrombosis of the arm: prospective cohort study. *BMJ* 329, 484-485.
Schoen N.; Netzsch, C. & Kröger K. (2007) Subclavian vein thrombosis and backpacking. *Clinical Research in Cardiology* 96, 42-44.
Sheeran, S.R.; Hallisey, M.J.; Murphy, T.P.; Faberman, R.S. & Sherman, S. (1997) Local thrombolytic therapy as part of a multidisciplinary approach to acute axillosubclavian vein thrombosis (Paget-Schroetter syndrome). *Journal of Vascular and Interventional Radiology* 8, 253-260.
Sheikh, M.A.; Topoulos, A.P. & Deitcher, S.R. (2002) Isolated internal jugular vein thrombosis: risk factors and natural history. *Vascular Medicine* 7, 177-179.
Shivakumar, S.P.; Anderson, D.R. & Couban, S. (2009) Catheter-associated thrombosis in patients with malignancy. *Journal of Clinical Oncology* 27, 4858-4864.
Sood, S.L. (2009) Cancer-associated thrombosis. *Current Opinion in Hematology* 16, 378-385.
Spencer, F.A.; Emery, C.; Lessard, D. & Goldberg, R.J. (2007) Upper extremity deep vein thrombosis: A community-based perspective. *American Journal of Medicine* 120, 678-684.
Thomas, I.H. & Zierler B.K. (2005) An integrative review of outcomes in patients with acute primary upper extremity deep venous thrombosis following no treatment or treatment with anticoagulation, thrombolysis, or surgical algorithms. *Vascular and Endovascular Surgery* 39, 163-174.
Timsit, J.F.; Farkas, J.C.; Boyer, J.M.; Martin, J.B.; Misset, B.; Renaud, B. & Carlet, J. (1998) Central vein catheter-related thrombosis in intensive care patients - Incidence, risks factors, and relationship with catheter-related sepsis. *Chest* 114, 207-213.
Urschel, H.C. & Razzuk, M.A. (1998) Neurovascular compression in the thoracic outlet - Changing management over 50 years. *Annals of Surgery* 228, 609-615.
Van Rooden, C.J.; Molhoek, S.G.; Rosendaal, F.R.; Schalij, M.J.; Meinders, A.E. & Huisman, M.V. (2004) Incidence and risk factors of early venous thrombosis associated with permanent pacemaker leads. *Journal of Cardiovascular Electrophysiology* 15, 1258-1262.
Van Rooden, C.J.; Tesselaar, M.E.T.; Osanto, S.; Rosendaal, F.R. & Huisman, M.V. (2005) Deep vein thrombosis associated with central venous catheters - a review. *Journal of Thrombosis and Haemostasis* 3, 2409-2419.
Van Stralen, K.J.; Blom, J.W.; Doggen, C.J.M. & Rosendaal, F.R. (2005) Strenuous sport activities involving the upper extremities increase the risk of venous thrombosis of the arm. *Journal of Thrombosis and Haemostasis* 3, 2110-2111.
Vargiami, E.G. & Zafeiriou, D.I. (2010) Eponym The Lemierre syndrome. *European Journal of Pediatrics* 169, 411-414.
Verso, M.; Agnelli, G.; Kamphuisen, P.W.;. Ageno, W.; Bazzan, M.; Lazzaro, A.; Paoletti, F.; Paciaroni, M.; Mosca, S. & Bertoglio, S. (2008) Risk factors for upper limb deep vein thrombosis associated with the use of central vein catheter in cancer patients. *Internal and Emergency Medicine* 3, 117-122.
Vik, A.; Holme, P.A.; Singh, K.; Dorenberg, E.; Nordhus, K.C.; Kumar, S. & Hansen, J.B. (2009) Catheter-directed thrombolysis for treatment of deep venous thrombosis in the upper extremities. *Cardiovascular and Interventional Radiology* 32, 980-987.
Wells, P.S.; Anderson, D.R.; Bormanis, J.; Guy, F.; Mitchell, M.; Gray, L.; Clement, C.; Robinson, K.S. & Lewandowski, B. (1997) Value of assessment of pretest probability of deep-vein thrombosis in clinical management. *Lancet* 350, 1795-1798.
Zimmermann, R.; Morl, H.; Harenberg, J.; Gerhardt, P.; Kuhn, H.M. & Wahl, P. (1981) urokinase therapy of subclavian-axillary vein-thrombosis. *Klinische Wochenschrift* 59, 851-856. Supported by grant P 20825-B05 of the Austrian Science Funds (FWF).

The Post Thrombotic Syndrome

Paolo Prandoni[1] and Susan R Kahn[2]
[1]*Department of Cardiothoracic and Vascular Sciences, Thromboembolism Unit, University of Padua, Padua*
[2]*Centre for Clinical Epidemiology and Community Studies, Sir Mortimer B. Davis Jewish General Hospital, Montreal, Quebec*
[1]*Italy*
[2]*Canada*

1. Introduction

Despite appropriate anticoagulant therapy, at least 1 of every 2-3 patients with deep-vein thrombosis (DVT) of the lower extremities will develop post-thrombotic sequelae. These vary from minor signs (i.e., stasis pigmentation, venous ectasia, slight pain and swelling) to severe manifestations such as chronic pain, intractable edema and leg ulcers (1). The established post-thrombotic syndrome (PTS) remains a significant cause of chronic illness, with considerable socio-economic consequences for both the patient and the health care services (2,3).

The precise incidence of the PTS following confirmed venous thrombosis is still controversial, as the rate of post-thrombotic sequelae reported in published studies has varied between 20% and 100%. In earlier studies, a surprisingly high rate of severe PTS complications was reported (50 to 100% of the patients within 4 to 10 years after the qualifying thrombotic episode) (4-6). This rate sharply decreased in studies performed in the last 25 years (7-39), which could be due to improved diagnostic and therapeutic approaches to patients with DVT. However, owing to large differences among studies in terms of study design, definition of PTS, sample size, length of follow-up, and use of compression elastic stockings, the reported incidence of both overall and severe PTS still shows considerable variability. In the absence of elastic stockings, PTS is expected to develop in approximately 50% of patients suffering an episode of DVT, and is severe in one fifth of patients (1). Of interest, PTS can develop, although to a lower extent, also after an asymptomatic episode of postoperative DVT (40,41).

According to the results of the most recent studies, most patients who develop post-thrombotic manifestations become symptomatic within two years from the acute episode of DVT (1,18-20,29-32,35-37,39). These findings challenge the general view that the PTS requires many years to become manifest.

2. Clinical diagnosis and objective diagnostic testing

2.1 Clinical diagnosis and scoring systems

The post-thrombotic syndrome is characterized by aching pain on standing, dependent edema, and the frequent development of brawny, tender induration of the subcutaneous tissues of the medial lower limb, a condition that has been termed "lipodermatosclerosis". Pruritus and eczematous skin changes are frequently present, and a proportion of patients develops secondary superficial varicose veins as the syndrome evolves. Ulceration, often precipitated by minor trauma, arises in a considerable number of patients and is characteristically chronic and indolent with a high recurrence rate, once healing has been achieved. Uncommonly, patients with persistent obstruction may experience venous claudication, a bursting pain in the leg during exercise, which, in some respects, mimics arterial claudication (42).

The clinical picture of the PTS is non-specific, as clinical conditions other than DVT may result in a similar set of symptoms and signs in the lower extremity, including superficial venous insufficiency, increased body mass index, and trauma (43-45).

The diagnosis of the PTS is made based on the development of the above mentioned clinical manifestations in patients with a history of DVT, irrespective of the presence of venous abnormalities as shown by invasive or non-invasive diagnostic procedures. In the absence of characteristic signs and symptoms, the demonstration of venous abnormalities (such as venous reflux, persistent venous obstruction, or both) does not, in itself, allow a patient with a history of DVT to be defined as having PTS.

Subjective Symptoms	**Objective Signs**
Heaviness	Pretibial edema
Pain	nduration of the skin
Cramps	Hyperpigmentation
Pruritus	New venous ectasia
	Redness
Paresthesia	Pain during calf compression
	Ulceration of the skin

*Each sign or symptom is graded with a score between 0 and 3. The presence of ulcer is only noted. PTS is classified as mild if the score is 5-9, moderate if the score is 10-14, and severe if the score is ≥ 15 or a venous ulcer is present.

Table 1. Villalta scale for the assessment of the PTS

Although the clinical picture of the PTS is classical, there is large variation among published studies as to its clinical classification. Among the suggested scoring systems, the Villalta scale and the CEAP classification are the most widely adopted (46). The former, based on clinical findings alone (Table 1), has high interobserver agreement (47,48), and good ability to discriminate patients with versus those without PTS and patients with mild versus those with severe PTS (1,47,49). In addition, this scale correlates well with the patient's perception of the interference of leg complaints with daily life (31,47,49). The Villalta scale has recently been recommended as a standard to define PTS for use in clinical investigations by the Scientific and Standardization Committee of the International Society on Thrombosis and Haemostasis (50). The latter, known as CEAP (Clinical, Etiologic, Anatomic, Pathophysiologic) classification, was developed as a result of the cooperative work of a panel of experts in the field of vascular disease, and combines clinical and objective findings into a sophisticated scoring system (Table 2) (51).

Clinical signs	Class 0	No visible or palpable signs of venous disease
	Class 1	Telangiectasia or reticular veins
	Class 2	Varicose veins
	Class 3	Edema
	Class 4	Skin changes ascribed to venous disease
	Class 5	Skin changes as described above with healed ulceration
	Class 6	Leg ulceration, skin changes as defined above
Etiologic classificatio	Congenital, primary, secondary	
Anatomic distribution	Superficial, deep, or perforator, alone or in combination	
Pathophysiologic dysfunction	Reflux or obstruction, alone or in combination	

Table 2. CEAP (clinical, etiologic, anatomic, pathophysiologic) classification of the PTS

2.2 Objective diagnostic testing

If a patient with a history of a previous (documented or highly suspected) DVT develops symptoms and signs compatible with PTS there is no need for further investigation. As the clinical picture may be non-specific (43-45), the need for objective confirmation arises in patients with leg complaints but without a likely or objectively proven previous DVT. Ascending phlebography is potentially useful to detect a previous DVT. Suggestive findings include narrowing or occlusion of the deep veins, contrast dye opacification of fewer veins (than normal) or perfusion of superficial or deep collateral veins. Recanalized veins show irregular margins, bizarre-appearing or multi-channeled lumen with webs, and usually have reduced caliber due to fibrotic thickening of their walls. Such veins may subsequently become dilated, probably because of loss of their elastic tissue (52). Despite the predictive value of these venographic patterns in patients with possible PTS, the invasive nature and cost of plebography makes such an approach inapplicable to most patients with a history of clinically suspected DVT.

We have shown that the combination of standardized clinical evaluation with compression ultrasonography and continuous-wave Doppler analysis can reliably diagnose or exclude a prior proximal-vein thrombosis in almost 90% of patients with a suggestive history (53). Compression ultrasonography should be performed first, checking the popliteal and the common femoral vein for compressibility. If either or both veins are incompressible, then a definite diagnosis of previous (proximal) DVT is made. Patients with normal ultrasound test results are interviewed and examined according to a standardized form (Table 1), and subsequently undergo continuous-wave Doppler analysis to test valve function, both in the common femoral and in the popliteal vein. The finding of both a popliteal reflux and/or of a clinical score > 8 is highly specific for the adjudication of a prior DVT in patients with a normal ultrasound test result. If ultrasound testing is normal, deep venous reflux is absent, and the clinical score is < 8, then previous proximal DVT is virtually excluded (53). The widespread availability of Duplex scanning renders our approach even more rapid and precise, as it permits venous flow sampling during direct visualization of the vessels.

Besides the demonstration of previous episodes of DVT, either invasive or non-invasive methods can be employed to document and quantify the presence of obstruction, reflux, or both, that are considered the major determinants of the PTS.

3. Pathophysiology of PTS development

It is generally believed that the PTS develops as a result of the combination of venous hypertension, due to persistent outflow obstruction and/or valvular incompetence, with abnormal microvasculature or lymphatic function. Long-standing venous hypertension in the deep-vein system ultimately leads to the onset of valve incompetence at the level of a constant series of perforating veins located in the medial ankle area. This allows the direct transmission of the high deep-venous pressures (especially during walking) to the venous end of subcutaneous capillaries, resulting in increased endothelial permeability. The escape of large molecules into the interstitial tissue may, in turn, explain the typical pattern of edema, hyperpigmentation and even ulcer formation (42,44,45). A few authors speculate that increased venous pressure with standing or walking causes a reduction in capillary flow rate, resulting in trapping of white blood cells in the leg and the subsequent release of free radical and proteolytic enzymes ultimately responsible for the venous ulceration (54,55).

The presence of reflux in the proximal veins is reputed to be crucial for the development of the PTS, and so is the persistence of venous obstruction, alone or in combination with venous reflux (15,35,56-61). However, this is an area of considerable uncertainty. Recently, we assessed the role of residual vein thrombosis and popliteal valve incompetence for the development of the PTS, as measured with the Villalta scale, in 180 consecutive patients who were followed for at least three years after an episode of acute proximal DVT (62). In the first six months following the thrombotic episode, venous abnormalities were detected in 104 patients (60%). The PTS developed in 18 of the 76 patients (24%) without vein abnormalities, and in 49 of the 104 (47%) with at least one abnormality: in 25 of the 52 (48%) with residual vein thrombosis alone, in 9 of the 24 (37.5%) with popliteal valve incompetence alone, and in 15 of the 28 (54%) with both abnormalities. The relative risk of the PTS was 1.0 (95% CI, 0.5 to 2.2) in patients with popliteal valve incompetence alone; 1.4 (0.9 to 2.3) in patients with transpopliteal reflux alone or combined with persistent venous obstruction; 1.6 (1.0 to 2.4) in patients with residual vein thrombosis alone; and 1.7 (1.2 to 2.3) in patients with persistent venous obstruction alone or combined with popliteal valve incompetence.

Roumen-Klappe and coworkers assessed the role of residual thrombosis, reflux and venous outflow resistance in 93 patients with proximal and distal DVT, followed for 6 years; the incidence of the PTS was 49% after 1 year, 55% after 2 years, without further increase up to 6 years. While the presence of reflux had only moderate predictive value, a strong increase in the predictive value was achieved by combining measures of residual thrombus, assessed by a thrombosis score, and venous outflow resistance, at three months (32). On the basis of these findings, a lack of recanalization within the first six months after the thrombotic episode appears to be an important predictor of PTS, while the development of transpopliteal venous reflux is not. However, incompetence of the popliteal valve increases the risk of the PTS when combined with residual vein thrombosis (32,62).

In a recent report, increased levels of inflammatory cytokines or adhesion molecules such as IL-6 and ICAM-1 were linked with the subsequent development of PTS (63). This suggests that inflammation at the time of, or consequent to the episode of acute DVT may play a role in the pathophysiology of PTS, a hypothesis that is being further explored in a large prospective study (64).

4. Predictors of PTS development

Among parameters that have been found to be associated with an increased risk of the PTS are proximal DVT (33,38,39,60), previous ipsilateral DVT (14,16,18,28,29,33,39), older age (29,65), obesity (38,39,65-67), and varicose veins (38). In one investigation the male gender was a predictor of the PTS (33), while in others the opposite was seen (38,39). Finally, whether the carriage of factor V Leiden or the prothrombin mutation are predictors of a lower risk or reduced severity of the PTS is controversial, as there are data in favor (31) and against (38,39) this association.

In order to determine the frequency, time course, and predictors of the PTS after acute DVT, we followed 387 patients for up to two years after an episode of acute symptomatic DVT (39). With the use of the Villalta score, greater postthrombotic severity category at the 1-month visit strongly predicted higher mean postthrombotic scores throughout 24 months of follow-up (1.97, 5.03, and 7.00 increase in Villalta score for mild, moderate, and severe 1-month severity categories, respectively, vs. none). Additional predictors of higher scores over time were venous thrombosis of the common femoral or iliac vein (2.23 increase in score vs. distal venous thrombosis), higher body mass index (0.14 increase in score per kg/m2), previous ipsilateral venous thrombosis (1.78 increase in score), older age (0.30 increase in score per 10-year age increase), and female sex (0.79 increase in score). Accordingly, appropriate strategies aimed at reducing the risk of recurrent DVT, and reducing the body weight in obese patients have the potential to help prevent late post-thrombotic sequelae.

Proximal DVT is associated with a higher frequency and more severe PTS than distal DVT. In the abovementioned study, patients with more extensive proximal (femoral or iliac vein) DVT had significantly worse PTS scores at all visits (adjusted average increase of > 2 points on the Villalta scale) than those with distal or popliteal vein DVT (39). Similarly, in another recent prospective study, proximal DVT was found to be associated with a 2-fold increased risk of PTS compared with distal DVT (33). As the rates of PTS in the control arms of trials of compression stockings to prevent PTS in patients with proximal DVT ranged from 40-50%, the rate of PTS after distal DVT is likely to be in the range of 20-25%, however in one study, symptoms of PTS after distal DVT were relatively mild (23).

Finally, an insufficient quality of oral anticoagulant therapy following the acute thrombotic episode has been found to be associated with an increased risk of the PTS (28,65). Accordingly, appropriate attention to the monitoring of oral anticoagulant therapy following the initial thrombotic episode, in terms of both adequate intensity and duration, has the potential to help prevent late post-thrombotic sequelae.

5. Treatment of the PTS

Once established, PTS, especially when complicated by leg ulceration, is a significant cause of disability with a considerable economic burden for both patients and the health care system (1,2). The management of this condition is demanding and oftentimes frustrating. Several treatment strategies, both conservative and surgical, have been tested, especially aimed at ulcer healing.

5.1 Conservative treatment

Compression therapy, either obtained with short stretch bandages, adhesive bandages, multiple layer bandages (with orthopedic wool plus compressive layers), stockings or zinc bandages, and frequent leg elevation are the cornerstones of the conservative management of venous ulcer (67). Irrespective of the choice, effective compression therapy is obtained with implements exerting a 35 to 40 mm Hg pressure at the ankle (68). Greater benefits (higher and faster healing rates, and low recurrence rates) are to be expected if compliance with compression therapy is monitored through ambulatory care programs, and if patients are encouraged to take regular exercise and to elevate the extremities while resting (69-71). According to the results of a survey conducted among Canadian physicians and patients, most patients with DVT reported being willing to comply with elastic stockings therapy and found them useful (72), although their use neither improves leg symptoms and signs during exercise nor increases exercise capacity (73).

In a randomized clinical trial conducted in a small number of patients with severe PTS, the adoption of cycles of intermittent pneumatic compression was found to reduce both intractable edema and leg swelling (74). In another randomized trial, a novel lower-limb venous-return assist device (VENOPTS) was found to considerably improve the clinical manifestations of severe PTS both alone and in combination with compression stockings (75). Finally, in a recent randomized clinical trial patients with PTS were found to benefit from an exercise training (a six-month trainer-supervised program that included aerobic, leg stretching and strengthening components) to a greater extent than those who had conventional treatment alone both in terms of severity of complaints and improvement in quality of life (76).

In addition to compressive therapy, a number of active compounds have been evaluated in a series of small randomized trials for the healing of venous ulcers. Among these oxpentifylline (77), aspirin (78), intravenous prostaglandin E1 (79), sulphydril-containing agents (DL-cysteine or DL-methionine) (80), radical scavengers (allopurinol or dimethyl sulfoxide) (81), and sulodexide (82) significantly improved the ulcer-healing rate.

With regards to other manifestations of the PTS, two small randomized trials demonstrated some beneficial effect of an anabolic steroid (stanozolol) plus elastic stockings on lipodermatosclerosis (83), and that of 0-(β-hydroxyethyl)-rutosides on edema and several milder PTS symptoms (84), respectively.

In a recent clinical trial, we evaluated the efficacy of elastic compression stockings, hydroxyethylrutosides or both for the treatment of PTS (85). In 120 consecutive patients with PTS who were randomized to receive below-knee elastic stockings (30-40 mm Hg at the ankle), oral administration of hydroxyethylrutosides (1000 mg b.i.d.) or both for one year, an improvement of PTS manifestations was observed in similar proportions of patients in each study group. According to these results, elastic stockings and hydroxyethylrutosides seem equally effective in patients with the PTS. The combination of the two remedies does not seem to improve the results obtained by each strategy alone.

5.2 Surgical treatment

Surgery is often advocated when severe clinical manifestations (e.g. ulcer) cannot be managed by conservative treatment: various strategies are available, among whom subfascial perforator ligation and valvuloplasty appear to be the most promising (86). A more recent trial on subfascial endoscopic perforator surgery plus correction of superficial venous reflux indicates that, although effective in improving symptoms and ulcer healing in patients with primary venous insufficiency, this procedure is not as effective in patients with PTS (87). Similarly, deep (femoral-popliteal) valve reconstruction surgery performed after unsuccessful endoscopic perforator surgery, and correction of superficial venous reflux, yields significantly better results in patients with primary venous insufficiency than in patients with PTS (88).

6. Prevention of the PTS

6.1 Initial treatment of DVT with thrombolytic drugs

Thrombolysis has been traditionally advocated as an alternative strategy to heparins for the initial treatment of DVT, based on the assumption that early vein recanalization will result in a more favorable long-term outcome. This assumption is in agreement with the findings from several recent studies, which have identified that proximal location of the initial thrombosis is among the strongest predictors of PTS development (33,38,60), especially when the thrombus involves the ilio-femoral segments (39). Consistent with this assumption is the demonstration that post-thrombotic complications develop predominantly in those patients in whom the initial complaints tend to persist (39). Both the intravenous infusion of thrombolytic drugs and the use of catheter-directed thrombolysis are likely to result in a higher frequency of early vein patency as compared to heparin (89-92). However, whether these therapeutic approaches improve the long-term patients' outcome as well is controversial, as there is data in favour (93-96) and against (97,98) this possibility. In addition, the use of either intravenous or catheter-directed thrombolysis is associated with a higher risk of complications compared with treatment with anticoagulants alone (90,100). Thus, the routine use of early thrombolytic therapy for the prevention of long-term sequelae of DVT does not seem to be currently justified, but is the subject of ongoing multicenter randomized trials (100).

6.2 Compression bandaging in the acute phase of DVT

In order to assess the influence of immediate multilayer compression bandages before application of elastic stockings in the acute phase of DVT on development of the PTS, 69 patients with acute symptomatic DVT were recently randomized to immediate bandaging or no bandaging (36). While bandaging resulted in a considerable improvement of clinical symptoms and decrease of leg circumference in the first week of treatment, no difference in the development of late sequelae was observed between the two groups after one year. Thus, the early application of bandages in patients with DVT is unlikely to improve the long-term patients' outcome.

6.3 Elastic compression stockings

Elastic compression stockings have long been utilized for the prevention of the PTS in patients with acute DVT (72). However, their efficacy had not been systematically investigated until a few years ago.

In 1997, the results of a prospective randomized Dutch study on the prevention of the PTS became available (19). In this trial, 194 consecutive patients with confirmed proximal DVT were allocated to wear or to not wear elastic compression stockings. A predefined scoring system was used to classify patients into three categories: no, mild-to-moderate, and severe PTS. After a median follow-up of 76 months, mild-to-moderate PTS occurred in 19 (20%) and severe PTS in 11 (11.5%) of the 96 patients with stockings, while these occurred in 46 (47%) and 23 (23.5%) of the 98 patients without stockings, respectively ($p<0.001$).

These results were recently confirmed by a prospective, controlled, randomized study performed in Italy (29), in which 180 consecutive patients with a first episode of symptomatic proximal DVT who were planned to receive conventional anticoagulant treatment were randomized to wear or to not wear below-knee compression (30-40 mm Hg at the ankle) elastic stockings for two years. Follow-up was performed for up to 5 years. Post-thrombotic sequelae, as assessed with the Villalta scale, developed in 44 of the 90 control patients (severe in 10), and in 23 of the 90 patients who were randomized to wear elastic stockings (severe in 3). After adjustment for baseline characteristics, the hazard ratio for the PTS in the stockings group as compared to the control group was 0.5 (0.3 to 0.8). A large, multicenter randomized trial is currently underway in North America to compare active versus placebo stockings to prevent PTS after proximal DVT (64).

Although the results of an investigation conducted in Canada (101) were not consistent with those of the above described studies (19,29,37), a recent meta-analytic review emphasized the role of graduated compression stockings for preventing long-term post-thrombotic sequelae (102). Accordingly, the latest edition of the American College of Chest Physicians has recently recommended elastic stockings beside conventional anticoagulation in all patients with acute symptomatic DVT, if feasible (99). While the effectiveness of compression stockings to prevent PTS after distal DVT has not been studied, it would be reasonable to offer compression stockings to patients with severe symptoms related to distal DVT.

Knee-length and thigh-length compression elastic stockings have similar physiologic effects in decreasing venous stasis of the lower limb, but the former are easier to apply and are more comfortable (103). A recent systematic review of knee versus thigh length graduated compression stockings for the prevention of DVT concluded that knee length were as effective as thigh length stockings and offer advantages in terms of patient compliance and cost (104). In order to directly compare the effectiveness and tolerability of below-knee versus thigh length stockings at the time of acute DVT to prevent PTS a randomized clinical trial has been conducted at our institution, whose results will be available soon (105).

The optimal duration of the treatment with elastic stockings has received little attention. In a recent trial, 169 patients with a first or recurrent proximal DVT who had received 6 months of standard compression treatment were randomized to wear or to not wear graduated elastic stockings for an additional 18 months (37). Overall, after 6 years of follow-up, prolongation of compression therapy failed to confer an additional advantage - according to the CEAP classification – over and above the initial 6-month period. However, when the analysis was confined to women, there was a statistically significant advantage to prolonging treatment with compression stockings. In a prospective cohort management study, the discontinuation of elastic stockings in patients free from PTS complaints who had been offered at least six months of compression therapy did not increase the rate of PTS development over patients in whom stockings had been used for at least two years irrespective of the presence of post-thrombotic manifestations (106). Further studies are needed to show whether compression therapy is or is not indicated in asymptomatic patients who have completed an initial 6-month period.

To our knowledge, there are no studies that have compared different compression strengths of stockings to prevent PTS. It would be worth studying the effectiveness of lighter compression (20-30 mm Hg) stockings as they are easier to apply, especially for elderly patients, than 30-40 mm Hg stockings. Of note, in a study of stockings to prevent recurrent venous ulcer, there was no difference in effectiveness between class 2 and class 3 stockings (107).

Interestingly enough, immediate mobilization in patients with acute DVT may reduce the rate of PTS development, provided that patients are provided with adequate compression therapy (108).

6.4 The potential of new anticoagulant drugs

An insufficient quality of oral anticoagulant therapy following the acute thrombotic episode has been found to be associated with an increased risk of the PTS (28,65). Conversely, the long-term use of LMWH has been found to reduce the PTS rate in comparison with vitamin K antagonists (35,109). We cannot exclude, therefore, the potential of a few emerging antithrombotic compounds (such as dabigatran etexilate and rivaroxaban), which can be administered orally in fixed daily dosage and have been found to be at least as effective and safe as conventional anticoagulation for the initial and long-term treatment of DVT (110,111), for further reducing the incidence and the severity of the PTS.

7. Prognosis

It is commonly believed that patients with established PTS have a poor prognosis, and that the majority will have sustained disability. In recent years, a few reports have suggested that prognosis of the PTS might not be as poor as previously reported (69-71). Indeed, when provided with elastic compression stockings and regularly supervised, more than 50% of patients either remain stable or improve during long-term follow-up, irrespective of the initial degree of PTS (69-71). Clinical presentation helps predict the prognosis, as the outcome of patients who have initially severe manifestations appears to be more favorable than that of patients whose symptoms progressively deteriorate over time (71). However, at present there is no way to reliably predict the course of PTS in individual patients.

8. Conclusion

PTS is a frequent, burdensome and costly complication of DVT. Currently, there are few effective treatments for PTS. Until such treatments are identified, prevention of PTS will have the greatest impact on reducing the overall burden of PTS on patients and society. Preventing DVT recurrence is likely to reduce the risk of PTS. Daily use of graduated ECS after DVT appears to reduce the risk of PTS. As of yet, there is no established role for thrombolysis in preventing PTS, but trials are underway to address this important question. Research is also underway to identify biologic markers that may predict the risk of PTS in individual patients. Finally, a few emerging antithrombotic compounds may have the potential to reduce the risk of PTS, however this requires further study.

9. Acknowledgements

Dr Kahn is a recipient of a Senior Clinical Research Scientist Award from the Fonds de la Recherche en Santé du Québec and received research funding from the Canadian Institutes of Health Research and the Heart and Stroke Foundation of Canada.

10. References

[1] Kahn SR, Ginsberg JS. Relationship between deep venous thrombosis and the postthrombotic syndrome. Arch Intern Med 2004; 164: 17-26.

[2] Bergqvist D, Jendteg S, Johansen L, Persson U, Ödegaard K. Cost of long term complications of deep venous thrombosis of the lower extremities: an analysis of a defined patient population in Sweden Ann Intern Med 1997; 126: 454-457.

[3] Kahn SR, M'Lan CE, Lamping DL, Kurz X, Bérard A, Abenhaim L. The influence of venous thromboembolism on quality of life and severity of chronic venous disease. J Thromb Haemost 2004; 2: 2146-2151.

[4] Bauer G. Roentgenological and clinical study of the sequelae of thrombosis Acta Chir Scand 1942; 86 (suppl 74): 1-110.

[5] Gjores JE. The incidence of venous thrombosis and its sequelae in certain districts of Sweden. Acta Chir Scand 1956; 206 (suppl 1): 1-88.

[6] O'Donnell TF, Browse NL, Burnand KG, Lea Thomas M. The socioeconomic effects of an ilio-femoral venous thrombosis. J Surg Res 1977; 22: 483-488.

[7] Strandness DE, Langlois Y, Cramer M, Randlett A, Thiele BL. Long-term sequelae of acute venous thrombosis. JAMA 1983; 250: 1289-1292.

[8] Widmer LK, Zemp E, Widmer T, Schmitt HE, Brandenberg E, Voelin R, Biland L, da Silva A, Magos M. Late results in deep vein thrombosis of the lower extremity. Vasa 1985; 14: 264-268.

[9] Lindner DJ, Edwards JM, Phinney ES, Taylor LM, Porter JM. Long-term hemodinamic and clinical sequelae of lower extremity deep vein thrombosis. J Vasc Surg 1986; 4: 436-442.

[10] Heldal M, Seem E, Snadset PM, Abildgaard U. Deep vein thrombosis: a 7-year follow-up study. J Intern Med 1993; 234: 71-75.

[11] Lagerstedt C, Olsson CG, Fagher B, Norgren L, Tengborn L. Recurrence and late sequelae after first-time deep vein thrombosis Relationship to initial signs. Phlebology 1993; 8: 62-67.

[12] Monreal M, Martorell A, Callejas JM, Valls R, Llamazares J,F Lafoz E, Arias A. Venographic assessment of deep vein thrombosis and risk of developing post-thrombotic syndrome: a prospective study. J Intern Med 1993; 233: 854-859.

[13] Eichlisberger R, Frauchiger B, Widmer MT, Widmer LK, Jager K. Late sequelae of deep venous thrombosis: a 13-year follow-up of 223 patients. Vasa 1994; 23: 234-243.

[14] Beyth RJ, Cohen AM, Landefeld CS. Long-term outcomes of deep-vein thrombosis. Arch Intern Med 1995; 155: 1031-1037.

[15] Johnson BF, Manzo RA, Bergelin RO, Strandness DE. Relationship between changes in the deep venous system and the development of the postthrombotic syndrome after an acute episode of lower limb deep vein thrombosis: a one- to six-year follow-up. J Vasc Surg 1995; 21: 307-313.

[16] Saarinen J, Sisto T, Laurikka J, Salenius JP, Tarkka M. Late sequelae of acute deep venous thrombosis: evaluation five and ten years after. Phlebology 1995; 10: 106-109.

[17] Franzeck UK, Schalch I, Jäger KA, Schneider E, Grimm J, Bollinger A. Prospective 12-year follow-up study of clinical and haemodynamic sequelae after deep vein thrombosis in low-risk patients (Zürich study). Circulation 1996; 93: 74-79.
[18] Prandoni P, Lensing AWA, Cogo A, Cuppini S, Villalta S, Carta M, Cattelan AM, Polistena P, Bernardi E, Prins MH. The long-term clinical course of acute deep venous thrombosis. Ann Intern Med 1996; 125: 1-7.
[19] Brandijes DPM, Büller HR, Heijboer H, Huisman MV, de Rijk M, Jagt H. Randomised trial of effect of compression stockings in patients with symptomatic proximal-vein thrombosis. Lancet 1997; 349: 759-762.
[20] Prandoni P, Villalta S, Bagatella P, Rossi L, Marchiori A, Piccioli A, Bernardi E, Girolami B, Simioni P, Girolami A. The clinical course of deep-vein thrombosis Prospective long-term follow-up of 528 symptomatic patients. Haematologica 1997; 2: 423-428.
[21] Biguzzi E, Mozzi E, Alatri A, Taioli E, Moia M, Mannucci PM. The post-thrombotic syndrome in young women: retrospective evaluation of prognostic factors. Thromb Haemost 1998; 80: 575-577.
[22] Masuda EM, Kessler DM, Kistner RL, Eklof B, Sato DT. The natural history of calf vein thrombosis: lysis of thrombi and development of reflux. J Vasc Surg 1998; 8: 67-74.
[23] McLafferty RB, Moneta GL, Passmann MA, Brant BM, Taylor LM, Porter JM. Late clinical and hemodynamic sequelae of isolated calf vein thrombosis. J Vasc Surg 1998; 27: 50-57.
[24] Haenen JH, Janssen MCH, van Langen H, van Asten WNJC, Wollersheim H, van't Hof MA, Skotnicki SH, Thien T. The postthrombotic syndrome in relation to venous hemodynamics as measured by means of duplex scanning and strain-gauge plethysmography. J Vasc Surg 1999; 29: 1071-1076.
[25] Holmström M, Åberg W, Lockner C, Paul C. Long term clinical follow-up in 256 patients with deep-vein thrombosis initially treated with either unfractionated heparin or dalteparin: a retrospective analysis. Thromb Haemost 1999; 82: 1222-1226.
[26] Saarinen J, Kallio T, Lehto M, Hiltunen S, Sisto T. The occurrence of the post-thrombotic changes after an acute deep venous thrombosis. A prospective two-year follow-up study J Cardiovasc Surg 2000; 41: 441-446.
[27] Mohr DN, Silverstein MD, Heit JA, Petterson TM, O'Fallon M, Melton LJ. The venous stasis syndrome after deep venous thrombosis or pulmonary embolism: a population-based study. Mayo Clin Proc 2000; 75: 1249-1256.
[28] Ziegler S, Schillinger M, Maca TH, Minar E. Post-thrombotic syndrome after primary event of deep venous thrombosis 10 to 20 years ago. Thromb Res 2001; 101: 23-33.
[29] Prandoni P, Lensing AWA, Prins MH, Frulla M, Marchiori A, Bernardi E, Tormene D, Mosena L, Pagnan A, Girolami A. Below-knee elastic compression stockings to prevent the post-thrombotic syndrome A randomized controlled trial. Ann Intern Med 2004; 141: 249-256.
[30] Gabriel F, Labios M, Portoles O, Guillen M, Corella D, Frances F, Martinez M, Gil J, Saiz C. Incidence of post-thrombotic syndrome and its association with various risk factors in a cohort of Spanish patients after one year of follow-up following acute deep venous thrombosis. Thromb Haemost 2004; 92: 328-336.
[31] Kahn SR, Kearon C, Julian JA, Mackinnon B, Kovacs MJ, Wells P, Crowther MA, Anderson DR, Van Nguyen P, Demers C, Solymoss S, Kassis J, Geerts W, Rodger M, Hambleton J, Ginsberg JS. Predictors of the post-thrombotic syndrome during long-

term treatment of proximal deep vein thrombosis. J Thromb Haemost 2005; 3: 718-723.

[32] Roumen-Klappe EM, den Heijer M, Janssen MCH, van der Vleuten C, Thien T, Wollersheim H. The post-thrombotic syndrome: incidence and prognostic value of non-invasive venous examinations in a six-year follow-up study. Thromb Haemost 2005; 94: 825-830.

[33] Stain M, Schönauer V, Minar E, Bialonczyk C, Hirschl M, Weltermann A, Kyrle PA, Eichinger S. The post-thrombotic syndrome: risk factors and impact on the course of thrombotic disease. J Thromb Haemost 2005; 3: 2671-2676.

[34] Schulman S, Lindmarker P, Holmstrom M, Larfars G, Carlsson A, Nicol P, Svensson E, Ljungberg B, Viering S, Nordlander S, Leijd B, Jahed K, Hjorth M, Linder O, Beckman M. Post-thrombotic syndrome recurrence and death 10 years after the first episode of venous thromboembolism treated with warfarin for 6 weeks or 6 months. J Thromb Haemost 2005; 4: 734-742.

[35] González-Fajardo JA, Martin-Pedrosa M, Castrodeza J, Tamames S, Vaquero-Puerta C. Effect of the anticoagulant therapy in the incidence of post-thrombotic syndrome and recurrent thromboembolism: Comparative study of enoxaparin versus coumarin. J Vasc Surg 2008; 48: 953-959.

[36] Roumen-Klappe EM, den Heijer M, van Rossum J, Wollersheim H, van der Vleuten C, Thien T, Janssen MC. Multilayer compression bandaging in the acute phase of deep-vein thrombosis has no effect on the development of the post-thrombotic syndrome. J Thromb Thrombolysis 2009; 27: 400-405.

[37] Aschwanden M, Jeanneret C, Koller MT, Thalhammer C, Bucher HC, Jaeger KA. Effect of prolonged treatment with compression stockings to prevent post-thrombotic sequelae: a randomized controlled trial. J Vasc Surg 2008; 47: 1015-1021.

[38] Tick LW, Kramer MH, Rosendaal FR, Faber WR, Doggen CJJ. Risk factors for post-thrombotic syndrome in patients with a first deep venous thrombosis. J Thromb Haemost 2008; 6: 2075-2081.

[39] Kahn SR, Shrier I, Julian JA, Ducruet T, Arsenault L, Miron MJ, Roussin A, Desmarais S, Joyal F, Kassis J, Solymoss S, Desjardins L, Lamping DL, Johri M, Ginsberg JS. Determinants and time course of the postthrombotic syndrome after acute deep venous thrombosis. Ann Intern Med 2008; 149: 698-707.

[40] Wille-Jorgensen P, Jorgensen LN, Crawford M. Asymptomatic postoperative deep vein thrombosis and the development of postthrombotic syndrome A systematic review and meta-analysis. Thromb Haemost 2005; 93: 236-241.

[41] Lonner JH, Frank J, McGuire K, Lotke PA. Postthrombotic syndrome after asymptomatic deep vein thrombosis following total knee and hip arthroplasty. Am J Orthop 2006; 35: 469-472.

[42] Immelman EJ, Jeffrey PC. The postphlebitic syndrome Pathophysiology prevention and management. Clin Chest Med 1984; 5: 537-550.

[43] Browse NL, Clemenson G, Lea Thomas M. Is the postphlebitic leg always postphlebitic? Relation between phlebographic appearances of deep-vein thrombosis and late sequelae. Br Med 1980; 281: 1167-1170.

[44] Raju S. Venous insufficiency of the lower limbs and stasis ulceration. Ann Surg 1983; 197: 688-697.

[45] Scott TE, LaMorte WW, Gorin DR, Menzoian JO. Risk factors for chronic venous insufficiency: a dual case-control study. J Vasc Surg 1995; 22: 622-628.

[46] Kolbach DN, Neumann HA, Prins MH. Definition of the post-thrombotic syndrome differences between existing classifications. Eur J Vasc Endovasc Surg 2005; 30: 404-414.
[47] Villalta S, Bagatella P, Piccioli A, Lensing AWA, Prins MH, Prandoni P. Assessment of validity and reproducibility of a clinical scale for the post-thrombotic syndrome. Haemostasis 1994; 24 (Suppl 1): 57a.
[48] Rodger MA, Kahn SR, Le Gal G, Solymoss S, Chagnon I,
[49] Anderson DR, Wells PS, Kovacs MJ. Inter-observer reliability of measures to assess the post-thrombotic syndrome. Thromb Haemost 2008; 100: 164-166.
[50] Kahn SR, Hirsch A, Shrier I. Effect of post-thrombotic syndrome on health-related quality of life after deep venous thrombosis. Arch Intern Med 2002; 162: 1144-1148.
[51] Kahn SR, Partsch H, Vedantham S, Prandoni P, Kearon C. Definition of post-thrombotic syndrome of the leg for use in clinical investigations: A recommendation for standardization. J Thromb Haemost 2009; 7: 879-883.
[52] Porter JM, Moneta GL. Reporting standards in venous disease: an update International Consensus Commitee on Chronic Venous Disease. J Vasc Surg 1995; 21: 635-645.
[53] Bettmann MA, Paulin, S. Leg phlebography: the incidence, nature, and modification of undesirable side effects Radiology 1977; 122: 101-104.
[54] Villalta S, Prandoni P, Cogo A, Bagatella P, Piccioli A, Bernardi E, Simioni P, Scarano L, Girolami A. The utility of non-invasive tests for detection of previous proximal-vein thrombosis. Thromb Haemost 1995; 73: 592-596.
[55] Coleridge Smith PD, Thomas P, Scurr JH, Dormandy JA. Causes of venous ulceration: a new hypothesis. Br Med J 1988; 296: 1726-1727.
[56] Shami SK, Shields DA, Scurr JH, Coleridge Smith PD. Leg ulceration in venous disease. Postgrad Med J 1992; 68: 779-785.
[57] Lindhagen A, Bergqvist D, Hallböök T, Efsing HO. Venous function five to eight years after clinically suspected deep venous thrombosis. Acta Med Scand 1985; 217: 389-395.
[58] Markel A, Manzo RA, Bergelin RO, Strandness DE. Valvular reflux after deep vein thrombosis: incidence and time of occurrence. J Vasc Surg 1992; 15: 377-384.
[59] Franzeck UK, Schalch I, Bollinger A. On the relationship between changes in the deep veins evaluated by Duplex sonography and the postthrombotic syndrome 12 years after deep vein thrombosis. Thromb Haemost 1997; 77: 1109-1112.
[60] Haenen JH, Janssen MC, Wollersheim H, Van't Hof MA, de Rooij
[61] MJ, van Langen H, Skotnicki SH, Thien T. The development of postthrombotic syndrome in relationship to venous reflux and calf muscle pump dysfunction at 2 years after the onset of deep venous thrombosis. J Vasc Surg 2002; 35: 1184-1189.
[62] Asbeutah AM, Riha AZ, Cameron JD, McGrath BP. Five-year outcome study of deep vein thrombosis in the lower limbs. J Vasc Surg 2004; 40: 1184-1189.
[63] Singh H, Masuda EM. Comparing short-term outcomes of femoral-popliteal and iliofemoral deep venous thrombosis: early lysis and development of reflux. Ann Vasc Surg 2005; 19: 74-79.
[64] Prandoni P, Frulla M, Sartor D, Concolato A, Girolami A. Vein abnormalities and the post-thrombotic syndrome. J Thromb Haemost 2005; 3: 401-402.
[65] Shbaklo H, Holcroft CA, Kahn SR. Levels of inflammatory markers and the development of the post thrombotic syndrome. Thromb Haemost 2009; 101: 505-12.

[66] Kahn SR, Shbaklo H, Shapiro S, Wells PS, Kovacs MJ, Rodger MA, Anderson DR, Ginsberg JS, Johri M, Tagalakis V. Effectiveness of compression stockings to prevent the post-thrombotic syndrome (the SOX Trial and Bio-SOX biomarker substudy): a randomized controlled trial. BMC Cardiovasc Disord 2007: 7: 21.

[67] Van Dongen CJ, Prandoni P, Frulla M, Marchiori A, Prins MH, Hutten BA. Relation between quality of anticoagulant treatment and the development of the postthrombotic syndrome. J Thromb Haemost 2005; 3: 939-942.

[68] Ageno W, Piantanida E, Dentali F, Steidl L, Mera V, Squizzato A, Marchesi C, Venco A. Body mass index is associated with the development of the post-thrombotic syndrome. Thromb Haemost 2003; 89: 305-309.

[69] Hafner J, Bounameaux H, Burg G, Brunner U. Management of venous leg ulcers. Vasa 1996; 25: 161-167.

[70] Evers EJ, Wuppermann T. Effect of different compression therapies on the reflux in deep veins with a post-thrombotic syndrome. Vasa 1999; 28: 19-23.

[71] Erickson CA, Lanza DJ, Karp DL, Edwards JW, Seabrook GR, Cambria RA, Freishlag JA, Towne JB. Healing of venous ulcers in an ambulatory care program: the roles of chronic venous insufficiency and patients compliance. J Vasc Surg 1995; 22: 629-636.

[72] Milne AA, Ruckley CV. The clinical course of patients following extensive deep venous thrombosis. Eur J Vasc Surg 1994; 8: 56-9.

[73] Prandoni P, Lensing AWA, Prins MH, Bagatella P, Scudeller A, Girolami A. Which is the outcome of the post-thrombotic syndrome? Thromb Haemost 1999; 82: 1196-1197.

[74] Kahn SR, Elman E, Rodger MA, Wells PS. Use of elastic compression stockings after deep venous thrombosis: a comparison of practices and perceptions of thrombosis physicians and patients. J Thomb Haemost 2003; 1: 500-506.

[75] Kahn SR, Azoulay L, Hirsch A, Haber M, Strulovitch C, Shrier I. Effect of graduated elastic compression stockings on leg symptoms and signs during exercise in patients with deep venous thrombosis: a randomized cross-over trial. J Thomb Haemost 2003; 1: 494-499.

[76] Ginsberg JS, Magier D, Mackinnon B, Gent M, Hirsh J. Intermittent compression units for severe post-phlebitic syndrome: a randomised crossover study. CMAJ 1999; 160: 1303-1306.

[77] O'Donnell MJ, McRae S, Kahn SR, Julian JA, Kearon C, Mackinnon B, Magier D, Strulovich C, Lyons T, Robinson S, Hirsh J, Ginsberg JS. Evaluation of a venous-return assist device to treat severe post-thrombotic syndrome (VENOPTS) A randomized controlled trial. Thromb Haemost 2008; 99: 463-464.

[78] Kahn SR, Shrier I, Shapiro S, Houweling AH, Hirsch AM, Reid RD, Kearon C, Rabhi K, Rodger MA, Kovacs MJ, Anderson DR, Wells PS. Six-month exercise training program to treat post-thrombotic syndrome: a randomized controlled two-centre trial. CMAJ 2011; 183: 37-44.

[79] Colgan MP, Dormandy JA, Jones PW, Schraibman IG, Shanik G, Young RA. Oxpentifylline treatment of venous ulcers of the leg. Br Med J 1990; 300: 972-975.

[80] Layton AM, Ibbotson SH, Davies JA, Goodfield MJ. Randomized trial of oral aspirin for chronic venous leg ulcer. Lancet 1994; 344: 164-165.

[81] Rudofsky G. Intravenous prostaglandin E1 in the treatment of venous ulcers - a double-blind placebo-controlled trial. Vasa 1989; 28 (Suppl): 39-43.

[82] Salim AS. Role of sulphydril-containing agents in the management of venous (varicose) ulceration A new approach. Clin Exp Dermatol 1992; 17: 427-432.

[83] Salim AS. The role of oxygen-derived free radicals in the management of venous (varicose) ulceration. A new approach World J Surg 1991; 15: 264-269.
[84] Coccheri S, Scandotto G, Agnelli G, Aloisi D, Palazzini E, Zamboni V. Randomised double blind multicentre placebo controlled study of sulodexide in the treatment of venous leg ulcers. Thromb Haemost 2002; 87: 947-952.
[85] Burnand K, Clemenson G, Morland M, Jarret PE, Browse NL. Venous lipodermatosclerosis: treatment by fibrinolytic enhancement and elastic compression. Br Med J 1980; 280: 7-11.
[86] de Jongste AB, Jonker JJC, Huisman MV, ten Cate JW, Azar AJ. A double blind three center clinical trial on the short-term efficacy of 0-(β-hydroxyethyl)-rutosides in patients with post-thrombotic syndrome. Thromb Haemost 1989; 62: 826-829.
[87] Frulla M, Marchiori A, Sartor D, Mosena L, Tormene D, Concolato A, Hartmann L, Prandoni P. Elastic stockings hydroxyethylrutosides or both for the treatment of post-thrombotic syndrome. Thromb Haemost 2005; 93: 183-185.
[88] Baste JC, Midy F. Surgery for post-thrombotic syndrome of the lower limbs Rev Prat 1994; 44: 781-785.
[89] Gloviczki P, Bergan JJ, Rhodes JM, Canton LG, Harmsen S, Ilstrup DM. Mid-term results of endoscopic perforator vein interruption for chronic venous insufficiency: lessons learned from the north American subfascial endoscopic perforator surgery registry. The north American study group J Vasc Surg 1999; 29: 489-502.
[90] Perrin M, Hiltbrand B, Bayon JM. Results of valvuloplasty in patients presenting deep venous insufficiency and recurring ulceration. Ann Vasc Surg 1999; 13: 524-532.
[91] Goldhaber SZ, Buring JE, Lipnick RJ, Hennekens CH. Pooled analyses of randomized trials of streptokinase and heparin in phlebographically documented acute deep venous thrombosis. Am J Med 1984; 76: 393-397.
[92] Sidorov J. Streptokinase vs heparin for deep venous thrombosis Can lytic therapy be justified? Arch Intern Med 1989; 149: 1841-1845.
[93] Rogers LQ, Lutcher CL. Streptokinase therapy for deep vein thrombosis: a comprehensive review of the English literature. Am J Med 1990; 88: 389-395.
[94] Alesh I, Kayali F, Stein PD. Catheter-directed thrombolysis (intrathrombus injection) in treatment of deep venous thrombosis: a systematic review. Catheter Cardiovasc Interv 2007; 70: 143-148.
[95] Comerota AJ, Aldridge SC, Cohen G, Ball DS, Pliskin M, White JV. A strategy of aggressive regional therapy for acute iliofemoral venous thrombosis with contemporary venous thrombectomy or catheter-directed Thrombolysis. J Vasc Surg 1994; 20: 244-254.
[96] Bjarnason H, Kruse JR, Asinger DA, Nazarian GK, Dietz CA Jr, Caldwell MD, Key NS, Hirsch AT, Hunter DW. Iliofemoral deep venous thrombosis: safety and efficacy outcome during 5 years of catheter-directed thrombolytic therapy. JVIR 1997; 8: 405-418.
[97] Comerota AJ, Paolini D. Treatment of acute iliofemoral deep venous thrombosis: a strategy of thrombus removal. Eur J Vasc Endovasc Surg 2007; 33: 351-360.
[98] Manninen H, Juutilainen A, Kaukanen E, Lehto S. Catheter-directed thrombolysis of proximal lower extremity deep vein thrombosis: A prospective trial with venographic and clinical follow-up. Eur J Radiol 2011; epub ahead of print
[99] Park YJ, Choi JY, Min SK, Lee T, Jung IM, Chung JK, Chung JW, Park JH, Kim SJ, Ha J. Restoration of patency in iliofemoral deep vein thrombosis with catheter-directed

thrombolysis does not always prevent post-thrombotic damage. Eur J Vasc Endovasc Surg 2008; 36: 725-730.
[100] Ghanima W, Kleven IW, Enden T, Rosales A, Wik HS, Pederstad L, Holme PA, Sandset PM. Recurrent venous thrombosis, post-thrombotic syndrome and quality of life after catheter-directed thrombolysis in severe proximal deep vein thrombosis. J Thromb Haemost. 2011; epub ahead of print.
[101] Kearon C, Kahn SR, Agnelli G, Goldhaber S, Raskob GE,
[102] Comerota AJ. Antithrombotic therapy for venous thromboembolic disease: American College of Chest Physicians evidence-based clinical practice guidelines (8th edition). Chest 2008: 133 (6 Suppl): 454S-545S.
[103] Enden T, Sandvik L, Klow NE, Hafsahl G, Holme PA, Holmen LO, Ghanima W, Njaastad AM, Sandbaek G, Slagsvold CE, Sandset PM. Catheter-directed Venous Thrombolysis in acute iliofemoral vein thrombosis-the CaVenT Study: rationale and design of a multicenter randomized controlled clinical trial. Am Heart J 2007; 154: 808-814.
[104] Ginsberg JS, Hirsh J, Julian J, Vander Laande Vries M, Magier D, MacKinnon B, Gent M. Prevention and treatment of postphlebitic syndrome Results of a 3-part study. Arch Intern Med 2001; 161: 2105-2109.
[105] Kakkos SK, Daskalopoulou SS, Daskalopoulos ME, Nicolaides AN, Geroulakos G. Review on the value of graduated elastic compression stockings after deep vein thrombosis. Thromb Haemost 2006; 96: 441-445.
[106] BenkoT, Cooke EA, McNally MA, Mollan RA. Graduated compression stockings: knee length or thigh length Clin Orthop Relat Res 2001; 383: 197-203.
[107] Sajid MS, Tai NR, Goli G, Morris RW, Baker DM, Hamilton G. Knee versus thigh length graduated compression stockings for prevention of deep venous thrombosis: a systematic review. Eur J Vasc Endovasc Surg 2006; 32: 730-736.
[108] Full-leg vs below-knee elastic stockings for prevention of the post-thrombotic syndrome. ClinicalTrials.gov identifier: NCT00426075
[109] Ten Cate-Hoek AJ, Ten Cate H, Tordoir J, Hamulyák K, Prins MH. Individually tailored duration of elastic compression therapy in relation to incidence of the postthrombotic syndrome. J Vasc Surg 2010; 52: 132-138.
[110] Nelson EA, Harper DR, Prescott RJ, Gibson B, Brown D, Ruckley CV. Prevention of recurrence of venous ulceration: randomized controlled trial of class 2 and class 3 elastic compression. J Vasc Surg 2006; 44: 803–808.
[111] Partsch H, Kaulich M, Mayer W. Immediate mobilisation in acute vein thrombosis reduces post-thrombotic syndrome. Int Angiol 2004; 3: 206-212.
[112] Hull RD, Pineo GF, Brant R, Liang J, Cook R, Solymoss S, Poon MC, Raskob G. Home therapy of venous thrombosis with long-term LMWH versus usual care: patient satisfaction and post-thrombotic syndrome. Am J Med 2009; 122: 762-769.
[113] Schulman S, Kearon C, Kakkar AK, Mismetti P, Schellong S, Eriksson H, Baanstra D, Schnee J, Goldhaber SZ. Dabigatran versus warfarin in the treatment of acute venous thromboembolism. N Engl J Med 2009; 361: 2342-52.
[114] The Einstein Investigators. Oral rivaroxaban for symptomatic venous thromboembolism. N Engl J Med 2010; 363: 2499-510.

10

Venous Thromboembolism in Orthopaedic Surgery

Justin R. Knight and Michael H. Huo
Department of Orthopaedic Surgery
University of Texas Southwestern Medical Center,
Dallas, Texas
USA

1. Introduction

Venous Thromboembolism (VTE) is a common complication following orthopaedic procedures. It is discussed most commonly as it relates to total hip arthroplasty (THA) and total knee arthroplasty (TKA), though this disease process can be seen after any orthopaedic surgery. It is associated with significant morbity and costs (Caprini et al., 2003). This chapter will provide an overview of the epidemiology, pathophysiology, and management of thromboembolic disease. This will include preventative strategies, evidence-based guidelines and a focus on newer drug agents currently being developed.

2. Epidemiology

Total joint arthroplasties remain some of the most common orthopaedic procedures performed worldwide. It is estimated that by 2015, over 500,000 total hip arthroplasties and 1.3 million total knee arthroplasties will be done in the United States alone (Kim, 2008). The aggregate costs in 2007 totaled over $15 billion (US Agency for Healthcare Research and Quality, 2007). Geerts et al. reported that VTE would occur in 40%-60% of the patients undergoing total joint arthroplasty if no prophylaxis was administered (Geerts et al., 2008). Despite appropriate chemophrophylaxis, one study noted asymptomatic proximal DVT found on ultrasound in 6.7% of THA and TKA patients at the time of transfer to a rehabilitation center (Schellong et al., 2005). As many as 80% of all clinical VTE events associated with arthroplasty patients occur within 3 months after surgery (Oster et al., 2004).

The costs of VTE are significant. Approximately 10% of the patients who develop VTE following THAs or TKAs require re-admission to the hospital within 3 months after their index surgery (Oster et al., 2004). The clinical sequelae are often significant and can include leg swelling, venous stasis ulcers, pulmonary hypertension, post-thrombotic syndrome, and recurrence (Heit, 2006). The one-year mortality following deep vein thrombosis (DVT) has been reported as high as 14.6%. Pulmonary embolism (PE) is associated with even higher mortality rate. Heit et al. reported as high as 52.3% in a recent cohort study (Heit et al., 1999).

3. Pathophysiology

The coagulation cascade is a complex system in which multiple components are activated to produce fibrin. An overview of the system along with the targets of various therapeutic interventions is shown in Figure 1. The coagulation pathway is separated into the intrinsic and the extrinsic pathways. The latter is activated in response to specific tissue injury. Both lead to the eventual formation of thrombin. Thrombin causes the conversion of fibrinogen to fibrin. Additionally, it activates factor XIII which stabilizes the fibrin. An endogenous fibrinolytic system balances this system. It consists of antithrombins, proteins C and S, and the plasmin-plasminogen system.

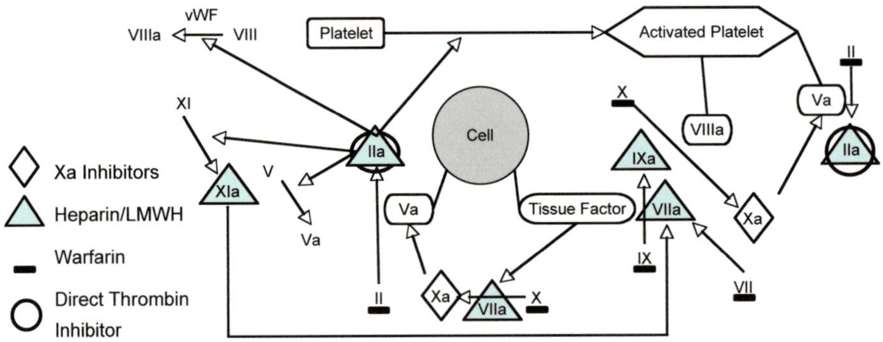

Fig. 1. Targets for anticoagulant drugs. LMWH = low-molecular-weight heparin. (Reference: Hoffman M, Dougald M. The action of high-dose factor VIIa in a cell-based model of hemostasis. *Disease a Month* 2003; 49: 14-21)

The primary pathophysiology factors that predispose any patient to VTE are the Virchow's Triad: endothelial injury, venous stasis (or turbulent blood flow), and hypercoagulability. Endothelial injury can occur due to manipulation, and retractor placement during surgery. Venous stasis can occur due to positioning and the use of a tourniquet. Hypercoagulability can occur as a result of depletion or dilution of endogenous anticoagulants. It is also associated with several pro-coagulant disease processes such as factor V Leiden deficiency, protein C and S deficiency, and others.

3.1 Natural history

The natural history of venous thromboembolism is variable. There are four potential outcomes when thrombosis occurs. The thrombus can propagate, embolize, organize, or undergo fibrinolysis. Proximal thrombi are more likely to propagate and embolize than the smaller distal thrombi in general. 80% of symptomatic DVTs involve the proximal veins (Conduah & Lieberman, 2007).

4. Prevention

Clinical VTEs occur due to many different causes, but one significant factor is inadequate prophylaxis (Amin et al., 2010). Several barriers exist for inadequate prophylaxis. These include: expense, bleeding concerns, availability of agents, and conflicting recommendations. The American College of Chest Physicians (ACCP) and the American

Academy of Orthopaedic Surgeons (AAOS) have each released separate guidelines regarding the prevention of VTE. This can be confusing to the providers.

Controversies exist regarding the two major practice guidelines for VTE prophylaxis. The ACCP has been updating its recommendations every 3 years for over 25 years (Hirsh et al., 2008). The AAOS guidelines have been a more recent development. Though the two have many similarities, there are a few significant differences. A major area of disagreement involves the use of DVT as a surrogate for PE in arthroplasty patients. The AAOS guidelines do not emphasize the correlation between DVT and pulmonary embolism (Eikelboom et al., 2009). In fact, the AAOS guidelines are for the prevention of PE following joint arthroplasty. The ACCP recommendations focus on the prevention of both VTE and PE as the goal rather than PE alone in the AAOS guidelines. Both guidelines focus on a balance between the risk of bleeding and the efficacy of anticoagulation. They both define risk-to-benefit ratio for different agents. Some of the most clinically relevant differences between the two guidelines are presented in Table 1. Neither guideline has been universally accepted. A recent survey was conducted by the American Association of Hip and Knee Surgeons regarding the practice standards among its member surgeons. The data demonstrated that 74% of the hospitals had adopted the ACCP guidelines, while 68% of the surgeons preferred the AAOS guidelines (Markel et al., 2010).

Furthermore, compliance with the current guidelines has been suboptimal. Many surgeons continue to under-appreciate the prevalence of VTE and remain concerned with postoperative bleeding. Additionally, patient factors can inhibit appropriate prophylactic treatment. Injectable agents are expensive. Moreover, some patients are not at ease or in compliance with their administration. Oral agents have the challenges including: titration, monitoring, and drug-drug, or drug-food interaction (Moyer et al., 2009).

4.1 Extended duration prophylaxis

The ACCP guidelines recommend the optimal duration of VTE prophylaxis to be 28 to 35 days following THAs, and 10 to 14 days following TKAs (Kolb et al., 2003). Currently, the mean length of hospital stay is between 3 to 4 days, therefore full compliance with this recommendation is difficult for both the patient and the provider. Several studies have reported that continuation of thromboprophylaxis beyond the hospitalization is efficacious and safe in the risk reduction of late VTE in surgical patients (Planes et al., 1996; Lassen et al., 1998; Comp et al., 2001; Bergqvist et al., 2002; Rasmussen et al., 2006).

Extended duration prophylaxis for VTE requires proper selection of pharmacological agent(s). The ideal anticoagulant should have the following characteristics: standard dosing with self-administration, no requirement for monitoring, established efficacy and safety profiles, acceptable tolerability in populations with co-morbid conditions, and few drug-drug or drug-foot interactions. The ACCP guidelines currently recommend warfarin, low-molecular weight heparins (LWMH), and fondaparinux. They specifically recommend against using aspirin alone in the high-risk orthopedic patient population as there are insufficient evidence-based data.

The AAOS guidelines recommend 2 to 6 weeks of prophylaxis with warfarin, 6 weeks using aspirin, or 7 to 12 days using LMWH or fondaparinux (AAOS 2007). The ACCP guidelines, in contrast, recommend pharmacological thromboprophylaxis for up to 35 days after THA and for 10 to 35 days after TKA. Moreover, they recommend against the use of aspirin in this patient population.

ACCP	AAOS		
Recommendation	**Risk**		**Reccommendation**
	PE	*Bleeding*	
Fondaparinux Warfarin LMWH	Standard	Standard	Aspirin LMWH Fondaparinux
	Elevated	Standard	LMWH Warfarin
	Standard	Elevated	Aspirin Warfarin Fondaparinux
	Elevated	Elevated	Aspirin Warfarin None

Table 1. Summary of ACCP and AAOS recommendations for pharmacologic thromboprophylaxis in patients undergoing elective hip or knee surgery. (Reference: Huo M. VTE prophylaxis after total joint arthroplasty: current challenges-potential solutions. *Current Orthopaedic Practice* 2011;22:193-197.)

4.2 Quality measures

Over the past 5 years, quality measures have been proposed and put into clinical application to monitor compliance with best practice guidelines in VTE prophylaxis. The Surgical Care Improvement Project (SCIP) was created in 2006 with reduction of VTE being one of its four primary focus areas. The Center for Medicare and Medicaid Services (CMS) has declared postoperative VTE as a "never event." As such, the CMS will no longer reimburse the hospital the costs associated with these complications. Other agencies and consumer groups have also declared VTE as a preventable complication.

Several important improvements have already occurred as a result of these outcome measures. Surgeons and administrators have collectively established hospital-wide or hospital system-wide prophylaxis protocols. They have also worked to establish training and education programs to deliver the best practice guidelines to all the staff involved in patient care. Several limitations still exist however. The AAOS and the ACCP guidelines should be modified to establish a consensus. Unmet needs and improvement in the safety profiles hopefully will be fulfilled by newer agents in clinical development (Huo, 2011a).

4.3 Specific modalities

A summary of specific oral pharmacologic agents currently in clinical application for orthopedic patients is in Table 2.

Drug	Mechanism	Dosing	Monitoring	Half Life	Renal Clearance
Warfarin	Vitamin K antagonist	Variable; Daily	Yes	40 hours	0%
Dabigatran etexilate	Factor IIa inhibitor	Fixed; Twice Daily	No	14-17 hours	100%
Apixaban	Factor Xa inhibitor	Fixed; Twice Daily	No	9-14 hours	25%
Rivaroxaban	Factor Xa inhibitor	Fixed; Once Daily	No	9 hours	65%

Table 2. Comparison of warfarin to new oral anticoagulants. (Reference: Eikelboom JW. Weitz JI. A replacement for warfarin: the search continues. *Circulation* 2007;116:131-133.)

4.3.1 Mechanical

Mechanical prophylaxis using sequential compressive devices (SCDs) or foot pumps can be used as a sole means of VTE prophylaxis. Their clinical efficacy and safety have been documented in multiple studies. This is particularly useful in a patient that is perceived to have an elevated bleeding risk (Geerts et al., 2008). In many practices, mechanical devices are often used in conjunction with pharmacological prophylaxis. Newer devices may be used in the outpatient setting upon hospital discharge. The clinical efficacy, safety, and compliance have been documented in a few studies. It is necessary to continue to follow larger cohorts of patients using outpatient mechanical prophylaxis alone to fully determine the efficacy and compliance.

4.3.2 Warfarin

Warfarin has been used as VTE chemoprophylaxis in high-risk orthopedic patients for decades. It is an efficacious agent. However, it requires close monitoring. It can be both difficult and costly in the outpatient setting (Eikelboom & Weitz, 2007). It also has numerous drug-drug and drug-food interactions. These interactions can be particularly challenging considering the issue of poly-pharmacy in the elderly joint arthroplasty patient population. It also has a delayed onset of action, which may require bridging with a shorter acting anticoagulant such as LMWHs or unfractionated heparin. A recent paper by Caprini et al. noted that physicians often used inadequate bridging protocols in the postoperative period. This can have important clinical implications. They found that the 30-day mortality rate was found to be 6% for DVT and 12% for PE in this cohort (Caprini et al., 2005).

4.3.3 Aspirin

The ACCP guidelines do not recommend using aspirin alone in any of the high-risk orthopedic patient populations. The AAOS guidelines do sanction its use in patients with standard risk profile for pulmonary embolism prevention (Geerts et al., 2008).

4.3.4 Unfractionated heparin

This has been included in the ACCP guidelines for patients undergoing general surgery procedures. However, the ACCP guidelines have recommended against using unfractionated heparin alone in total joint arthroplasty or hip fracture patients due to inadequate evidence-based data to support its efficacy in these patient populations (Geerts et al., 2008).

4.3.5 Low-molecular-weight heparin

In contrast to warfarin, LMWHs have a predictable dose response with few interactions. Self-administration is generally well-tolerated and acceptable patient compliance has been documented in several studies. Additionally, there is no need for monitoring (Noble & Finlay, 2005). Dose adjustment may be necessary in the elderly, in particular in those with compromised renal clearance. LMWHs have considered to be the standard-of-care in many medical communities (Geerts et al., 2008).

5. Newer agents

There are several new oral anticoagulants in various stages of clinical development. These new classes target the inhibition of either thrombin or factor Xa. Most of the clinical trial data have demonstrated equal or even superior efficacy in comparison to LMWH. However, bleeding complications remain the primary concern. There are several other potential complications that have been reported.

5.1 Newer agents of historic importance

Ximelagatran was the first direct-thrombin inhibitor, and was approved initially by the European regulatory agencies. The initial trials showed no signs of liver toxicity in short-term use of up to 11 days (Eriksson et al., 2003). However, extended treatment (greater than 35 fays) was found to be associated with an increased risk of liver toxicity in one study (Agnelli et al., 2009). The liver toxicity was unpredictable, and the product was later withdrawn from the market (Vaughan, 2005).

Razaxaban was the first oral Factor Xa inhibitor to be developed. Data from phase I clinical trials demonstrated adequate efficacy and safety (Spyropoulos, 2007). A phase II trial involving TKA patients demonstrated significantly higher bleeding complication rates when compared with enoxaparin (Lassen et al., 2003). The trial was terminated prematurely and the drug development was discontinued.

5.2 Current oral anticoagulants

Dabaigatran etexilate is a pro-drug of the direct thrombin inhibitor, dabigatran (Eriksson et al., 2004). There have been four phase III clinical trials comparing this drug to enoxaparin. In addition, a meta-analysis of three of these has been conducted (Wolowacz et al., 2009). It demonstrated non-inferiority to once-daily enoxaparin 40mg dose in one clinical trial involving THA, but failed to do so when compared to twice-daily enoxaparin dosing with 30mg Additionally, it demonstrated non-inferiority to once-daily enoxaparin 40mg dose in two clinical trials involving THA patients (Eriksson et al., 2007a; Eriksson et al., 2007b). It was approved in the European Union and in Canada in 2008 for use in total joint arthroplasty patients as VTE prophylaxis. In the United States, it was approved for use in certain atria fibrillation patients for stroke prevention (Huo, 2011b).

Rivaroxaban and apixabab are both inhibitors of factor Xa. Their mechanism involves the inhibition of circulating factor Xa as well as bound factor Xa within the prothrombinase complex (Weitz, 2006). There have been four phase III clinical trials comparing rivaroxaban to enoxaparin (Eriksson et al., 2008). It also is approved in the European Union and Canada for VTE prophylaxis in patients undergoing THAs and TKAs. It has recently been approved in the United States.

Apixaban has been evaluated in several phase III clinical trials as well. It has not been approved for use anywhere (Lassen et al., 2010a). It was found to be more efficacious than once-daily dosing of enoxaparin, but failed to demonstrate non-inferiority to twice daily dosing of enoxaparin (Lassen et al., 2009; Lassen et al 2010b).

5.2.1 Potential problems with the newer agents

Bleeding events are the most important complication. A recent survey reported that 50% or more orthopaedic surgeons in the United States stated that they were more concerned with bleeding than the risk of VTE (Anderson et al., 2009). Major bleeding has occurred with all of these agents as it has with other pharmacological agents. LMWHs have been studied for over 20 years, and the incidents of significant bleeding complications ranges from 0.9% to 9.3% (Leizorovicz et al., 1992). A major difference between LMWH and the newer agents is that enoxaparin can be at least partially reversed using protamine in certain situations (Crowther et al., 2002). The thrombin and factor Xa inhibitors have no such reversal agents yet (Ng & Crowther, 2006). An overview of the bleeding in clinical trials involving new agents is included in Table 3. It is also important to note the effect of drug-drug interactions. There have been trials showing prolonged bleeding when rivaroxaban was taken with clopidogrel or aspirin (Perzborn et al., 2007). Though there may be a relationship between bleeding and infection, the use of anticoagulation has not specifically been associated with a higher infection rate (Parvizi et al., 2007; Saleh et al., 2002).

Aside from bleeding risk, there are other adverse effects that have been documented with the thrombin and factor Xa inhibitors. Drug-induced liver toxicity is the most common reason cited for the withdrawal of a drug from the market (Lee, 2003). The exact mechanism has not been identified. There have been several trials with dabigatran that reported elevated liver enzymes, but all returned to baseline within 2 months (Eriksson et al., 2007b). Dabigatran is a substrate for the cellular transporter P-glycoprotein which could be a mechanism of drug interaction (Aszalos, 2007). CYP240 enzymes are involved in the metabolism of both factor Xa inhibitors (Bayer Inc, 2010). Both factor Xa and thrombin inhibitors are excreted through the renal system, so this could potentially lead to complications.

Both types of drugs are promising alternatives due to several characteristics. They have predictable pharmacokinetics, few drug interactions, and no monitoring is required (Weitz et al., 2008). It is important to note that a perfect anticoagulant does not exist at this point. The thrombin and facto Xa inhibitors have been shown to be effective and safe in multiple trials, but there still is a lack of data from community practice.

Drug	Study	Number of Patients	Arthroplasty	Duration (Days)	Regimine (mg)	Major Clinically Significant Bleeding	Surgical Site Bleeding	Non-Major Clinically Relevant Bleeding
Dabigatran etexilate (Dab)	BISTRO I (Eriksson, 2004)	289	Hip	6-10	Dab 12.5-, 25-, 50-, 100-, 150-, 200-, 300-BID; and 150-, 300-QD	2.4% Dab 150-QD	N/A	2.4% Dab 150-QD
	BISTRO II (Eriksson, 2005)	1949	Hip and Knee	6-10	Dab 50-, 150-, 225-BID; and 300-QD; Enox 40-QD	8.2% Dab 150-BID; 8.3% Dab 300-QD; 4.6% Enox	N/A	4.1% Dab 150-QD; 4.9% Dab 300-QD; 2.6% Enox
	RE-NOVATE (Eriksson, 2007a)	3463	Hip	28-35	Dab 150-, 220-QD; Enox 40-QD	6.0% Dab 150-QD; 6.2% Dab 220-QD; 5.1% Enox	N/A	4.7% Dab 150-QD; 4.2% Dab 220-QD; 3.5% Enox
	RE-MODEL (Eriksson, 2008b)	2076	Knee	6-10	Dab 150-, 220-QD; Enox 40-QD	8.1% Dab 150-QD; 7.4% Dab 220-QD; 6.6% Enox	N/A	6.8% Dab 150-QD; 5.9% Dab 220-QD; 5.3% Enox
	RE-MOBILIZE (Ginsberg, 2009)	2596	Knee	12-15	Dab 150-, 220-QD; Enox 30-BID	3.1% Dab 150-QD; 3.3% Dab 220-QD; 3.8% Enox	N/A	2.5% Dab 150-QD; 2.7% Dab 220-QD; 2.4% Enox
Rivaroxaban (Riv)	ODIXa-KNEE (Turpie, 2005)	613	Knee	5-9	Riv 2.5-, 5-, 10-, 20-, 30-BID; Enox 30-BID	2.9% Riv 5-BID; 4.8% Enox	0% Riv 5-BID; 1.9% Enox	2.9% Riv 5-BID; 2.9% Enox
	ODIXa-OD-HIP (Eriksson, 2006a)	845	Hip	5-9	Riv 5-, 10-, 20-, 30-, 40-QD; Enox 40-QD	2.8% Riv 10-QD; 5,1% Enox	N/A	2.1% Riv 10-QD; 3.2% Enox
	ODIXa-HIP (Eriksson, 2006b)	704	Hip	5-9	Riv 2.5-, 5-, 10-, 20-, 30-BID; Enox 40 QD	8.1% Riv 5-BID; 1.5% Enox	2.2% Riv 5-BID; 0.8% Enox	5.9% Riv 5-BID; 0% Enox
	Dose-escalation study (Eriksson, 2007c)	625	Hip	5-9	Riv 2.5-, 5-, 10-, 20-, 30-BID; 30-QD; Enox 40 QD	3.8% Riv 5-BID; 1.9% Enox	2.5% Riv 5-BID; 0% Enox	1.3% Riv 5-BID; 1.9% Enox
	RECORD1 (Eriksson, 2008)	4433	Hip	31-39	Riv 10-QD; Enox 40-QD	3.2% Riv; 2.5% Enox	N/A	2.9% Riv; 2.4% Enox
	RECORD2 (Kakkar, 2008)	2457	Hip	31-39 Riv; 10-14 Enox	Riv 10-QD; Enox 40-QD	3.4% Riv; 2.8% Enox	N/A	3.3% Riv; 2.7% Enox
	RECORD3 (Lassen, 2008)	2459	Knee	10-14	Riv 10-QD; Enox 40-QD	3.3% Riv; 2.8% Enox	N/A	2.7% Riv; 2.3% Enox
	RECORD4 (Turpie, 2009)	3034	Knee	10-14	Riv 10-QD; Enox 30-BID	3.0% Riv; 2.3% Enox	N/A	2.6% Riv; 2.0% Enox
	RECORD1-3 (Eriksson, 2009)	9349	Hip and Knee	10-39	Riv 10-QD; Enox 40-QD	3.3% Riv; 2.7% Enox	N/A	3.0% Riv; 2.5% Enox
	RECORD1-4 (US FDA, 2009)	12383	Hip and Knee	10-39	Riv 10-QD; Enox 40-QD or 30-BID	3.19% Riv; 2.55% Enox	1.8% Riv; 1.37% Enox	N/A
Apixaban (Apix)	APROPOS (Lassen, 2007)	1217	Knee	10-14	Apix 5-, 10-, 20-QD; 2.5-, 5-, 10-BID; Enox 30-BID or Warfarin (INR 1.8-3.0)	0% Apix 2.5-BID; 1.3% Enox; 0% Warfarin	N/A	N/A
	ADVANCE-1 (Lassen, 2009)	3184	Knee	10-14	Apix 2.5-BID; Enox 30-BID	2.9% Apix; 4.3% Enox	0.5% Apix; 0.9% Enox	2.2% Apix; 3.0% Enox
	ADVANCE-2 (Lassen, 2010b)	3009	Knee	10-14	Apix 2.5-BID; Enox 40-QD	3.5% Apix; 4.8% Enox	0.5% Apix; 0.7% Enox	2.9% Apix; 3.8% Enox
	ADVANCE-3 (Lassen, 2010a)	5332	Hip	N/A	Apix 2.5-BID; Enox 40-QD	4.8% Apix; 5.0% Enox	0.7% Apix; 0.6% Enox	4.1% Apix; 4.5% Enox

Table 3. Major bleeding rates in VTE prophylaxis clinical trails in THA and TKA. (Reference: Huo, M. New oral anticoagulants in venous thromboembolism prophylaxis in orthopaedic patients: Are they really better? *Thromb Haemost* 2011;106:45-57.

6. Conclusion

VTE remains a challenging problem that complicates many orthopaedic procedures. The incidence has been found to be particularly high following TKA and THA. Governmental and consumer governing bodies are beginning to recognize it as a "never-event" indicating that increased emphasis will be placed on prophylaxis in the years to come. Recommendations have been released by both the ACCP and the AAOS and there remains some disagreement as to the optimal management of VTE. Warfarin and LMWH remain the standard of care in many practices, but newer agents show increasing promise.

The authors have several recommendations regarding the duration and type of therapy. Patients should be anticoagulated for 25-30 days postoperatively following total hip arthroplasty and for 14 days following a total knee arthroplasty. Certain patients with high risk of VTE (obese, low mobility, prior VTE, family history of VTE, or protein C/S deficiency) should be treated for 25-30 days as well following hip or knee replacement. At our institution, we generally use enoxaparin for postoperative anticoagulation. For inpatients, either 30mg twice daily or 40mg daily may be used following total hip arthroplasty. The FDA has approved only the twice daily dosing after total knee arthroplasty. For outpatients, enoxaparin 40mg daily is our regimen of choice.

7. References

Agnelli G, Eriksson BI, Cohen AT, et al. Safety assessment of new antithrombotic agents: lessons from the EXTEND study on ximelagatran. *Thromb Res* 2009; 123:488–497.

AHRQ. Diagnosis and treatment of deep venous thrombosis and pulmonary embolism; US Agency for Healthcare Research and Quality. 2007.

American Academy of Orthopaedic Surgeons. American Academy of Orthopaedic Surgeons clinical guideline on prevention of symptomatic pulmonary embolism in patients undergoing total hip or knee arthroplasty. *www.aaos.org/Research/guidelines/PE_guideline pdf* 2007.

Amin A, Spyropoulos AC, Dobesh P *et al.* Are hospitals delivering appropriate VTE prevention? The venous thromboembolism study to assess the rate of thromboprophylaxis (VTE start). *J Thromb Thrombolysis* 2010;29:326–339.

Anderson FA, Lieberman J, Pellegrini VD, et al. Practices in prevention of venous thromboembolism in primary hip and knee arthroplasty vary with surgeon operative volume: findings from a survey of US orthopedic surgeons. *J Thromb Haemost* 2009; 7 (Suppl 2): Abstract PP-MO-248.

Aszalos A. Drug-drug interactions affected by the transporter protein, P-glycoprotein (ABCB1, MDR1) II. Clinical aspects. *Drug Discov Today* 2007;12:838–843.

Bergqvist D, Agnelli G, Cohen AT, et al., for the ENOXACAN II Investigators. Duration of prophylaxis against venous thromboembolism with enoxaparin after surgery for cancer. *N Engl J Med.* 2002;346:975–980.

Burnett RS, Clohisy JC, Wright RW, et al. Failure of the American College of Chest Physicians-1A protocol for Lovenox in clinical outcomes for thromboembolic prophylaxis. *J Arthroplasty* 2007;22:317–324.

Caprini JA, Botteman MF, Stephens JM *et al.* Economic burden of long-term complications of deep vein thrombosis after total hip replacement surgery in the United States. *Value Health* 2003;6:59–74.

Caprini JA, Tapson VF, Hyers TM *et al.*; NABOR Steering Committee. Treatment of venous thromboembolism: adherence to guidelines and impact of physician knowledge, attitudes, and beliefs. *J Vasc Surg* 2005;42:726–733.

Comp PC, Spiro TE, Friedman RJ, et al., for the Enoxaparin Clinical Trial Group. Prolonged enoxaparin therapy to prevent venous thromboembolism after primary hip or knee replacement. *J Bone Joint Surg Am.* 2001;83-A:336–345.

Conduah, AH; Lieberman JR (2007). Thromboembolism and Pulmonary Distress in the Setting of Orthopaedic Surgery. In TA Einhorn, RJ O'Keefe, JA Buckwalter (Eds.), *Orthopaedic Basic Science: Foundations of Clinical Practice* (3rd edition, pp. 105-113). Rosemont, IL: AAOS.

Crowther MA, Berry LR, Monagle PT, et al. Mechanisms responsible for the failure of protamine to inactivate low-molecular-weight heparin. *Br J Haematol* 2002;116:178–186.

Eikelboom JW, Karthikeyan G, Fagel N *et al.* American Association of Orthopedic Surgeons and American College of Chest Physicians guidelines for venous thromboembolism prevention in hip and knee arthroplasty differ: what are the implications for clinicians and patients? *Chest* 2009;135:513–520.

Eikelboom JW, Weitz JI. A replacement for warfarin: the search continues. *Circulation* 2007;116:131–133.

Eriksson BI, Agnelli G, Cohen AT, et al. Direct thrombin inhibitor melagatran followed by oral ximelagatran compared with enoxaparin for prevention of venous thromboembolism after total hip or knee replacement. *Thromb Haemost* 2003;89: 288–296.

Eriksson BI, Dahl OE, Ahnfelt L, et al. Dose escalating safety study of a new oral direct thrombin inhibitor, dabigatran etexilate, in patients undergoing total hip replacement: BISTRO I. *J Thromb Haemost* 2004; 2: 1573–1580.

Eriksson BI, Dahl OE, Buller HR, et al. A new oral direct thrombin inhibitor, dabigatran etexilate, compared with enoxaparin for prevention of thromboembolic events following total hip or knee replacement: the BISTRO II randomized trial. *J Thromb Haemost* 2005; 3:103–111.

Eriksson BI, Borris LC, Dahl OE, et al. A once-daily, oral, direct Factor Xa inhibitor, rivaroxaban (BAY 59-7939), for thromboprophylaxis after total hip re- placement. *Circulation* 2006; 114: 2374–2381.

Eriksson BI, Borris L, Dahl OE, et al. Oral, direct Factor Xa inhibition with BAY 59-7939 for the prevention of venous thromboembolism after total hip replacement. *J Thromb Haemost* 2006; 4: 121–128.

Eriksson BI, Dahl OE, Rosencher N, et al. Dabigatran etexilate versus enoxaparin for prevention of venous thromboembolism after total hip replacement: a randomised, double-blind, non- inferiority trial. *Lancet.* 2007; 370:949--956.

Eriksson BI, Dahl OE, Rosencher N, et al. Oral dabigatran etexilate versus subcutaneous enoxaparin for the prevention of venous thromboembolism after total knee replacement: the RE-MODEL randomized trial. *J Thromb Haemost.* 2007; 5: 2178--2185.

Eriksson BI, Borris LC, Dahl OE, et al. Dose-escalation study of rivaroxaban (BAY 59-7939)--an oral, direct Factor Xa inhibitor--for the prevention of venous thromboembolism in patients undergoing total hip replacement. Thromb Res 2007; 120: 685–693.

Eriksson BI, Borris LC, Friedman RJ, et al. Rivaroxaban versus enoxaparin for thromboprophylaxis after hip arthroplasty. *N Engl J Med* 2008; 358: 2765–2775. 30.

Eriksson BI, Kakkar AK, Turpie AG, et al. Oral rivaroxaban for the prevention of symptomatic venous thromboembolism after elective hip and knee replacement. *J Bone Joint Surg Br* 2009; 91: 636–644.

Freedman KB, Brookenthal KR, Fitzgerald RH Jr, et al. A meta-analysis of thromboembolic prophylaxis following elective total hip arthroplasty. *J Bone Joint Surg Am* 2000; 82-A: 929–938.

Geerts WH, Bergqvist D, Pineo GF *et al.* Prevention of venous thromboembolism: American College of Chest Physicians Evidence-Based Clinical Practice Guidelines (8th ed). *Chest* 2008;133(6 suppl):381S–453S.

Ginsberg JS, Davidson BL, et al. RE-MOBILIZE Writing Committee. Oral thrombin inhibitor dabigatran etexilate vs North American enoxaparin regimen for prevention of venous thromboembolism after knee arthroplasty surgery. *J Arthroplasty* 2009; 24: 1-9.

Heit JA. The epidemiology of venous thromboembolism in the community: implications for prevention and management. *J Thromb Thrombolysis* 2006;21:23–29.

Heit JA, Silverstein MD, Mohr DN, Petterson TM, O'Fallon WM, Melton LJ III. Predictors of survival after deep vein thrombosis and pulmonary embolism: a population-based, cohort study. *Arch Intern Med* 1999;159:445–453.

Hirsh J, Guyatt G, Lewis SZ. Reflecting on eight editions of the American College of Chest Physicians antithrombotic guidelines. *Chest* 2008;133:1293–1295.

Hoffman M, Dougald M. The action of high-dose factor VIIa in a cell-based model of hemostasis. Disease a Month 2003; 49: 14-21

Huo, M. Prevalence and Economic Burden of Venous Thromboembolism Following Total Joint Arthroplasty. *Current Orthopaedic Practice* 2011:22:193–197.

Huo M. New oral anticoagulants in venous thromboembolism prophylaxis in orthopaedic patients: are they really better? *Thromb Haemost* 2011; 106:45-57.

Imperiale TF, Speroff T. A meta-analysis of methods to prevent venous thromboembolism following total hip replacement. *J Am Med Assoc* 1994; 271: 1780–1785.

Kakkar AK, Brenner B, Dahl OE, et al. Extended duration rivaroxaban versus short-term enoxaparin for the prevention of venous thromboembolism after total hip arthroplasty: a double-blind, randomised controlled trial. *Lancet* 2008;372: 31–39.

Kim S. Changes in surgical loads and economic burden of hip and knee replacements in the US: 1997–2004. *Arthritis Rheum* 2008;59:481–488.

Kolb G, Bodemer I, Galster H *et al.* Reduction of venous thromboembolism following prolonged prophylaxis with the low molecular weight heparin Certoparin after endoprosthetic joint replacement or osteosynthesis of the lower limb in elderly patients. *Thromb Haemost* 2003;90:1100–1105

Lassen MR, Borris LC, Anderson BS, et al. Efficacy and safety of prolonged thromboprophylaxis with a low molecular weight heparin (dalteparin) after total hip arthroplasty—the Danish Prolonged Prophylaxis (DaPP) Study. *Thromb Res.* 1998;89:281–287.

Lassen MR, Davidson BL, Gallus A, et al. A phase II randomized, double-blind five-arm parallel-group, dose-response study of a new oral directly-acting factor Xa inhibitor, razaxaban, for the prevention of deep vein thrombosis in knee replacement surgery. *Blood* 2003; 102: Abstract 41.

Lassen MR, Davidson BL, Gallus A, et al. The efficacy and safety of apixaban, an oral, direct factor Xa inhibitor, as thromboprophylaxis in patients following total knee replacement. *J Thromb Haemost* 2007; 5: 2368–2375.

Lassen MR, Ageno W, Borris LC, et al. Rivaroxaban versus enoxaparin for thromboprophylaxis after total knee arthroplasty. *N Engl J Med* 2008; 358: 2776–2786.

Lassen MR, Raskob GE, Gallus A, et al. Apixaban or enoxaparin for thromboprophylaxis after knee replacement. *N Engl J Med* 2009;361:594–604.

Lassen MR, Gallus A, Raskob GE, Pineo G, Chen D, Ramirez LM; ADVANCE-3 Investigators. Apixaban versus enoxaparin for thromboprophylaxis after hip replacement. *N Engl J Med* 2010; 363: 2487–2498.

Lassen MR, Raskob GE, Gallus A, Pineo G, Chen D, Hornick P; ADVANCE-2 investigators. Apixaban versus enoxaparin for thromboprophylaxis after knee replacement (ADVANCE-2): a randomised double-blind trial. *Lancet* 2010; 375: 807–815.

Lee WM. Drug-induced hepatotoxicity. *N Engl J Med* 2003;349:474–485.

Leizorovicz A, Haugh MC, Chapuis FR, et al. Low molecular weight heparin in prevention of perioperative thrombosis. *Br Med J* 1992; 305: 913–920.

Markel DC, York S, Liston MJ Jr, Flynn JC, Barnes CL, Davis CM 3rd; AAHKS Research Committee. Venous thromboembolism: management by American Association of Hip and Knee Surgeons. *J Arthroplasty* 2010;25:3–9.

Mega JL, Braunwald E, Mohanavelu S, et al. Rivaroxaban versus placebo in patients with acute coronary syndromes (ATLAS ACS-TIMI 46): a randomised, double-blind, phase II trial. *Lancet* 2009; 374: 29–38.

Moyer TP, O'Kane DJ, Baudhuin LM, *et al.* Warfarin sensitivity genotying: a review of the literature and summary of patient experience. *Mayo Clin Proc* 2009:84:1079–1094.

Ng HJ, Crowther MA. New anti-thrombotic agents: emphasis on hemorrhagic complications and their management. *Semin Hematol* 2006; 43 (1 Suppl 1): S77–83.

Noble SI, Finlay IG. Is long-term low-molecular-weight heparin acceptable to palliative care patients in the treatment of cancer related venous thromboembolism? A qualitative study. *Palliat Med.* 2005;19:197–201.

Nurmohamed MT, Rosendaal FR, Büller HR, et al. Low-molecular-weight heparin versus standard heparin in general and orthopaedic surgery: a meta-analysis. *Lancet* 1992; 340: 152–156.

Oster G, Ollendorf DA, Vera-Llonch M, Hagiwara M, Berger A, Edelsberg J. Economic consequences of venous thromboembolism following major orthopedic surgery. *Ann Pharmacother* 2004;38:377–382.

Parvizi J, Ghanem E, Joshi A, et al. Does "excessive" anticoagulation predispose to periprosthetic infection? *J Arthroplasty* 2007;22:24-28.

Perzborn E, Fischer E, Lange U. Concomitant administration of rivaroxaban - an oral, direct Factor Xa inhibitor - with clopidogrel and acetylsalicylic acid enhances antithrombosis in rats. Pathophysiol Haemost Thromb 2007/2008; 36 (Suppl 1): 157–200: Abstract P060.

Planes A, Vochelle N, Darmon JY, et al. Risk of deep-venous thrombosis after hospital discharge in patients having undergone total hip replacement: Double-blind randomized comparison of enoxaparin versus placebo. *Lancet*. 1996;348:224–228.

Rasmussen MS, Jorgensen LN, Wille-Jørgensen P, et al., for the FAME Investigators. Prolonged prophylaxis with dalteparin to prevent late thromboembolic complications in patients undergoing major abdominal surgery: A multicenter randomized open-label study. *J Thromb Haemost*. 2006;4:2384–2390.

Saleh K, Olson M, Resig S, et al. Predictors of wound infection in hip and knee joint replacement: results from a 20 year surveillance program. *J Orthop Res* 2002; 20:506-515.

Schellong S, Hesselschwerdt HJ, Paar WD, von Hanstein KL. Rates of proximal deep vein thrombosis as assessed by compression ultrasonography in patients receiving prolonged thromboprophylaxis with low molecular weight heparin after major orthopedic surgery. *Thromb Haemost*. 2005;94:532–536.

Spyropoulos AC. Investigational treatments of venous thromboembolism. *Exp Opin Investig Drugs* 2007; 16: 431–440.

Turpie AG, Fisher WD, Bauer KA, et al. BAY 59-7939: an oral, direct factor Xa inhibitor for the prevention of venous thromboembolism in patients after total knee replacement. A phase II dose-ranging study. *J Thromb Haemost* 2005; 3: 2479–2486.

Turpie AG, Lassen MR, Davidson BL, et al. Rivaroxaban versus enoxaparin for thromboprophylaxis after total knee arthroplasty (RECORD4): a randomized trial. *Lancet* 2009; 373: 1673–1680.

U.S. Food and Drug Administration, Center for Drug Evaluation and Research, Meeting of the Cardiovascular and Renal Drugs Advisory Committee March 19, 2009. Available at: http://www.fda.gov/downloads/AdvisoryCommittees/CommitteesMeetingMaterials/Drugs/CardiovascularandRenalDrugsAdvisoryCommittee/UCM143660.pdf. Accessed September 23, 2011.

Vaughan C. Ximelagatran (Exanta): alternative to warfarin? Proc (Bayl Univ Med Cent) 2005; 18: 76–80.

Weitz JI. Emerging anticoagulants for the treatment of venous thromboembolism. *Thromb Haemost* 2006; 96: 274–284.

Weitz JI, Hirsh J, Samama MM. New antithrombotic drugs. American College of Chest Physicians Evidence-Based Clinical Practice Guidelines (8th ed). *Chest* 2008;133:234S–256S.

White RH, Romano PS, Zhou H, et al. Incidence and time course of thromboembolic outcomes following total hip or knee arthroplasty. *Arch Intern Med*. 1998;158:1525–1531.

Wolowacz SE, Roskell NS, Plumb JM, Caprini JA, Eriksson BI. Efficacy and safety of dabigatran etexilate for the prevention of venous thromboembolism following total hip or knee arthroplasty. A meta-analysis. *Thromb Haemost* 2009; 101: 77–85.

Xarelto product monograph, Bayer Inc., Canada, September 10, 2008. Available at: www.bayer.ca/files/XARELTO-PM-ENG-10SEP2008–119111.pdf. Accessed September 29, 2010.

11

Deep Venous Thrombosis After Radical Pelvic Surgery

Bedeir Ali-El-Dein
Mansoura University, Urology and Nephrology Center
Egypt

1. Introduction

Deep venous thrombosis or DVT is a blood clot formation in one or more of the deep veins. The blood clot does not break down and therefore, it can become larger and occlude the blood flow within the affected vein. The most frequent sites are the leg veins (femoral and popliteal) and the deep pelvic veins. Rarely, the arm veins are affected (Paget-Schrötter disease). Pulmonary embolism (PE) is the most dangerous complication of DVT. PE occurs when the clot breaks into small pieces (emboli) and travel to the lung. The embolus may travel to other vital organs and cause life-threatening complications such as stroke or heart attack.

The etiology of thrombosis is exactly unknown, however, the Virchow's triad of slow circulation (stasis), increased blood coagulability and vessel wall intimal injury is the alleged mechanism.

DVT and PE developing after trauma and pelvic surgery are of a major concern to surgeons of all subspecialties. Therefore, proper assessment of the patient risk to develop DVT is of paramount importance. The risk of DVT can be decreased significantly by adopting some appropriate prophylactic procedures.

Although adopting anti-DVT prophylactic measures is not debatable, the use of these measures has not yet been a universal issue, even in patients having no contraindications to their use.

In this chapter, the term "radical pelvic surgeries" mean all types of major surgeries performed to treat malignancies developing in the pelvis, such as radical cystectomy, salvage cystectomy, radical prostatectomy, radical or pan-hysterectomy, radical surgery for colo-rectal cancer and excision of a local tumor recurrence after primary radical surgery or after definitive radiotherapy

2. Incidence

DVT constitutes a major health problem, especially among the elderly. In comparison with previous era, the incidence of DVT remains the same among men and possibly increasing in elderly females (Silverstein et al., 1998). On the other hand, the incidence of PE is decreasing over years (Silverstein et al., 1998). However, the incidence of DVT and PE may be underestimated because of the missed diagnosis, absence of pertinent symptoms or the absence of laws to permit routine autopsies in sudden post-operative mortalities in most centers (Dalen & Alpert, 1975; Clagett, 1994). Furthermore, unexplained DVT may be the first presentation in some malignancies, such as prostate, colorectal and bladder (Monreal & Prandoni, 1999).

In a series of 2373 patients, the incidence of DVT was 0.87% after urologic surgeries for prostate and bladder tumors, 2.8% in general surgery and 2% in gynecological surgeries (Scarpa etal., 2007).

The incidence of DVT may be as low 2% after radical cystectomy (Ali-El-Dein et al., 2008; Ghoneim et al., 2008), or as high as 40% following prolonged gynecological or obstetrical surgery (Walsh et al., 1974; Clarke-Pearson et al., 1983). Patients undergoing large bowel surgery also have a considerable risk of DVT and pulmonary embolism. The incidence of DVT following radical cystectomy in our hospital is 2% to 2.6% and PE following DVT or without prior DVT has long been a leading cause of post-operative death (Ali-El-Dein et al., 2008; Ghoneim et al., 2008). In patients undergoing surgery or radiotherapy for treatment of localized prostate cancer the incidence of DVT was 2% for pelvic lymphadenectomy alone and 1.9% following prostatectomy, while fatal PE occurred in 2 patients (3.7%) after prostatectomy (Bratt et al., 1994).

The incidence of DVT after gynecologic and obstetrical surgeries varies according to the presence or absence of the known risk factors among patients and according to the methods of diagnosis. It has been reported that this incidence is 14% after benign gynecological surgeries (Walsh et al., 1974), while the rate has been higher (38%) for patients undergoing surgery for gynecological tumors (Crandon & Knotts, 1983). In addition, among all causes of death following gynecologic surgeries, PE has been a leading cause of postoperative mortality in high risk women with gynecologic malignancy (Clarke-Pearson et al., 1983). Following laparoscopic radical hysterectomy for cervical carcinoma the incidence of DVT has been 3% (Chen et al., 2008).

In the study of yang et al. on 3645 patients undergoing surgery for colorectal cancer, 31 (0.85%) developed symptomatic venous thromboembolism or VTE (Yang et al., 2011).

3. Pathogenesis and risk factors

The traditional Virchow's triad of hypercoagulability, Stasis of the venous stream and vessel wall (endothelial) trauma is still the basis of description of the pathophysiology of DVT.

One or more of these three factors may explain DVT in patients with radical pelvic surgeries. The risk factors and the underlying pathogenetic mechanisms of DVT are shown in table (1).

A major factor is immobilization (prolonged bed rest), which can impair venous drainage from the lower limb with subsequent venous stasis (Clark & Cotton, 1968).

The other reasons that can induce venous stasis as well as other risk factors for DVT/PE are enlisted in table (1).

Stasis:	-Immobilization. -Pelvic masses. - A gravid uterus - Surgically induced hematomas. - lymphocysts also can lead to venous stasis
Vessel wall injury:	-Surgical trauma. -Intravascular catheters. -Malignant involvement of the vessels of the tumor.
Thrombophilia	-Factor V Leiden mutation. -Prothrombin gene mutation. -G20210A. -Antithrombin deficiency -Factors I, V, VIII, IX, X, and XI. -The presence of activated intermediate coagulation products such as thrombin-antithrombin III complexes . -Abnormalities of the platelets . -Tissue factor and cancer procoagulant -Factors that influence vascular endothelial permeability such as vascular endothelial growth factor. -Protein C deficiency -Protein S deficiency
General factors:	-Obesity -Prior history of DVT -Hormonal therapy, -Chemotherapy, or radiotherapy for cancer -Old age -Oral contraceptive pills or hormonal replacement therapy -Pregnancy and the postpartum period -Burns -Sepsis -Systemic lupus erythematosus -Polycythemia rubra vera -Thrombocytosis -Erythropoiesis-stimulating agents -Dysfibrinogenemias and disorders of plasminogen activation -Intravenous (IV) drug abuse -Acute medical illness -Inflammatory bowel disease -Myeloproliferative disorders -Paroxysmal nocturnal hemoglobinuria -Nephrotic syndrome -Positive family history of DVT/PE -Smoking

Table 1. Risk factors in DVT following radical pelvic surgeries

Endothelial injury of the vessel wall may be induced by surgical dissection in various radical pelvic surgeries (e.g. radical cystectomy) or from infiltration of the vessel wall by the tumor. In addition, catheters placed distally or proximally in the venous system are among the risk factors (Evans et al., 2010). However, in this situation, the risk of DVT/PE is determined by multiple factors including catheter size (Evans et al., 2010), degree of vein trauma during catheter insertion and dwell and hypercoagulability of the patient' blood.

Hypercoagulability or thrombophilia or prothrombotic state is a blood coagulation disorder with a subsequent increase in the incidence of thrombosis (Heit, 2007). There are multiple genetic and acquired risk factors that influence thrombophilia. The presence of these inherited risk factors alone usually does not cause thrombosis unless an additional risk factor is present (Heit, 2007; Kyrle et al., 2010).

Antithrombin deficiency, which is the first major form of thrombophilia, was identified in 1965, while the most common defects, such as factor V Leiden mutation and prothrombin gene mutation G20210A were described in the 1990s (Dahlbäck, 2008; Rosendaal & Reitsma, 2009). The risk of developing DVT/PE increases significantly if one of these abnormalities is present in patients undergoing radical pelvic surgery.

There are various possibilities, which can induce a hypercoagulable state during major radical pelvic surgeries. These possibilities include decreased fibrinolytic activity associated with surgery (Egan et al., 1974), increased level of coagulation factors I, V, VIII, IX, X, and XI, the presence of activated intermediate coagulation products such as thrombin-antithrombin III complexes and abnormalities of the platelets (Piccioli et al., 1996). In addition, the malignant cells may secrete a substance promoting coagulation, such as tissue factor and cancer procoagulant or factors that influence vascular endothelial permeability such as vascular endothelial growth factor and subsequently stimulate fibrin deposition (Goad & Gralnick, 1996).

In the prospective study of Duke University Medical Center 411 patients undergoing major abdominal and pelvic gynecologic surgery were evaluated for DVT and the related possible risk factors (Clarke-Pearson et al., 1987). In this study, the important factors, which maintained statistical significance in stepwise logistic regression model were age, edema of the ankle, type of surgery, nonwhite race, presence of varicose veins, history of radiation preoperatively, past DVT and duration of surgery.

It has been found that the risk factors for distal DVT are different from those of proximal DVT. In the national (France) multicenter prospective OPTIMEV study, out of 6141 patients with symptoms suggestive of DVT, diagnosis was objectively confirmed in only 1643 and isolated distal DVT was more common than proximal one (Galanaud et al., 2009). In this study, acute or transient risk factors, such as recent surgery, recent plaster immobilization and recent travel, were more frequently discovered in distal DVT. On the other hand, in proximal DVT chronic risk factors such as active cancer, congestive heart failure or respiratory insufficiency and age above 75 years were more frequent.

Active cancer and related chemotherapy can increase the incidence of DVT by multiple mechanisms. In chronic lymphocytic leukemia patients, studies showed a link between lenalidomide associated DVTs and inflammation, upregulation of TNFα and endothelial cell dysfunction (Aue etal., 2011).

4. Diagnosis of DVT/PE

The majority of cases of DVT/PE have one or more risk factor. Many cases of DVT/PE are asymptomatic. Suspected pulmonary embolism is a medical emergency and can be fatal. In symptomatic DVT cases, the patient may present with lower limb pain, unilateral leg swelling, redness and sometimes prominent superficial veins. A tender calf, especially with dorsiflexion (Homan's sign) and rarely a palpable venous cord are among the possible physical signs. However, the presence of these manifestations is nonspecific, because in more than 50% of the cases presenting with these symptoms, DVT is absent (Dainty et al., 2004). Therefore, diagnosis of DVT based on symptoms only is problematic and proper hospital assessment and further diagnostic tools are needed for accurate diagnosis._Similarly, most of the symptoms and signs of PE are nonspecific and simulate post-surgery pulmonary complications. However, physicians should maintain a high degree of suspicion if the patient is complaining of pleuritic chest pain, hemoptysis, dyspnea, tachycardia and tachypnea.

4.1 Laboratory testing

The use of a simple prediction tool, together with the laboratory tests of D-dimers and arterial blood gases (ABG) in cases of suspected PE are useful tools to exclude or prove DVT (Crisan et al., 2011). D-dimers are fibrinogen degradation products which are generally present at higher concentrations than normal in the blood of people with DVT.

4.2 Imaging in DVT

Imaging for DVT includes B-mode duplex Doppler ultrasound, impedance plethysmography, contrast venography, and magnetic resonance venography (MRV). Doppler ultrasound is currently the most common technique for the diagnosis of symptomatic DVT. B-mode ultrasonography allows a bi-dimensional image of the vessels of the lower extremity and when compression techniques are used, a sensitivity of up to 90% and a specificity of 96% to 100% can be achieved in the detection of DVT (Cronan et al., 1987; O'Leary et al., 1988).

In duplex ultrasonography B-mode is combined with Doppler flow, therefore, providing information about flow velocity. When color Doppler flow is used with compression B-mode ultrasonography (color duplex ultrasonography), additional data on the direction of flow is gained (Cronan et al., 1987; O'Leary et al., 1988).

Impedance plethysmography is a noninvasive diagnostic test that has a good accuracy in the detection of proximal DVT, when the results are analyzed in combination with positive clinical data (Kearon et al., 1998). However, false positive results may be obtained with this test and if the results of this test are non-diagnostic or not coping with the clinical data, venography should be performed (Kearon et al., 1998).

Contrast venography is still the gold standard for the diagnosis of DVT and is used by investigators as a reference standard for testing the new noninvasive diagnostic DVT measures (Tapson et al., 1999).

The technique is done as classically described (Rabinov & Paulin, 1972). A misdiagnosis is expected if all the deep veins from the leg up to the vena cava are not seen. When there is a persistent filling defect in the lumen of 2 or more veins, the diagnosis of DVT is confirmed

(Rabinov & Paulin, 1972). Currently, contrast venography is rarely indicated nowadays and has been replaced by the noninvasive measures. It is sometimes performed to confirm the diagnosis of a clinically suspected DVT. However, if noninvasive imaging is normal or inconclusive and still DVT is clinically suspected, venography is done to confirm the diagnosis. In the cases of clinical suspicion of DVT, a negative contrast venography rules out the need for anticoagulant treatment (Hull et al., 1981). The test has certain limitations and complications.

Magnetic resonance venography (MRV) is an accurate noninvasive venographic technique for the detection of DVT. It has a sensitivity and specificity comparable to contrast venography (Carpenter et al., 1993). Furthermore, it can detect thrombi places not seen by the conventional venography, such as pelvic, ovarian veins or vena cava. Two major limitations for MRV are present, namely, the expensive cost and prolonged time necessary (Carpenter et al., 1993).

Scintigraphy has been described as a diagnostic tool for DVT (Knight, 1993). However, the data of its clinical efficacy compared to the standard methods are still lacking.

4.3 Imaging in PE

The diagnosis of PE may be made by a variety of imaging techniques, including chest X-ray, ventilation-perfusion scan, computed tomography (CT) of the chest vessels and pulmonary angiography.

On clinical suspicion of PE, the initial evaluation is made using chest X-ray, Electrocardiography (ECG) and ABG. Further evaluation is made by ventilation-perfusion scan, CT of the chest vessels (Gulsun Akpinar & Goodman, 2008).

Currently, CT venography combined with pulmonary CT angiography for the detection of PE is increasingly used to confirm the diagnosis of suspected PE and the results have been extremely promising (Krishan et al., 2011).

5. Prophylaxis of DVT/PE

The incidence of DVT and subsequent PE can be decreased by adopting certain prophylactic mechanical and/ or pharmacologic measures, which have been proved to be safe and effective in most types of major surgeries (Martino et al., 2007; Geerts et al., 2008). Mechanical methods act by reducing stasis of venous blood and may stimulate endogenous fibrinolysis, while pharmacologic agents act by clot prevention through the various steps of the clotting cascade (Martino et al., 2007; Geerts et al., 2008).

5.1 Mechanical measures

Mechanical prophylaxis is usually simple to conduct and relatively less costy. It may be achieved through the use of graduated compression stockings, anti-embolism stocking, electrical stimulation of the leg muscles, intermittent external pneumatic calf compression and/ or the use of specific tables (Martino et al., 2007; Geerts et al., 2008; Miller, 2011).

5.2 Pharmacologic measures

These measures are very effective in most surgeries and therefore, should be made a routine practice (Agnelli, 2004). Low-dose unfractionated heparin or low-molecular-weight heparin

(LMWH) are the drugs of choice in patients undergoing radical pelvic operations in the fileds of general, vascular, major urologic and gynecologic surgeries (Agnelli, 2004). In urologic patients judged as low-risk, early postoperative mobilization is the only measure needed. On the other hand, higher-risk patients should receive vitamin K antagonists, LMWH and/ or fondaparinux (Agnelli, 2004).

Some investigators recommended a double prophylaxis of mechanical measures as well as pharmacologic measures using pre- and post-operative anticoagulation, usually in the form of LMWH (Whitworthet al., 2011). They found that the use of preoperative anticoagulation seems to significantly decrease the risk of DVT in high-risk patients undergoing major gynecologic surgeries. In addition, there was no significant change in the rates of complications secondary to this protocol.

5.3 Dual prophylaxis

DVT may develop while the patient is on prophylaxis, therefore, the idea of dual prophylaxis (mechanical and pharmacologic) has emerged (Dainty et al., 2004; Whitworthet al., 2011).

This combination has been evaluated in patients undergoing colorectal operations. A combination of low-dose unfractionated heparin and graduated compression stockings has been found to be 4-fold more effective than low-dose unfractionated heparin alone in DVT/PE prophylaxis (Wille-Jorgensen et al., 2003). Similarly, this dual prophylaxis has been found to be cost-effective in high-risk patients undergoing surgeries for gynecologic tumors (Dainty et al., 2004).

5.4 Duration of prophylaxis during radical pelvic surgeries

Following radical pelvic surgery, mechanical prophylaxis may be started before the operation, while pharmacologic prophylaxis is usually started after the operation and continued daily for 5–10 days or until the patient was fully mobile (Geerts et al., 2008; unpublished data by the author).

6. Treatment of DVT/PE

The goals of treatment of patients with DVT and PE are to prevent local growth of the thrombus, prevent the thrombus from breaking down into small pieces (emboli) and traveling to other places, prevent complications of DVT, prevent recurrence of the thrombus and in some clinical situations accelerate fibrinolysis (Hirsh & Hoak, 1996).

DVT is treated by immediate institution of anticoagulant therapy. Treatment is given as either unfractionated heparin or low molecular weight heparins, followed by few weeks to 6 months of oral anticoagulant therapy (Clarke-Pearson & Abaid, 2008). However, life-long anticoagulation has been recommended in some patients with active cancers after partial improvement or failure of treatment, because they remain at very high risk to recurrent DVT (Clarke-Pearson & Abaid, 2008).Low concentrations of heparin can inhibit the early stages of blood coagulation. However, higher concentrations are needed to inhibit the much higher concentrations of thrombin that are formed if the DVT process is not modulated (Hirsh & Hoak, 1996).

When unfractionated heparin is used, we usually start by a bolus injection followed by continuos infusion and the dose is then adjusted to maintain the level of activated partial thromboplastin time (APTT) at 1.5–2.5 times the control value (Clarke-Pearson & Abaid, 2008). Oral anticoagulation (warfarin) should be started on the first day of the heparin infusion aiming to achieve an international normalized ratio (INR) of 2.0-3.0. IV heparin may be discontinued in 5 days if an adequate INR level has been established (Clarke-Pearson & Abaid, 2008). Studies have demonstrated that some of the new anticoagulants, such as hirudin and its fragments, are effective inhibitors of clot-bound thrombin and therefore, they may provide a better efficacy than heparin in neutralizing the procoagulant effects of the fibrin-bound thrombin (Weitz et al., 1990).

Low molecular weight heparins such as enoxaparin and dalteparin have been proved to be as effective and safe as unfactionated heparin in the treatment and recurrence prophylaxis of DVT/PE (Quinlan et al., 2004). They have the advantage of the possibility to be given in the outpatient setting (Clarke-Pearson & Abaid, 2008).

Fibrinolysis can be performed by one of the fibrinolytic enzymes, such as streptokinase, urokinase and TPA, all of them can increase the dissolution rate of the thromus or embolus (Hirsh & Hoak, 1996). They are not routinely recommended in the treatment of DVT/PE, because of their cost and the high risk of bleeding (Hirsh & Hoak, 1996). Thrombolytic therapy is indicated in all patients with massive pulmonary embolism and in some selected cases of proximal DVT or with severe obstruction (Hirsh & Hoak, 1996). Thrombolytic therapy has the advantage of preserving the pulmonary microcirculation after PE and decreasing the possibility of post-thrombotic syndrome (PTS) following DVT (Linn et al., 1988). Intrapulmonary artery infusion of urokinase in extensive PE has been found to be safe and effective in treatment of patients with and without contraindication to the use of systemic thrombolytic therapy (McCotter et al., 1999). With the recommended dose, thrombolytic therapy produces significant and rapid resolution of pulmonary emboli with a low morbidity and mortality rate. However, in lower extremity DVT, therapeutic thrombolysis is still controversial.

In PE immediate anticoagulant therapy is given and respiratory support is maintained. In addition, pulmonary artery catheterization with the administration of thrombolytic agents has been tried as previously mentioned (McCotter et al., 1999).

Surgical intervention of the thrombus or embolus is rarely indicated. However, surgical extirpation of the thrombus (venous thrombectomy), of the embolus (pulmonary embolectomy) and endovascular therapies to treat DVT have been reported with promising results (Lindow et al., 2010; Jenkins, 2011).

Long-term results after transfemoral venous thrombectomy for iliofemoral DVT has shown that the technique is safe and effective and can prevent the development of severe post-thrombotic syndrome in the long term (Lindow et al., 2010).

Inferior vena cava filters have been introduced to prevent PE in patients in whom anticoagulation therapy is contraindicated, has failed or has been associated with complications and in patients with extensive free-floating thrombi or residual thrombi following massive PE (Chung et al., 2008; Kalva et al., 2008).

7. Conclusion

Deep venous thrombosis and pulmonary embolism are among the major post-operative complications that develop after radical pelvic surgeries. Pulmonary embolism is one of the leading causes of post-operative mortality in these patients. Most of the cases are asymptomatic and in the majority of patients dying from pulmonary embolism the embolism is diagnosed at autopsy. Treatment is essentially prophylactic and the primary treatment objectives are to prevent PE, decrease morbidity and to prevent the risk of developing the post-thrombotic syndrome (PTS). High-risk patients may be subject for dual mechanical and pharmacologic prophylaxis with good results. Anticoagulation provides the main stay of treatment. Thrombolytic therapy is currently used for massive pulmonary embolism and some selected cases of deep venous thrombosis. Surgical (thrombectomy or embolectomy) or endovascular techniques have been tried with promising results.

8. References

Ali-El-Dein, B., Shaaban, A.A., Abu-Eideh, R.H., El-Azab, M., Ashamallah, A. & Ghoneim, M.A. (2008). Surgical complications following radical cystectomy and orthotopic neobladders in women. *J Urol*,180,1,206-10.

Agnelli, G. (2004). Prevention of venous thromboembolism in surgical patients. Circulation, 110, (24 Suppl 1), IV4-12.

Aue, G., Nelson Lozier, J., Tian, X., Marie Cullinane, A., Soto, S., Samsel, L., McCoy, P. & Wiestner, A. (2011). Inflammation, TNFα and endothelial dysfunction link lenalidomide to venous thrombosis in chronic lymphocytic leukemia. *Am J Hematol*, Jun 27. doi: 10.1002/ajh.22114. [Epub ahead of print][http://www.ncbi.nlm.nih.gov/pubmed/21812019]

Bratt, O., Elfving, P., Flodgren, P. & Lundgren, R. (1994). Morbidity of pelvic lymphadenectomy, radical retropubic prostatectomy and external radiotherapy in patients with localised prostatic cancer. *Scand J Urol Nephrol*, 28,3,265-71.

Carpenter, J.P., Holland, G.A., Baum, R.A., Owen, R.S., Carpenter, J.T. & Cope, C. (1993). Magnetic resonance venography for the detection of deep venous thrombosis: comparison with contrast venography and duplex Doppler ultrasonography. *J Vasc Surg*, 18,5, 734-41.

Chen, Y., Xu, H., Li, Y., Wang, D., Li, J., Yuan, J. & Liang, Z. (2008). The outcome of laparoscopic radical hysterectomy and lymphadenectomy for cervical cancer: a prospective analysis of 295 patients. *Ann Surg Oncol*, 15,10,2847-55.

Chung, J. & Owen, R.J.T. (2008). Using inferior vena cava filters to prevent pulmonary embolism. *Can Fam Physician*, 54,1, 49 – 55 .

Clagett, G.P. (1994) Prevention of postoperative venous thromboembolism: An update. *Am J Surg*, 168,6, 515-22.

Clark, C. & Cotton, L.T. (1968). Blood-flow in deep veins of leg: Recording technique and evaluation of methods to increase flow during operation. *Br J Surg*,55,3, 211-4.

Clarke-Pearson, D.L., Jelovsek, F.R. & Creasman, W.T. (1983). Thromboembolism complicating surgery for cervical and uterine malignancy: Incidence, risk factors and prophylaxis. *Obstet Gynecol*, 61,1, 87-94.

Clarke-Pearson, D.L., DeLong, E.R., Synan, I.S., Coleman, R.E. & Creasman, W.T. (1987). Variables associated with postoperative deep venous thrombosis: a prospective study of 411 gynecology patients and creation of a prognostic model. *Obstet Gynecol*,69,2, 146-50.

Clarke-Pearson, D. & Abaid, L. (2008). Venous Thromboembolism in Gynecologic Surgery. *Glob. libr. women's med., (ISSN: 1756-2228)* 2008; DOI 10.3843/GLOWM.10069

Crandon, A.J. & Knotts, J. (1983). Incidence of post-operative thrombosis in gynaecological oncology. *Aust NZ J Obstet Gynaecol*, 23,4, 216-9.

Crişan, S., Vornicescu, D., Crişan, D., Pop, T. & Vesa, S. (2011). Concomitant acute deep venous thrombosis and superficial thrombophlebitis of the lower limbs. *Med Ultrason*, 13,1, 26-32.

Cronan, J.J., Dorfman, G.S., Scola, F.H., Schepps, B. & Alexander, J. (1987). Deep venous thrombosis: US assessment using vein compression. Radiology, 162,1, 191-4.

Dahlbäck, B. (2008). Advances in understanding pathogenic mechanisms of thrombophilic disorders. *Blood*,112,1, 19-27.

Dainty, L., Maxwell, G.L., Clarke-Pearson, D.L. & Myers, E.R. (2004). Cost-effectiveness of combination thromboembolism prophylaxis in gynecologic oncology surgery. *Gynecol Oncol*, 93,2, 366-73.

Dalen, J.E. & Alpert, J.S. (1975). Natural history of pulmonary embolism. *Prog Cardiovasc Dis*, 17,4, 259-70.

Egan, E.L., Bowie, E.J.W., Kazmier, F.J., Gilchrist, G.S., Woods, J.W. & Owens, C.A. Jr. (1974). Effect of surgical operations on certain tests used to diagnose intravascular coagulation and fibrinolysis. *Mayo Clin Proc*, 49,9, 658-64.

Evans, R.S., Sharp, J.H., Linford, L.H., Lloyd, J.F., Tripp, J.S., Jones, J.P., Woller, S.C., Stevens, S.M., Elliott, C.G. & Weaver, L.K. (2010). Risk of symptomatic DVT associated with peripherally inserted central catheters. *Chest*, 138,4, 803-10.

Galanaud, J.P., Sevestre-Pietri, M.A., Bosson, J.L., Laroche, J.P., Righini, M., Brisot, D., Boge, G., van Kien, A.K., Gattolliat, O., Bettarel-Binon, C., Gris, J.C., Genty, C., Quere, I. & OPTIMEV-SFMV Investigators. (2009). Comparative study on risk factors and early outcome of symptomatic distal versus proximal deep vein thrombosis: results from the OPTIMEV study. *Thromb Haemost*, 102,3, 493-500.

Geerts, W.H., Bergqvist, D., Pineo, G.F., Heit, J.A., Samama, C.M., Lassen, M.R., Colwell, C.W. & American College of Chest Physicians. (2008). Prevention of venous thromboembolism: American College of Chest Physicians Evidence-Based Clinical Practice Guidelines (8th Edition). *Chest*, 133(6 Suppl), 381S-453S.

Ghoneim, M.A., Abdel-Latif, M., el-Mekresh, M., Abol-Enein, H., Mosbah, A., Ashamallah, A. & el-Baz, M.A (2008). Radical cystectomy for carcinoma of the bladder: 2,720 consecutive cases 5 years later. *J Urol*, 180,1,121-7.

Goad, K.E. & Gralnick, H.R. (1996). Coagulation disorders in cancer. *Hematol Oncol Clin North Am*, 10,2, 457-84.

Gulsun Akpinar, M. & Goodman, L.R. (2008). Imaging of pulmonary thromboembolism. Clin Chest Med, 29,1, 107-16.

Heit, J.A. (2007). Thrombophilia: common questions on laboratory assessment and management. *Hematology Am Soc Hematol Educ Program*, 2007(1), 127-35. doi:10.1182/asheducation-2007.1.127. PMID 18024620. http://asheducationbook.hematologylibrary.org/cgi/content/full/2007/1/127

Hirsh, J. & Hoak, J. (1996). Management of deep vein thrombosis and pulmonary embolism. A statement for healthcare professionals. Council on Thrombosis (in consultation with the Council on Cardiovascular Radiology), American Heart Association. Circulation, 15,93,12, 2212-45.

Hull, R., Hirsh, J., Sackett, D.L., Taylor, D.W., Carter, C., Turpie, A.G., Powers, P. & Gent, M. (1981). Clinical validity of a negative venogram in patients with clinically suspected venous thrombosis. Circulation, 64,3, 622-5.

Jenkins, J.S. (2011). Endovascular therapies to treat iliofemoral deep venous thrombosis. Prog Cardiovasc Dis, 54,1, 70-6.

Kalva, S.P., Chlapoutaki, C., Wicky, S., Greenfield, A.J., Waltman, A.C. & Athanasoulis, C.A. (2008). Suprarenal inferior vena cava filters: a 20-year single-center experience. J Vasc Interv Radiol, 19,7, 1041-7.

Kearon, C., Julian, J.A., Newman, T.E. & Ginsberg JS. (1998). Noninvasive diagnosis of deep venous thrombosis. McMaster Diagnostic Imaging Practice Guidelines Initiative. Ann Intern Med, 128,8, 663-77.

Knight, L.C. (1993). Scintigraphic methods for detecting vascular thrombus. *J Nucl Med*, 34,3 Suppl, 554-61.

Krishan, S., Panditaratne, N., Verma, R. & Robertson, R. (2011). Incremental value of CT venography combined with pulmonary CT angiography for the detection of thromboembolic disease: systematic review and meta-analysis. AJR Am J Roentgenol, 196,5, 1065-72.

Kyrle, P.A., Rosendaal, F.R. & Eichinger, S. (2010). Risk assessment for recurrent venous thrombosis. *Lancet*, 376(9757), 2032-9. doi:10.1016/S0140-6736(10)60962-2. PMID 21131039.

Lindow, C., Mumme, A., Asciutto, G., Strohmann, B., Hummel, T. & Geier B. (2010). Long-term results after transfemoral venous thrombectomy for iliofemoral deep venous thrombosis. *Eur J Vasc Endovasc Surg*, 40,1, 134-8.

Linn, B.J., Mazza, J.J. & Friedenberg, W.R. (1988). Treatment of venous thrombotic disease. *Postgrd Med*, 79,6, 171-80.

Martino, M.A., Williamson, E., Rajaram, L., Lancaster, J.M., Hoffman, M.S., Maxwell, G.L. & Clarke-Pearson, D.L. (2007). Defining practice patterns in gynecologic oncology to prevent pulmonary embolism and deep venous thrombosis. Gynecol Oncol, 106,3, 439-45.

McCotter, C.J., Chiang, K.S. & Fearrington, E.L. (1999). Intrapulmonary artery infusion of urokinase for treatment of massive pulmonary embolism: a review of 26 patients with and without contraindications to systemic thrombolytic therapy. Clin Cardiol, 22,10, 661-4.

Miller, J.A. (2011). Use and wear of anti-embolism stockings: a clinical audit of surgical patients. Int Wound J, 8,1, 74-83.

Monreal, M, & Prandoni, P. (1999). Venous thromboembolism as first manifestation of cancer. *Semin Thromb Hemost*,25,2,131-6.

O'Leary, D.H., Kane, R.A. & Chase, B.M. (1988). A prospective study of the efficacy of B-scan sonography in the detection of deep venous thrombosis in the lower extremities. J Clin Ultrasound, 16,1, 1-8.

Piccioli, A., Prandoni, P., Ewenstein, B.M. & Goldhaber, S.Z. (1996). Cancer and venous thromboembolism. *Am Heart J*, 132,4, 850-5.

Quinlan, D.J., McQuillan, A. & Eikelboom, J.W. (2004). Low-molecular-weight heparin compared with intravenous unfractionated heparin for treatment of pulmonary embolism: a meta-analysis of randomized, controlled trials. Ann Intern Med, 140,3, 175-83.

Rabinov, K. & Paulin, S. (1972). Roentgen diagnosis of venous thrombosis in the leg. *Arch Surg*, 104,2, 134-44

Rosendaal, F.R. & Reitsma, P.H. (2009). Genetics of venous thrombosis. *J Thromb Haemost*, 7, Suppl 1,301-4.

Scarpa, R.M., Carrieri, G., Gussoni, G., Tubaro, A., Conti, G., Pagliarulo, V., Mirone, V., De Lisa, A., Fiaccavento, G., Cormio, L., Bonizzoni, E., Agnelli, G. @RISTOS Study Group (2007). Clinically overt venous thromboembolism after urologic cancer surgery: results from the @RISTOS Study. *Eur Urol*,51,1,130-5

Silverstein, M.D., Heit, J.A., Mohr, D.N., Petterson, T.M., O'Fallon, W.M.& Melton, L.J .3rd. (1998). Trends in the incidence of deep vein thrombosis and pulmonary embolism: a 25-year population-based study. *Arch Intern Med*, 158, 6,585-93.

Tapson, V.F., Carroll, B.A., Davidson, B.L., Elliott, C.G., Fedullo, P.R. & Hales, C.A., Hull, R.D., Hyers, T.M., Leeper, K.V. Jr., Morris, T.A., Moser, K.M., Raskob, G.E., Shure, D., Sostman, H.D. & Taylor Thompson, B. (1999). The diagnostic approach to acute venous thromboembolism. Clinical practice guideline. American Thoracic Society. *Am J Respir Crit Care Med*, 160, 3, 1043- 66.

Walsh, J.J., Bonnar, J. & Wright, F.W. (1974). A study of pulmonary embolism and deep leg thrombosis after major gynecologic surgery using labeled fibrinogen phlebography and lung scanning. *J Obstet Gynaecol Br Commonw*, 81,4, 311-6.

Weitz, J.I., Hudoba, M., Massel, D., Maraganore, J. & Hirsh, J. (1990). Clot-bound thrombin is protected from inhibition by heparin-antithrombin III but is susceptible to inactivation by antithrombin III-independent inhibitors. J Clin Invest, 86,2, 385-91.

Whitworth, J.M., Schneider, K.E., Frederick, P.J., Finan, M.A., Reed, E., Fauci, J.M., Straughn, J.M. Jr. & Rocconi, R.P. (2011). Double prophylaxis for deep venous thrombosis in patients with gynecologic oncology who are undergoing laparotomy: does preoperative anticoagulation matter? Int J Gynecol Cancer, 21,6, 1131-4.

Wille-Jorgensen, P., Rasmussen, M.S., Andersen, B.R. & Borly, L. (2003). Heparins and mechanical methods for thromboprophylaxis in colorectal surgery. *Cochrane Database Syst Rev*, 2003(4), CD001217.

Yang, S.S., Yu, C.S., Yoon, Y.S., Yoon, S.N., Lim, S.B. & Kim, J.C. (2011). Symptomatic venous thromboembolism in Asian colorectal cancer surgery patients. *World J Surg*, 35,4, 881-7.